A MILESTONE
IN MEDICAL REPORTING

Barbara Seaman is a leading women's health expert. Her husband, Gideon Seaman, is a psychiatrist and psychopharmacologist. Together they have written the one book that reveals the true facts about what sex hormones do to human health. And they offer safe and sane alternatives.

DID YOU KNOW:

- Most of us unknowingly consume sex hormones in our daily meat
- Many doctors consider the ginseng herb a safe and reliable remedy for hot flashes
- Vitamins can improve your complexion and your gums, soothe nerves, help prevent osteoporosis and much, much more
- Many DES (diethylstilbestrol) babies are being treated for vaginal cancer
- There is a birth control pill for men

WOMEN AND THE CRISIS
IN SEX HORMONES

WOMEN AND THE CRISIS
IN SEX HORMONES

"It is a practical book, not simply an exercise in popular science, and one from which many women (and men) could learn things to their advantage."

—*Washington Post*

"People consider Barbara Seaman the Ralph Nader of contraception."

—*The New York Times*

"Highly readable and authoritative consideration of birth control, of interest not only to women but to men who don't want to father a larger portion of their country."

—Roger Kahn

"A delightful frankness pervades every chapter of this exhilarating work."

—*Nutritional Health Review*

Women and the Crisis in Sex Hormones

Barbara Seaman
and
Gideon Seaman, M.D.

BANTAM BOOKS · TORONTO · NEW YORK · LONDON

This book is for our children
Noah, Elana and Shira Seaman—
and for everyone's children.

This low-priced Bantam Book
has been completely reset in a type face
designed for easy reading, and was printed
from new plates. It contains the complete
text of the original hard-cover edition.
NOT ONE WORD HAS BEEN OMITTED.

WOMEN AND THE CRISIS IN SEX HORMONES
A Bantam Book / published by arrangement with
Rawson Associates Publishers, Inc.

PRINTING HISTORY
Rawson edition published August 1977
2nd printing . . . September 1977   4th printing . . . December 1977
3rd printing . . . September 1977   5th printing . . . January 1978
Book-of-the-Month Club edition published Fall 1977
Bantam edition / September 1978

Cover photograph by Schiavone/Alpha

ISBN 0-553-11476-X

Published simultaneously in the United States and Canada

Bantam Books are published by Bantam Books, Inc. Its trade-
mark, consisting of the words "Bantam Books" and the por-
trayal of a bantam, is registered in the United States Patent
Office and in other countries. Marca Registrada. Bantam
Books, Inc., 666 Fifth Avenue, New York, New York 10019.

PRINTED IN THE UNITED STATES OF AMERICA

Acknowledgments

A book of this scope would not have been possible without the generous cooperation and support of several dozen persons. Patricia Curtis has been a most devoted, creative and central contributor to the whole development of this book, while Ellen Weiss and Linda O'Callaghan, medical librarians, assisted us greatly in our research and the preparation of page notes. Janice Mitchell, Michael Ossias, Rachel Paine and Ann Wilson performed yeoman service in preparation of the manuscript, and also made valuable suggestions.

Others who helped with research or manuscript preparation include Peggy Brooks, Roger Mason, Wendy Palitz, Lynn Faught, Ann O'Shea, Janet Milton, Kacy Cook, Michael Horowitz and Houston Stationers. Shira Seaman helped with the preparation of the vitamin tables, while Elana Seaman and Jon Mosenson provided input and case histories on the health concerns of adolescents. Noah Seaman made editorial suggestions.

The entire women's health network has been of support, especially Belita Cowan, Drs. Michelle Harrison and Pauline Bart, Carol Downer and Lorraine Rothman of the Feminist Women's Health Center in Los Angeles, Judy Norsigian, Esther Rome and Norma Swenson of the Boston Women's Health Book Collective, Alice Wolfson, Doris Haire, Fran Fishbane of DES-Action and Martha Aldridge.

For help in understanding nutrition and food chemistry we are especially grateful to Beatrice Trum Hunter, Dr. William Seaman, Dr. Emmanuel Cheraskin, and Rosalind La Roche, at the Brain Bio Center. We also wish to thank Dr. Victor and Jan Struber.

This book literally would not have been possible without the cooperation, far beyond her line of duty, of Mary Carol Kelly, formerly of the FDA. We also wish to thank Dr. J. Richard Crout, director of the Bureau of Drugs.

Many dozens of physicians, scientists, and government officials have generously provided us with interviews, as well as their published and unpublished research. These are too numerous to list here, but are cited throughout the book and page notes. However, we wish to mention the following nine individuals who, through the years, have been unfailingly generous and patient in responding to any and all of our inquiries: Dr. Philip Corfman at the National Institutes of Health, Dr. Christopher Tietze at the Population Council, Dr. Jean Pakter at the New York City Health Department, Richard Lincoln at Planned Parenthood, and gynecologists William Spellacy, Sarah Roshan, Arthur Davids, and Charles Debrovner. Debrovner, in particular, has devoted a great deal of time to this manuscript. Additionally, we wish to thank the Department of Medical and Public Affairs at George Washington University for providing us with their invaluable *Population Reports*.

In Washington, we wish to thank Ben Gordon of Senator Gaylord Nelson's staff, and Morton Mintz of the *Washington Post* who supplied information we would not otherwise have obtained.

In England, we wish to thank Drs. William Inman, C. Michael Besser, Clifford Kay, Michael Thorner, Stephen Johnson, Sir Edwin Bickerstaff, Victor Wynn, and the late Sir Charles Dodds.

Dr. Peter Greenwald clarified many complex issues concerning DES.

We are grateful to Shirley Fingerhood and Paul Rheingold for legal information and advice; to Shirley Fisher, our literary agent, and, at our publishers, to Eleanor Rawson and Alice Fleming for their support.

We wish to thank Dr. Maurice Nadelman, Leon Savage, the late Joseph Nemecek, and the many friends and relatives who gave us emotional reinforcement and various kinds of assistance. Judith Rossner, Alix Kates Shulman and her daughter Polly, Betty Friedan, Heidi Toffler, Lois Gould, Katharine Balfour, and Ray Pike all made valuable suggestions.

We are indebted to Drs. George and Olive Smith and Dr. Robert Wilson for granting us interviews. They could not have expected to figure heroically in this book, but they still allowed us to tape-record their views.

Above all we are indebted to the eight thousand women and men who have shared with us their personal experiences of birth control and hormones. We especially wish to thank Jim Luggen, a gallant pill widower, and to mention his late wife, Dona Jean Walter.

The wisdom in this book derives from many sources; the errors are ours alone.

Preface

What This Book Is About, What It Can Do for You

If doctors were paid for keeping people well, instead of curing them once they are sick, our medical school curricula would be quite different. They would include a more thorough study of nutrition, physical therapy, public health, and occupational medicine, as well as time-tested home remedies. In a recent front page article, the financially minded *Wall Street Journal* pointed out: ". . . the returns from scientific advances are diminishing . . . nothing that emerges from a clinic or a test tube will contribute nearly so much to better health generally as a little individual self-care in the form of wiser living."

Dr. John Knowles, president of the Rockefeller Foundation agrees: *"The next major advance in the health of the American people will result only from what the individual is willing to do for himself."*

Or herself. Since the end of World War II, millions upon millions of American women have faithfully swallowed sex hormones, prescribed by their physicians. In recent Senate testimony Dr. Dwight Janerich of New York State's Cancer Control Bureau explained: *"Natural semisynthetic and synthetic forms of estrogen and progesterone are used in many ways in medicine. These substances are potent modifiers of biological function. Unlike many other drugs which have a narrow function, these drugs produce simultaneous effects in many systems of the body."*

Do women want their natural functions "potently modified," and the "many systems" of their bodies "simultaneously affected"? Not anymore. Doctors used to complain, with some justice, that patients begged them for Premarin or the pill. Now patients beg their doctors for alternatives, but it's easy to write a pill prescription and push it across a desk, and harder to fit a diaphragm correctly. Gynecologist Louis Hellman, former top population officer at HEW, admits that *he* finds diaphragms distasteful, and *he* prefers instructing women in other methods. When a reporter asked: "What about the patients' preference?" he brushed her aside.

Amazingly, in this age of omnipresent TV ads for "personal products" like jockey shorts and vaginal deodorants, Hellman testified *against* the changing of TV codes to permit contraceptive advertising. Drug store methods such as condoms and spermicidal foam are *not doctor controlled*, which may have colored Hellman's thinking.

Some physicians act as if hormone panic is an invention of the lay press. "We all have to take chances," they shrug. Perhaps these doctors don't read their own bluest-ribbon publications. In England, the *Lancet* had cooled on the pill by 1969, when it stated in an editorial: ". . . the metabolic changes associated with this treatment may modify biochemical processes in all body tissues. More than fifty metabolic changes have been recorded . . . these changes are unnecessary for contraception and their ultimate effect on the health of the user is unknown. . . . the wisdom of administering such compounds to *healthy* women for many years must be seriously questioned."

Here in the United States, the *New England Journal of Medicined* echoed *Lancet* by 1976: "The pill abolishes the normal cycle, distorts metabolism, and causes serious disorders in some users. . . . The whole question of the use of drugs to alter normal metabolism must be raised."

The longer a woman stays on hormones, the more each cell in her body is poisoned. Does poison sound like too strong a word? A woman must decide for herself. As the years pass, her sugar metabolism may test out like a diabetic's. Her blood fats, including cholesterol and tri-glycerides, resemble those of a coronary-prone middle-aged male. At Hunter College in New York City, a young scientist named Chris Chilvers, who screened the lipid levels (blood fats) of pill-using students, found that 85 *percent had elevated cholesterol and triglycerides. Of those not taking the pill, only 5 percent had such elevation.* Chilvers had less opportunity to study Premarin users, but these showed a similar trend.

How many women on hormones know that their bile is saturated with cholesterol, a near-universal effect that can and sometimes does produce gall-bladder disease?

How many are told that their bodies are deficient in essential vitamins and minerals—including folic acid, vitamin C, vitamin B_6, and zinc—or that their blood plasma has a greenish tinge due to increased copper?

How many know of the growing concern—and evidence—that pill use may produce infertility and birth defects?

It's *not* just that "a few" women die or are crippled in the aftermath of hormones. *Every* woman who takes these products is walking around in an altered biochemical state. Sir Charles Dodds, the British scientist who synthesized orally effective estrogen in 1938, lived to see—and to deplore—the applications of his discovery.

Sir Charles was as sanguine about the casual use of hormones as Einstein was about the nuclear weapons race. When we interviewed Sir Charles in 1969, he could hardly believe that the pill was so in vogue. "When a clock is working," he said glumly, "you don't tinker with it."

That hormones taken in pregnancy cause birth defects was established in 1960. Thirteen years later, in 1973, our FDA issued a tardy warning against the use of hormones for diagnostic pregnancy tests or preventing miscarriages. Finally, in 1975, *the agency withdrew approval of any use of hormones during pregnancy*.

Many physicians didn't notice or care. Recently, Dr. Sidney Wolfe of the Public Citizens Health Research Group gathered some astonishing statistics. He ascertained that in 1972, before the ban, 588,000 hormone prescriptions were written for *pregnant* women in the United States. In 1975 the figure dropped but slightly, to 533,000 prescriptions.

Adjusting for our declining birth rate, the proportional use of hormones by pregnant women may actually be going up. The major drugs involved are progesterone-like substances, including Provera, Depo Provera, Delalutin, Duphaston, Norlutin, and Norlutate. Consequently, as recently as 1975, more than half a million unborn babies were exposed to artificial hormones.

Thus, doctors who speak of "hormone therapy" usually take a license with language, for *therapy means treatment of disease*. Pregnancy or non-pregnancy are hardly diseases; and neither is menopause. The latter is a normal developmental state wherein reproductive capacity is *winding down;* the temporary hot flashes some women experience may be compared to the high-to-low voice-register changes adolescent boys evidence when their reproductive capacity is *gearing up.*

We no longer castrate young boys to preserve their male sopranos, nor should we treat hot flashes with a cancer-and-cholesterol pill.

Which is not to suggest that women need endure menopause symptoms, or the fear of pregnancy. There are plenty of safe alternatives to hormones, which this book will explore. Women need not make guinea pigs of themselves, nor have they any obligation to support the pharmaceutical industry.

If couples can manage the harmless methods of birth control, they make an important contribution to the health of their own and future generations. If women treat menopause symptoms nutritionally, they conserve both their pocketbooks and lives.

Proverbs 17:22 reminds us: "A joyful heart is the health of the body, but a depressed spirit dries up the bones." To your heart, your spirit, your health and longevity, we dedicate our work.

Contents

The Amazing Story of DES

One day, a Virginia woman named Grace M. was reading the newspaper when she noticed an article concerning a drug called DES—diethylstilbestroi, often called simply stilbestrol. The article pointed out a newly discovered danger associated with this drug: The daughters of some of the women who had taken it during their pregnancies had developed vaginal cancer as a result, said the author of the report, Dr. Arthur Herbst.

"I became alarmed and called my doctor immediately," recalls Mrs. M. "I had first taken DES in 1949 when I was pregnant with one daughter, and again in 1955 before the birth of another. So I took both my daughters to the doctor, and from the examinations, Marilyn, the 14-year-old, was found to have cancer of the vagina.

"Three weeks later, she had vaginal surgery in New York City. She was four weeks in the hospital. The doctors told me they had gotten all of it, there was no problem, everything was taken care of, this type of cancer rarely ever spread beyond the female organs.

"And so, reassured, we went back to Virginia. A year later, Marilyn developed cancer of the lung and also three tumors on her trachea and her bronchial tubes. The doctors operated and removed the lung and the tumors.

"About four months later, Marilyn started having severe head pains. The cancer had spread into her head. She had whole-head radiation, and her hip started to hurt, and she had hip radiation and from hip radiation she went on to the arms and legs, and eventually she went blind and died, two and half years after we had discovered the cancer. It is a horrible, terrible thing to watch your child suffer, and eventually, when she dies, you think it is a blessing—the death is far easier to accept than the actual suffering."

Today, Mrs. M.'s other daughter, Patty, who is in her twenties, is under constant care. She is checked every three months because she has adenosis, an abnormal condition in her vaginal tract associated with prenatal exposure to DES and thought to be a possible precursor of cancer of the vagina.

On December 16, 1975, a 21-year-old woman named Sherry L. spoke on the steps of the Food and Drug Administration in Rockville, Maryland, at a National Women's Health Network memorial service that was held for all the women who have died from unnecessary estrogen products. Sherry herself is a "DES daughter"—like Marilyn M., *and an estimated 1.5 million other young United States women.* She has cervical abnormalities that were discovered in a routine checkup at a women's health center and in tests at Massachusetts General Hospital's DES screening program. She has to undergo continual monitoring. Sherry is anxious about the outcome of her life.

"I relieve a lot of my anxiety by working on DES projects, but it's still hard to live with," she says.

Mothers suffer equally. On Long Island, New York, many are active in an organization called DES-Action. This is a group of mothers and daughters who were exposed to the drug and who have banded together for mutual support, advice, and possible action. Similar activist groups are organizing in other areas. DES women in California have prodded the state health department to publish material alerting women and doctors to the dangers of DES, and to offer doctors one-day courses in the use of the colposcope, an instrument that aids in the discovery of vaginal abnormalities. Other women exposed to DES have themselves filed suits against the drug companies who make it—or have joined in filing class-action suits.

Why are these tragedies, connected to a relatively small group of people, receiving so much attention? In terms of the population as a whole, the cause of a group of mothers and daughters who, over a thirty-year span, were given a drug that proved dangerous to many does not seem of imminent concern to the rest of us.

But these women are not the only ones at risk. Abnormalities are now beginning to show up in some of the sons of women who were given DES during pregnancy. And in spite of the alarming track record of this synthetic hormone in after-the-fact testing, *DES is still being given today in the form of the morning-after pill, a favorite contraceptive handed out at many university health services. It is also being given as a milk suppressant to new mothers* who do not wish to nurse their babies.

And on top of all that, this known carcinogen *is in the meat we eat.* The fact is that today—man, woman, or child *—we are all chemically medicated to some degree with DES, without our permission and usually without our knowledge.*

CHAPTER 1

More Normal than Normal

We have always done our work with human material. We've used animals, of course, but we thought human material was the most interesting.
Dr. Olive Watkins Smith, 1976

DES is the grandmother product of all synthetic estrogens, as well as being the loss leader. (Leader to the pharmaceutical industry, loss to the women who have taken it.)

Synthesized by Sir Charles Dodds in England in 1938, it was the first hormone product that was both cheap to manufacture and effective to take by mouth. DES has been defined by Dr. Robert H. Furman, vice-president of Eli Lilly, as "a synthetic compound capable of producing feminizing effects similar to those of the naturally occurring feminizing hormone estrogen." *Similar to*, but not identical with, as Dodds himself pointed out.

Nearly thirty years later, in 1965, Sir Charles made this comment about his brainchild: "It is interesting . . . to speculate on the difference in attitude toward new drugs thirty years ago and today. Within a few months of the first publication of the synthesis of stilbestrol, the substance was being marketed throughout the world. No long-term toxicity tests on animals such as dogs were ever done with stilbestrol. . . . It is really surprising that we escaped major pharmacological disasters until a few years ago."

According to Dr. Furman, the following are the four medical conditions for which DES is presently most often prescribed:

• as replacement therapy for women in menopause, or whose ovaries have been removed or never developed

• for the prevention of post-partum breast engorgement in mothers who decline to breast feed

- to treat certain cases of cancer of the prostate
- to treat certain breast cancers

DES is commercially in hale and hearty shape. But many women who have been exposed to it are not so hale —and some are dead.

The Boston Disease: Its Origins

Paul Rheingold is an attorney specializing in malpractice and drug-liability cases. Rheingold's office, in New York's skyscraper Pan Am building, affords sweeping views of the city. But the visitor's eye is riveted to an enormous picture on the wall—a blown-up x-ray of a human patient with a surgical retractor visible in his abdomen. The picture graphically illustrates Rheingold's type of practice.

Rheingold is planning a class-action suit against the drug companies to pay for the health care of the daughters of women who were given DES while they were pregnant. He also handles individual DES lawsuits. "You know," he mused when we interviewed him in 1976, "it's almost like a Boston disease. The closer you get to Boston, the more DES daughters you find, and the farther away you get, the fewer."

He could have said Harvard because, in point of fact, the tragic story of DES begins at Harvard University. The first promoters of DES as a therapy for pregnant women were Dr. George Van Siclen Smith, head of Harvard's gynecology department from 1942 to 1967 and now professor emeritus, and his wife, biochemist Dr. Olive Watkins Smith.

George and Olive Smith married in 1930, when he was a Fellow in gynecology at Harvard Medical School, and she was a young Ph.D. out of Radcliffe. Today they are a handsome enough couple to star in a leisure village advertisement, except that leisure is the one thing they don't have. He is still in private practice, and she performs research—seventy hours a week—at the Fearing Research Laboratory of the Free Hospital for Women in Brookline.

They are tall, the two of them, and blue-eyed. Dr. George's hair is faded brown and parted in the middle, 1920s fashion. He wears austere clothes and highly polished shoes. Dr. Olive wore her usual lab coat and sneakers when we interviewed them. Her abundant white hair was brushed back from her face. They chuckle a lot together, and they are proud of their grown daughter and son. They also adopt a parental attitude toward the doctors they trained—"our boys"—including some who will appear later in this story, such as DES investigators Arthur Herbst, Philip Corfman, and John Lewis.

Philip Corfman, of the National Institutes of Health's Division of Child Health and Human Development, has given grants for several studies on the aftermath of DES. Dr. George said of Corfman, "He's too young to be an administrator. He was a good resident. We wanted to keep him here."

George and Olive Smith "started right in on the ovary" in 1928, and have been working on it ever since. As Dr. George puts it, "We have just *lived* ovarian hormones—pituitary and placental—for years and years." The Smiths were among the first to demonstrate how pituitary and ovarian hormones function over the course of the normal menstrual cycle, and, with the help of a tip from their friend Dr. Gregory Pincus, inventor of the birth control pill, were the first to demonstrate estradiol as one of the naturally occurring forms of estrogen.

The First DES Study

The Smiths' natural conservatism made them cautious about treatments such as radical mastectomy, so their espousal of DES is all the more poignant.

From the mid-1930s on, Dr. George and Dr. Olive, together and separately, published many important papers on estrogen excretion in normal pregnancy. It was in 1941, based on their observation of low hormone levels in mothers spontaneously aborting, that they conceived the idea of using the newly developed DES to help pregnancies that seemed threatened by miscarriage. Dr. Olive stated in her landmark report, published in the *American Journal of Obstetrics and Gynecology* in November 1948, "It was found . . . that diethylstilbestrol . . . might theoretically . . . provide an ideal agent for progesterone deficiency in pregnancy."

The report described a study of 632 DES-treated

pregnancies, which dated back to 1943. The earliest DES mothers were not all Bostonians, for 117 obstetricians from 48 cities and towns in New York, New Jersey, Pennsylvania, the District of Columbia, Illinois, North Carolina, Virginia, Texas, New Mexico, California, and all of the New England states cooperated in the study by following the Smiths' regimen and sending them a record of each treated case. Presumably the cooperating doctors gave the pills to pregnant patients who seemed in danger of miscarrying, although possibly some gave them to women who merely had had problems with previous pregnancies.

The obstetricians supplied the records, and E.R. Squibb & Sons supplied the DES pills, which were given in the following dosages: "Five milligrams daily by mouth, starting during the sixth or seventh week (counting from the start of the last menstrual period). The daily dosage is increased by 5 milligrams at two-week intervals to the fifteenth week, when 25 milligrams daily are being taken. Thereafter, the daily dosage is increased by 5 mg at weekly intervals. Administration is discontinued at the end of the thirty-fifth week, since a drop in estrogen and progesterone normally precedes the onset of labor."

By 1948 the Smiths were convinced that DES could be effective against many complications of pregnancy, including threatened miscarriage and diabetes. In addition, the babies of DES-treated mothers were said to be unusually rugged; the placentas were found to be "grossly more healthy-looking."

The Big Boston Success

The following year the Smiths completed their second major study at Boston Lying-In—then, as now, one of the world's most prestigious maternity hospitals. This study, which had begun in April 1947, included 387 women who received DES throughout pregnancy, compared to 550 who did not. All of these women—the stilbestrol mothers as well as the unmedicated—were observed to be having *normal first pregnancies*. Those who did not receive DES got no special treatment, or even a placebo. Only 28 of the 387 treated patients dropped out of the study. Possibly the high level of cooperation could be accounted for by the fact that the women taking DES were given extra attention and encouragement. Women with known illnesses such as diabetes or hypertension were excluded from the study, in spite of the Smiths' claims that DES had proved effective in pregnancies threatened by diabetes. Those in the study were all normal and healthy first-time mothers. What was the reason for giving them a powerful drug, except in the name of research?

Yet the women who were given DES were never informed that they were part of a highly controversial experiment. Some DES mothers now recall that they were told the pills were "vitamins."

"The babies of treated mothers," wrote the Smiths, "gave evidence of having been in a better maternal environment. . . . The explanation appears to be that the drug stimulated better placental function and hence bigger and healthier babies. . . . Although stilbestrol was expected to keep more gestations normal . . . we did not anticipate that it could render normal gestation 'more normal,' as it were."

The Smiths had a dream—a dream of helping women with problem pregnancies achieve motherhood, and then, as their experiment unfolded, a yet more daring dream of making normal pregnancies more normal! There was understandable excitement and controversy when they reported their Boston Lying-In study at the Seventy-second Annual Meeting of the American Gynecological Society in Hot Springs, Virginia.

Not only was the research not conclusive—by today's standards it wasn't even good. The untreated group was simply that—an untreated group. On the other hand, the DES mothers had been given that extra attention and support.

Nowadays a well-designed drug study must handle both treated and untreated patients in exactly the same way. The untreated patients are given placebos and the same kind of care as the treated. Codes are kept secret so that the doctors and staff (as well as the patients) never know who has received the real medication until it's all over.

The first discussant, Dr. Ernest W. Page of San Francisco, reacted skeptically. "Dr. Olive Smith and Dr. George Smith have been among the most astute and assiduous observers in this field for over fifteen years, [but] it is difficult to believe that such a potent drug as stilbestrol will prove to be like an essential vitamin—necessary for the most successful outcome of normal pregnancies."

Dr. Willard M. Allen of St. Louis, an authority on ovulation in rabbits, was puzzled. He pointed out that, in rabbits at least, "the administration of estrogen is very deleterious to the fetus. In early pregnancy estrogen will *prevent implantation or produce abortion,* and during the later stages it leads to death of the fetus."

(Dr. Allen was on to something. Humans may have turned out to be more like rabbits than the Smiths expected, and the use of DES today as a morning-after contraceptive makes up for some of the loss the drug industry must have suffered when its popularity as a miscarriage preventive fell off. But we're getting ahead of our story.)

The regional battle lines concerning DES were drawn on that day in 1949 in Hot Springs, Virginia. In general, the New Englanders supported the Smiths—and Harvard —while the midwesterners did not. Dr. William J. Dieckmann of the University of Chicago and Chicago Lying-In Hospital pointed out that the untreated control group in the Smiths' study *was not given a placebo,* which he considered essential for scientific accuracy. He proposed a plan for testing DES at Chicago Lying-In, using a placebo as a control, and recommended that other obstetricians who had large clinic services do the same.

Troublesome News from New Orleans and Chicago

Dr. Dieckmann was as good as his word, and he began a DES study. Before his work was completed, a New Orleans obstetrician, Dr. John Henry Ferguson of Charity Hospital and Tulane University, also attempted to replicate the Harvard DES work. Like Dieckmann, Ferguson believed that the Smiths had erred in not giving their control patients an inert pill. Alternate pregnant patients at Charity Hospital were given tablets called "white stilbestrol" and "yellow stilbestrol," but only the white ones contained the real stuff.

Close to half of the women dropped out of Ferguson's

study. Luckily for them (and their fetuses!), 46 of the "real" stilbestrol mothers missed their appointments, 35 disappeared, 41 would not cooperate, and 33 provided inadequate data or delivered at home. Ferguson was left with only 184 obedient DES mothers, and 198 controls. Nonetheless, his study was important, for it was the first to show stilbestrol had no more effect than the placebo. In fact, more DES patients than placebo patients had miscarriages and premature births, while the control group babies (and placentas) were slightly bigger and healthier. The only diabetic patient in the study, a DES mother, lost her baby! Dr. Ferguson had, in the words of one admiring contemporary, "driven a very large nail into the coffin that we will use someday to bury some of the extremely outsized claims for the beneficial effects of stilbestrol."

The Dieckmann Chicago study was begun on September 29, 1950. This time Eli Lilly & Company had provided the carefully prepared DES pills and placebos, while we, out of our tax dollars, provided the money, for the study was sponsored by our National Institutes of Health. All 2,162 Chicago Lying-In clinic patients were included— first-time mothers and experienced ones, the healthy and the sick, women who had miscarried previously and those who had not. Every patient was offered a box of tablets, without charge, and was told that "the tablets were of value in preventing some of the complications of pregnancy and would cause no harm to [the patient] or the fetus." Coding was properly kept top secret. Most of the staff didn't know what drug was being studied, and none knew which patients got DES and which a placebo. Five hundred sixteen women dropped out of the study, leaving 840 DES mothers and 806 in the placebo group.

The Dieckmann Chicago study was completed on November 20, 1952, and reported at Lake Placid, New York, in 1953, at the annual meeting of American gynecologists. The DES babies in this study did not do better in any respect. To the contrary: Twice as many of the DES mothers had miscarriages; they had more hypertension (high blood pressure) and smaller babies than the mothers on placebos. Dr. Dieckmann and his associates concluded that DES *actually favors premature labor*, as in rabbits. "We think that the number of patients studied and the methods used showed that stilbestrol has no therapeutic value in pregnancy," they announced firmly.

It was now fifteen years after Charles Dodds perfected the first oral estrogen in London, and twelve years after the Smiths of Boston started to treat pregnant women with it. The Chicago and even the New Orleans studies were scientifically more valid than the study performed at Boston Lying-In. In both later studies, DES was shown to be not helpful, and possibly deleterious.

But even more serious in its implications was the testing of DES for carcinogenicity by animal researchers. At the National Cancer Institute, for example, Michael B. Shimkin and Hugh C. Grady dissolved the new DES in sesame oil and fed it to male mice. These mice were of a strain called C_3H, which is so highly susceptible to cancer that most of the virgin females develop breast cancer spontaneously, though males do not.

The DES-fed males *did*. They also developed serious abnormalities of the spleen and sex organs. By 1940, when the Smiths were conceiving their human experiments, DES had already been proven carcinogenic in mice.

The Smiths were aware of this research, for as Dr. Olive told us in 1976, "Before we even started any clinical work at all, we went through all the literature."

"However," said her husband, "you can do all kinds of things to rats and mice by giving them overdoses."

The New Orleans and Chicago reports, if not the mouse studies, must have convinced many obstetricians that there was no value in using DES, though apparently not some of the sons of Harvard. In 1953, when the bad news from Chicago was brought to the Lake Placid meeting, one doctor was quick to quip: "As a former Bostonian, I would be entirely lacking in . . . loyalty if I had not used stilbestrol in my private practice."

CHAPTER 2

The Time-Bomb Effect

Iatrogeny: An abnormal state or condition produced by the physician in a patient by inadvertent or erroneous treatment.
Stedman's Medical Dictionary,
22nd Edition

The Herbst Report

Back in Boston, while the Lake Placid meeting was taking place, a young New Yorker named Arthur Herbst was graduating cum laude from Harvard College, class of '53. After serving as a line officer in the navy, Herbst got his M.D. from Harvard Medical School in 1959, trained in obstetrics and gynecology, and became one of George Smith's "boys." In 1966, at Massachusetts General Hospital, a 15-year-old girl with clear-cell adenocarcinoma of the vagina came to his attention. It was the first time that this type of cancer had ever been seen at Massachusetts General Hospital in any woman under twenty-five.

(Adenocarcinoma is cancer that occurs in *glandular tissue*. In normal women, the vaginal lining has no such tissue, but we now know that the vaginas of most daughters of women who took DES while pregnant, including those who are thus far free from cancer, have many tiny glands. We have learned only after thirty years of widespread use in humans that DES interferes with the formation of normal genital tissue at a critical time in the early development of the fetus.)

Within the next three years, 6 similar cases of clear-cell adenocarcinoma in young women turned up at Massachusetts General Hospital. The youngest patient was 15, the oldest 22. These 7 cases were more than had been reported in such young women *in all of the world's medical literature*. Arthur Herbst and his colleague Howard Ulfelder, in a study designed by David C. Poskanzer, began a careful search for the source of this mysterious cancer. The patients and their mothers all were questioned about possible causes, such as douches, tampons, birth control pills, and sexual activity. "Finally," says Herbst, "*one of the mothers made an intuitive guess that the cause might be the DES she was given in pregnancy.*" The researchers then added prenatal hormones to their list of questions.

And that was the connection. The mothers of the young women with adenocarcinoma all had taken DES while pregnant.

Today George Smith says sadly, "We've been in on that from the beginning because we're close friends with Dr. Herbst. Of course he felt terrible about it, but a lot is being learned as the result of it, and who could predict thirty years ago that anything like this would develop? I mean, regardless of the rat and mouse work."

Herbst's relationship with the Smiths did not prevent him from publishing his findings in the *New England Journal of Medicine* on April 22, 1971, in an article co-authored with Drs. Ulfelder and Poskanzer. At this point Herbst had examined 8 cases of adenocarcinoma in young women. All but one were DES daughters.

The frightening implications of these findings go far beyond DES because, for the first time, Herbst showed that estrogen products can be cancer-producing in humans. It had been known since 1896, when surgeons started removing the ovaries of breast-cancer patients, that hormones—even the hormones produced by a woman's own body—could *speed* up the growth of an existing malignancy.

It had been known since 1932 that breast cancer could be produced in *male* mice by giving them estrogen injections, that sex hormones could *produce* cancer in laboratory animals, serving as "seed" as well as "fertilizer" in *susceptible* strains.

Like our distant mouse relative, we humans vary in

our cancer thresholds, but unlike mice, we haven't been bred for susceptibility or resistance. We just have to take pot luck with our own genes, and we never know where we stand personally. Then too, we don't live in cages in a scientifically controlled environment, so we may be randomly exposed to a great many carcinogens we're unaware of. Finally, a cancer that takes four or five months to develop in a mouse takes years or decades to develop in a human being. In terms of the human cancer span, most estrogen products have not been in widespread use long enough for us to chart all the returns.

DES was the first hormone product to be named a human carcinogen. Young women exposed in the womb to DES in the 1940s and 1950s developed cancer in the 1960s and 1970s. The work of Herbst and his colleagues was a crucial "missing link" concerning estrogens and the *initiation* of cancer in humans, for all estrogens have a similar way of behaving biologically. Mice who get cancer from DES *also get it from other estrogen products*. In 1971, the millions of hormone-using women all over the world should have been warned of the significance of Herbst's DES findings. They should have been warned that a scientist had found that estrogens *cause* cancer as well as *help it to grow*.

They were not. Only in 1975, when additional hormone products, such as Premarin and the sequential pill, were also linked to cancer, did the U.S. Food and Drug Administration start to acknowledge that estrogen products must be viewed as a group. There *are* differences among them, but it isn't clear what all of them are. The risks established for any one product must be assumed to apply to the others.

Herbst himself—and the editors of the *New England Journal of Medicine*—understood the sweeping implications of his 1971 report concerning the DES link among the young women with cancer. In March, several weeks before publication, Dr. Franz Ingelfinger, then editor of the *New England Journal of Medicine*, sent galleys of Herbst's article to the FDA. On April 14, Herbst also shipped the FDA his raw data sheets. Then he waited . . . and waited.

The Greenwald Report

But while the FDA dallied, health officials of one state—New York—swung promptly into action. Dr. Peter Greenwald, the 34-year-old director of New York's Cancer Control Bureau, was a 1967 graduate of the Harvard School of Public Health. His specialty was epidemiology. He quickly collected data on 5 young New York women (aged 15 to 19 at the time of diagnosis) who had adenocarcinoma of the vagina. Three had died of advanced disease, and 2 were doing well post-operatively. The mothers of 4 of the young women had taken DES, and the fifth a series of different estrogens and progesterones.

In Dr. Greenwald's opinion, the symptoms of abnormal pregnancy in some of these mothers had been minimal. One mother had no symptoms, only a history of a previous miscarriage. Greenwald and his colleagues, Drs. J. J. Barlow, P. C. Nasca, and W. S. Burnett, quickly submitted their findings to the *New England Journal of Medicine*, which published them on August 12.

Meanwhile, on June 22, 1971, Dr. Hollis S. Ingraham, New York's Commissioner of Health and Greenwald's boss, sent an individual letter to every physician in his state telling of the Herbst findings and the confirming evidence collected by Greenwald. New York physicians were urged to report all similar cases immediately (Greenwald's phone number was enclosed) and to stop prescribing DES to pregnant women at once. Dr. George Himler, president of the Medical Society of the State of New York, and Dr. Eli Stark, president of the New York State Osteopathic Society, both endorsed Ingraham's appeal.

Though New York saw the situation as urgent, Washington did not. Earlier in June, Ingraham had written a letter to Dr. Charles Edwards, commissioner of the FDA, which said in part:

A study in the *New England Journal of Medicine* associating adenocarcinoma of the vagina in seven young women with administration of diethylstilbestrol to their mothers during pregnancy suggests a new mechanism in the development of congenital neoplastic disease. The *Journal* also noted editorially the great scientific importance and serious social implications of these findings.

The Cancer Control Bureau of the New York State Department of Health has surveyed its extensive statewide cancer registry to determine whether department records confirm the association report. The registry records five cases of vaginal cancer; the mothers of all five girls had received synthetic estrogens during pregnancy.

We feel this is adequate documentation that the administration of synthetic estrogens during pregnancy leads to an increased incidence of vaginal adenocarcinoma in female children resulting from that pregnancy. It appears from the data that adenocarcinoma of the vagina is extremely rare except when induced by estrogen administration *in utero,* since our registry discloses no case of this cancer which did not have such a history.

On the basis of our findings, we are officially notifying all physicians in New York State of the danger of estrogen administration during pregnancy.

We also recommend most urgently that the Food and Drug Administration initiate immediate measures to ban the use of synthetic estrogens during pregnancy. . . .

The Fountain Committee

It was *two months* before Commissioner Edwards so much as acknowledged Ingraham's letter. In November, when Congressman L. H. Fountain held a congressional committee hearing on DES, he asked Edwards *why* he had dallied. Edwards said, "Well, I have no response to the delay . . . obviously when I received it, I sent it on to the Bureau of Drugs. I must however say that I do not agree with Dr. Ingraham's action. I think he was premature . . . not that his actions are necessarily wrong, but I think he could well have studied it a little bit more than he did."

Herbst had to wait even longer. The FDA did not get back to him until late October, some seven months after receiving galleys of his "missing link" report. During that seven months, many thousands of pregnant women continued to get DES.

The FDA took no steps to restrict DES use in pregnancy until November 10, 1971, *the day before Congressman Fountain opened hearings to investigate the delay.* Dr. Edwards explained, "We have a significant responsibility to be certain about what we are acting upon. . . . There were lots of analyses to be carried out on these figures before we were prepared to act." Dr. Edwards's statement was affirmed by Dr. Henry Simmons, director of the FDA's Bureau of Drugs: "We sought advice from experts throughout the country."

No matter how the Fountain subcommittee pressed the FDA for written reports or memoranda pertaining to their "analyses" of the Herbst and Greenwald data, the FDA was unable to produce a single record or document. On March 12, 1972, it conceded to the subcommittee that "We have not been able to locate any memoranda pertaining to the . . . review of the raw data Dr. Herbst provided with his letter of April 14, 1971." On March 29, the FDA further acknowledged, "The Bureau of Drugs advises us that there are no written evaluations of these case studies."

Attorney Peter Barton Hutt, then general counsel of the FDA, accompanied Edwards and Simmons to the Fountain hearings. Hutt had come to the FDA from Covington and Burling, a major Washington law firm, where he had specialized in food and drug law. Among his clients had been Continental Baking, the Cosmetic, Toiletry, and Fragrances Association, the Institute of Shortening and Edible Oils, the Carnation Company, and the National Association of Chewing Gum Manufacturers. Hutt's appointment as FDA general counsel had met with bitter criticism from consumer advocates and several congressmen.

(It seems fitting that after his time with the FDA, Peter Hutt returned to employment at Covington and Burling, his old law firm. Former commissioner Edwards is today vice-president of Becton-Dickinson, a hospital supply corporation, while former drug bureau director Simmons went on to work for a period as senior vice-president of J. Walter Thompson, an advertising agency that handles hormone products.)

The result of all these maneuvers was that although DES was known to be both dangerous *and* ineffective for threatened miscarriage, the FDA took no action until a congressman called a hearing. Thanks to the Kefauver-Harris legislation of 1962, the FDA now does have some real authority (which is not always exercised) over the pharmaceutical industry. But this was not the case in the early 1940s, when Lilly, Squibb, and other drug companies started to market DES. Then manufacturers could promote a drug without really having to prove safety or efficacy, and without any long-term toxicity tests in animals.

In the 1960s, when regulations were tightened up, the National Academy of Sciences–National Research Council (NAS–NRC) was asked to help re-evaluate many thousands of old drugs. Those shown to be *effective* were left on the market, and those deemed *ineffective* were taken off. Then there were two intermediate categories: *probably effective* and *possibly effective*. Here the burden was supposed to fall on the manufacturer to supply proof that a product worked. With drugs rated *possibly effective*, manufacturers were given *six months* to respond. After that, failing proof of effectiveness, the drug was to be prohibited.

In 1967, the NAS–NRC had rated DES *possibly effective* and had sent the FDA the following report:

> The panel feels that estrogens are not harmful in conditions such as threatened abortion, but that their effectiveness can't be documented by literature or its own experience. The company should be asked to supply further evidence to substantiate the claims in question.

In retrospect, these NAS–NRC scientists sound casual about safety; after all, this was long after the thalidomide tragedy had convinced most pregnant women, at least, that they should be extremely careful about what drugs they take. And, as we cannot say too often, by 1967 the carcinogenicity of DES in animals had already been established. As Dr. Umberto Saffiotti, Associate Scientific Director for Carcinogenesis, National Cancer Institute, was to state a few years later: "There is no question about the carcinogenicity . . . of DES in animals. This is well established. It is one of the chapters in a textbook on cancer research."

Nonetheless, the statement *"effectiveness can't be documented by literature or experience"* gave the FDA a clear mandate, and obligation, in 1968 to prohibit DES in pregnancy cases *unless* the manufacturers came up with new evidence.

They did not. At the Fountain hearings, four years after the NAS–NRC report, Dr. Delphis Goldberg of the subcommittee staff asked Commissioner Edwards: "Have the companies provided further evidence to FDA leading you to believe that this is not an ineffective drug?"

The commissioner admitted they had not.

To recapitulate: Our FDA commissioner, who testified that he felt Dr. Ingraham's warning letter to physicians was "premature," should have restricted DES for use in pregnancy cases (indeed, his predecessors should have!)— even though it was not yet known to be lethal—simply because it didn't work. Under the circumstances, with the proof of the drug's effectiveness three and a half years overdue, it is astonishing the FDA did not take action the moment that the Herbst galleys were received.

Let us examine the results of the FDA's inaction: During the 1940s and especially the early 1950s (after the Boston studies had been published, but before they were challenged in Chicago and New Orleans), DES was enormously popular as a pregnancy treatment. It has been estimated that estrogens were prescribed for nearly 6 million pregnant women between 1943 and 1959, resulting in the birth of at least 3 million children who had been exposed *in utero* to estrogens. Use of stilbestrol in pregnancy declined by the 1960s (probably because doctors became aware that it didn't work). On the basis of research that has been done on pharmacy records from 1960 to 1970, let's assume that some 30,000 unborn females were exposed to DES in 1971, an average of 2,500 a month. Had the FDA acted decisively upon receiving the Herbst galleys in March, instead of waiting until November, when Congressman Fountain forced their hand, more than 20,000 young women who are now in danger of developing adenocarcinoma could have been spared. Four out of every thousand, or a total of 80, may be diagnosed as having vaginal or cervical cancer before the age of 30. How many will develop cancer in later years is anybody's guess.

Peter Greenwald has stated: "Four per 1,000 is . . . 44 times higher than the annual incidence rate for leukemia, and considerably higher than the annual incidences of breast cancer and colon cancer. . . . If this rate is unimportant, then I think a number of researchers should seek other occupations."

Two DES Women Speak

If cancer happens to *you*, the rate seems like 100 percent. Here are two women who have been affected by DES. Their stories bring the statistics into perspective. Janice L. is a young bride who lost her womb to DES; Helen G. lost her daughter.

Janice L. of Los Angeles, whose mother was treated with DES:

"I went to a gynecologist for what I supposed was a routine exam. At that time he told me that he had found what he described as an irritation, and made another appointment for me to come back. So I did.

"I was operated on last August. The repercussions of this operation are still strong in my life. . . . Assuming that I will live a long, full life, there is always the chance that the cancer will appear again, and meanwhile I have to live with the fact that it has rendered me sterile. Family life is very important to me. The fact that I can never have a child matters terribly. . . .

"I have talked to many other women who have had hysterectomies, and I understand it is common knowledge that you go through a transition period where you feel like you are not a woman. I am still trying to adjust.

"And added to this is the constant fear hanging over my head—the suspicion that the cancer will crop up again.

"Not only has it affected me, but naturally it has affected my family—especially my mother. Sometimes I can just cry when I see her. She feels so guilty."

About one-quarter of the young women who have developed DES cancer have died. One of them was 18-year-old Susan G.

Helen G. of Glen Cove, Long Island:

"My daughter was born on February 9, 1951, and she was fine until she was 15. Then one day she hemorrhaged, and the doctors told me she had a very rare form of cancer.

"In Glen Cove, no one had ever treated it, no one had ever even seen it. They recommended a doctor in New York City, which is about twenty-five miles away. The doctor who treated Susan there was wonderful to her. He was treating one other case like hers, from California.

"She was fine for a while, and then the cancer spread. She died when she was 18, in March 1969.

"About two years later, I received a call from a Dr. Herbst, I think it was, asking about Susan, and telling me there was some connection between diethylstilbestrol, DES, and my daughter's vaginal cancer. I could not believe that something with any inherent danger would be given out as indiscriminately as that drug was given out in the 1950s.

"The other thing that bothers me is that many friends contacted me when this became publicly known and said they had taken it, and asked me what I would suggest they do. I suggested . . . they take their daughters and have them checked immediately. And many of them were told by gynecologists, 'Oh, do not worry. The chances of your daughter developing cancer—well, you can get hit by an automobile faster.'

"That bothered me, the attitude of some of the doctors.

"You know, statistics are meaningless, unless one of the statistics is one of your own children."

Don Harper Mills, a physician and lawyer who serves as a medico-legal expert on the editorial board of the *Journal of the American Medical Association* (*JAMA*), advises all physicians who have ever used DES in pregnancy to search their records and send a notice to all such patients at their last known address. Few physicians are complying. Janice L.'s condition was spotted by *her own* gynecologist; the doctor her mother had used denied, at first, that he had given her DES. Grace M. took her daughters in for a checkup after reading a newspaper article. Helen G.'s daughter died before the connection between DES and cancer was established.

We have not yet located one DES mother whose prescribing physician has complied with the Mills recommendation published by the AMA on July 22, 1974. Still earlier, in May 1973, the American College of Obstetricians and Gynecologists (ACOG) issued a technical bulletin to its members, with an editorial that emphasized the need for early examination of girls at risk. All ACOG members were urged to "notify patients who have been treated with stilbestrol during pregnancy so that their daughters can be examined."

Paul Rheingold, the attorney, has not heard of many doctors who have complied either. He guesses there are three reasons for this lack of cooperation: fear of lawsuits, laziness, and sloppy record-keeping. In Rheingold's experience, many doctors do not begin to keep the kinds of records they should.

Pantell and the Idaho Women

Incredibly, not only have a great many doctors failed to notify their patients but some still prescribe DES for pregnant women. At Senate hearings on DES, Dr. Robert Pantell, a pediatrician, gave the following testimony:

> All drugs are potentially dangerous. In this respect, diethylstilbestrol is no different from any other drug. However, I feel there are several characteristics peculiar to diethylstilbestrol which make it unique in the annals of hazardous drugs. A number of drugs have been used in pregnancy with tragic consequences in the newborn. In these instances . . . the drugs taken in the previous months could be readily identified and their risks investigated rapidly.
>
> Diethylstilbestrol is far more sinister. It strikes more than a decade later. Many persons will never know if they are at risk and if they should be seeking special early detection services. Other families will live in a perpetual state of anxiety, guilt and fear. . . .
>
> In August 1972, I began work as a pediatrician for Community Health Clinics, a nonprofit organization that provided health care to migrant farmworkers and rural residents in southwestern Idaho. . . .
>
> One of the questions asked routinely of all women who came to us was whether they received drugs during pregnancy. . . . It soon became apparent that . . . patient recall of events occurring many years ago is especially difficult. . . .
>
> In the winter of 1973, Mrs. A.G. came to our clinic. In 1971 she had received a medication from an obstetrician to help her maintain her pregnancy. Because of our concern that Mrs. A.G. had received diethylstilbestrol, a drug posing potential risks to her 3-year-old daughter, we requested her records. . . . After several mail and phone

requests, a note was received from the obstetrician stating that her pregnancy had been normal. No mention of drugs was made. Upon further questioning, Mrs. G. recalled the pharmacy in Homedale, Idaho, where the medication had been dispensed. The pharmacist identified the drug as des-Plex, a preparation manufactured by Amfre-Grant, containing 25 mg diethylstilbestrol. . . .

At the same time, another patient, Mrs. M.S., also came to our office for care. Mrs. S. was currently being seen for prenatal care by the same obstetrician who formerly had cared for Mrs. G. Mrs. S. was at that time taking des-Plex and had been on this medication continuously for the first six months of her pregnancy. Mrs. S. was unaware of this risks of diethylstilbestrol to pregnancy. She was taking this drug two years after the November 1971 FDA bulletin stated that diethylstilbestrol was contraindicated in pregnancy. Mrs. S. . . . subsequently delivered a female child.

Because of our inability to establish an effective line of communication with the obstetrician who was prescribing diethylstilbestrol, a letter was sent in conjunction with Dr. Thomas McMeekin to . . . the Idaho State Board of Pharmacy and to . . . the Idaho State Board of Medicine, on March 25, 1974. We described our experience and suggested (1) an independent party negotiate with the obstetrician to identify those patients at risk, (2) an effort be made by the Board of Pharmacy and/or Medicine to educate this physician as to the dangers of diethylstilbestrol and current recommendations for its usage. The reply from the State Board of Pharmacy was that this was not in their jurisdiction. . . . Neither Dr. McMeekin nor I have received any further communication concerning this issue. The physician under consideration, besides maintaining a private practice, was then, and to my knowledge still is, an obstetrical consultant for the state.

Neither the drug companies, nor the government, nor professional medical societies such as the AMA or ACOG have offered to finance the search for and treatment of DES daughters. Who will?

CHAPTER 3

Who Pays the Piper and for What?

Kristin S. is a 29-year-old Albany, New York, woman who learned about DES several years ago from newspaper accounts. Her mother remembered that she had taken the drug. Kristin discussed it with her gynecologist, who said, "I wish the papers would stop printing these things. It only scares women." He assured Kristin that being a DES daughter was not significant, and no special examinations were necessary. Yet on one visit he informed Kristin that because he had just "zapped a thingumajig" on her "whatchamacallit," she shouldn't have intercourse for two weeks.

"It was a bad time to have zapped a thingumajig—we women call it a cauterized cervix—because by the time the two weeks were over, my husband would be away for summer reserve camp," Kristin commented later. "If my doctor had asked me before he zapped, I would have made an appointment for a few weeks later.

"Another thing disturbed me. He told me that on my previous visit he had noticed a lesion. He said he had decided to 'watch it and see if it was there on this visit.' He hadn't told me about it then, he said, because unlike the newspapers, he was interested in my peace of mind.

"What if I hadn't come back for this next visit, and what if it had been something serious? So, I didn't trust him when he told me that being a DES daughter was not significant, and no special examinations were necessary. By this time I trusted myself enough to find another doctor."

Kristin had been reading everything about DES she could lay her hands on. She had learned, from *Ms.* magazine and other sources, that the "thingumajig" on her cervix might have been a DES effect. She had learned that Arthur Herbst and others recommend colposcopic examination (a method of magnifying the vagina and cervix for examination) and iodine staining (areas that do not stain are more apt to have abnormal tissue) at every checkup.

Kristin went to Peter Greenwald, the Avis, so to speak, of DES prevention—Arthur Herbst being the Hertz. She asked Greenwald for the name of a gynecologist who had worked with DES and who had a colposcope.

He referred her to Dr. Ben Hahn, whom Kristin sees twice a year. Kristin's colposcopic examination costs $75, and the Pap smear an additional $6. She writes: "I lie in the usual position for a gynecologic exam. The doctor sits on a stool and examines me. The whole thing lasts about twenty minutes. I can feel the speculum move once in a while, and I can feel slight pressure from the swab.

"Most of the time my doctor takes a few biopsies. The vagina and cervix have almost no feeling. The most I can feel during the exam is a dislocated pressure.

"This lack of feeling makes biopsies more difficult. The doctor uses a long, thin metal implement which pinches small pieces of tissue. Until I hear the metal click, I do not know if the cut will go deep enough for me to feel anything. If it hurts, the pain is not intense, but again comes from somewhere that cannot be located. The first sharp pain spreads out. My mind cannot find it and soothe it. It is like trying to stop menstrual cramps by massaging your abdomen—it doesn't work.

"My doctor is very good to me. He shows me the instruments he is using and explains how they work, 'You see?' he says, and he shows me the tiny clips which pinch my tissues.

"He tells me that 'very few' DES daughters develop cancer, but he does not tell me it is silly to worry. He does not say it would be better if the newspapers hadn't told me about DES.

"After each biopsy, I try not to worry about the results. I basically believe that nothing really bad can happen to me. Then, when I call him for the report, I realize that in this little speck of time my world could be devastated. He comes on the line and says, 'Everything's fine, don't worry.' And it's all over until next time."

Kristin is relatively fortunate. Her mother remembered *for certain* that she had taken DES, and upon deciding to remove her "zapped thingumajig" to an expert, Kristin called a good source. It takes money and causes some discomfort, but Kristin now receives the careful follow-up every DES daughter should be getting.

In contrast to Kristin, who lucked into Peter Greenwald, consider what might happen to an Idaho DES family seeking advice from the State Board of Medicine.

Townsend and Those Office Fires

How *does* a DES mother find out for certain that she was exposed, and how does a daughter know whether she is getting a thorough checkup? Dr. Duane Townsend of the DES registry at the University of Southern California Medical Center acknowledges: "If the physician who has administered the DES to prevent a miscarriage is retired or has died"—or, Townsend might have added, if he is lying low—"it becomes very difficult to trace these records. And, of course, some records have been destroyed by fires in offices and hospitals."

Townsend estimates the number of DES-exposed daughters to be "anywhere" from 500,000 to 2 million. He doesn't explain those fires in obstetricians' offices, nor does he acknowledge that too many doctors and hospitals simply don't save their records, and that, where records do exist, a search is extremely costly.

It has now been clarified that the earlier in pregnancy a mother received DES, the greater the chances that her daughter will develop one of the abnormalities associated with this syndrome. Of the daughters examined thus far, almost 100 percent of those whose mothers took DES before the eighth week of pregnancy have revealed vaginal and cervical abnormalities, but these rarely occur if exposure was at eighteen weeks or later. Most of the girls and women in current treatment at our four national DES registries (located at the Mayo Clinic, Baylor University in Houston, and Massachusetts General, as well as at the University of Southern California) were exposed before the eighteenth week of fetal life. Two-thirds of these were exposed to DES specifically and another 10 percent to unidentifiable hormone preparations.

Herbst's Cancer Registry

With funding from the National Cancer Institute and the American Cancer Society, Herbst and his colleagues established an international DES information center that lists women born after 1940 who have had DES-related cancer. The patients, now numbering several hundred, were aged 7 to 29 at the time of diagnosis. Two-thirds of their cancers originated in the vagina, and one-third in the cervix. The number of cases diagnosed each year has been rising. In 1975, Herbst stated: "Although the first reported cases of DES-related carcinoma occurred in New England, cases have now been submitted to the registry from throughout the United States, as well as from other countries, including Australia, Belgium, Canada, France, and Mexico. In countries such as Denmark, where DES was not used, no recent outbreak of these tumors has been noted, nor have DES-associated cancers been observed thus far in countries, such as Great Britain, where the exposed population numbers only a few thousand individuals."

Canada and Australia used DES in pregnancy cases, but not England. Sir Charles Dodds, a physician as well as a biochemist, served as president of the Royal College of Physicians in 1961. On his own turf, at least, his cautionary finger was longer than Harvard's arm.

Back now to Arthur Herbst, who reports, "The dosages to which cancer patients were exposed *in utero* have varied widely. One mother took as little as 1.5 mg daily, while others received as much as 225 mg of DES daily. The duration of treatment also varied, from as short as one week to as long as almost the entire length of pregnancy. In all the cases in which the precise dates of treatment are available, the drug was initiated before the eighteenth week."

Thus far, one-quarter of the DES daughters with diagnosed cancer have had recurrences, or have died. The typical adenocarcinoma measures between one and three centimeters in diameter (about 1/3 to 1 inch), but some are smaller, while others "fill the vagina." The prognosis is much better *if* the diagnosis is made before the first symptoms—usually abnormal vaginal bleeding—occur.

By failing to search their records and notify patients for whom they prescribed DES, obstetricians are sealing the fates of many young women. They have placed the daughters of their patients in double jeopardy—by prescribing DES in the first place, and by failing to act responsibly about it now.

Finally, it is disheartening to note that some obstetricians are actually lying to their patients, denying that they administered DES or other hormones. A not unusual story was told to us by Ruth M., a member of DES-Action.

"I still go to the same doctor who delivered Tammy, my 20-year-old daughter. During the pregnancy I had some staining, and he gave me medication which—I was almost sure—he had referred to as 'stilbestrol.'

"Tammy's away at college. I'd been avoiding the issue; but the more I learned, the more I realized how imperative checkups are. I had to find out for certain, and I had to tell her.

"So I asked my doctor—I'll call him 'Sam,' because he and I are on a first name basis. I'm such an old patient, and we even see each other socially. Well, 'Sam' said I was mistaken; he'd not given me the drug.

"I didn't quite believe him, so I tricked the nurse. 'By the way,' I said to her offhandedly as I was leaving, 'I forgot to ask doctor if he prescribed diethylstilbestrol during my pregnancy with Tammy. Could you take a peek at my chart?'"

"It was right on her desk and she showed it to me. 'Yes,' she said. Sure enough, the dates and the dosages were all there, in Sam's familiar handwriting. . . . And, by the way, Tammy does have abnormalities of her vagina and cervix. She gets a checkup every four months. She was also taking the birth-control pill, prescribed by her student health service, but now the DES specialist she goes to has advised her to stop."

"Did you tell 'Sam' you had caught him in his lie?" we asked.

"No, I didn't. He would fire the nurse. Right now I'm looking for a new doctor, and it's all so difficult since we're friends. But I want to advise other mothers to obtain their own records if they can, by hook or crook."

DES *Abnormalities*

There is no precedent in medical history for the early developing vaginal and cervical abnormalities observed in today's DES daughters. We are speaking here not of cancer but of the much more common and possibly unimportant (only time will tell) aberrations that seem to occur in *all females* exposed to DES before the eighth week of uterine life as well as many who were exposed between the eighth and eighteenth weeks.

On February 13, 1975, a report by Herbst on the DES vagina appeared in the *New England Journal of Medicine.* This was by no means the first such discussion, for a number of other investigators, such as Adolf Stafl and his colleagues at the Medical College of Wisconsin in Milwaukee, had also been studying the DES vagina since 1971.

But the Herbst study of "normal" (i.e., noncancerous) DES daughters has special pertinence to our story, for it was a follow-up of 110 women, aged 18 to 25, whose mothers had been patients at the Smiths' clinic at Boston Lying-In. These were matched with 82 comparable young women whose mothers had not taken DES. The research analysts who identified and communicated with the mothers and daughters knew which had been exposed to DES, but the doctors performing the physical, pathological, and cytologic examinations did not know.

No evidence of cancer was found in any of the 110 DES daughters. The appearance of the external genitalia was entirely normal, and the uterus and ovaries were also normal in size. However, vaginal and cervical examination revealed "highly significant" *differences* between the 110 DES daughters and the 82 comparison patients. DES daughters are apt to have some or all of the following structural abnormalities, which divide into two groups:

One: DES ABNORMALITIES VISIBLE TO THE NAKED EYE: These occur (singly or together) in about 1 in 3 of the women exposed to DES in the first three or four months of uterine life. They include:

• *Vaginal or cervical ridges,* sometimes appearing as a ring around the cervix. Some doctors have coined names for these new conditions, such as cock's-comb cervix, cervical pseudopolyp, or vaginal hood. Specifically, a vaginal hood is a circular fold in the recesses at the vault of the vagina which partially covers the cervix. In such cases, it may be necessary to use a spatula to displace the hood for examination of the cervix and portions of the vagina.

• *Erythroplakia*, or reddish areas on the cervix or the vagina, not unlike a "strawberry" birthmark.

Two: DES ABNORMALITIES NOT USUALLY VISIBLE TO THE NAKED EYE:

• *Cervical "erosion,"* identifiable on biopsy, which occurs in non-DES women also, but not to nearly the same extent.

• *Abnormal mucosa*, as evidenced by failure to stain with iodine solution.

• *Adenosis*, or glandular structures in the vagina. When adenocarcinoma *does* occur, it is usually found near the adenosis or intermingled with it. Thus adenosis is considered a possible "precursor" of malignancy.

Adenosis was first described in Germany in 1877 by a Dr. F. van Preuschen, whose report of four cases (discovered at autopsy) was barely believed, as the vagina is a glandless organ. By 1964 a total of 45 cases of adenosis had been described in all of the world's medical literature.

Adenosis is no longer rare. In Staff's Milwaukee study of 63 young women whose mothers took DES *in the first three months of pregnancy*, 91 percent had adenosis. Herbst found adenosis in 30 percent of the Boston Lying-In daughters, but some of their mothers had not registered at the clinic until well after the third month of pregnancy. In most cases, adenosis cannot be spotted in a routine pelvic exam. Of Staff's 63 DES daughters, who ranged in age from 12 to 23, about half had been examined by gynecologists previously, and all but 7 were erroneously reassured that they had no such abnormality.

Aside from the mental anguish and the costly checkups engendered by a DES vagina, does it also create discomfort and symptoms? This has not yet been fully elucidated. Some DES daughters have a profuse mucus discharge, while others complain of dyspareunia (painful or difficult coitus), burning, and a feeling of heat in the vagina after intercourse. There are tentative reports of fertility problems in some DES daughters, which will be discussed in the next chapter.

If the question of DES exposure cannot be settled, the daughter should certainly be examined with a colposcope. If adenosis, cock's-comb cervix or other characteristic DES markers are found, it can be assumed that the daughter was exposed.

At what age should the checkups begin? Since a pelvic examination can be traumatic to a young girl, and since 90 percent of the cancers associated with DES do not occur until after puberty, Herbst advises that, in the absence of symptoms, checkups need not be started until age 14, or when the girl begins to menstruate. The procedure he recommends is the one that Kristin S. has described from a patient's point of view. The doctor looks and feels (palpates), stains with iodine, explores with a colposcope, and then takes biopsies of any abnormal areas.

However, there is a second school of thought, represented by, among others, cancer specialist John Lewis of Sloan-Kettering Memorial Institute for Cancer Research, who is also an alumnus of the Smiths'. Lewis describes himself as "a little more aggressive" in his approach because he thinks parents should get their daughters in early.

But how do you examine a little girl? Even teen-agers may have to wear tampons for a few months to stretch themselves before a satisfactory view of their interiors can be obtained. With tiny children, John Lewis does a rectal exam and feels inside the abdomen. As they get older, he employs a cystoscope, which is ordinarily used to examine the interior of the bladder and can be applied through an intact hymen. After that he uses a small speculum. Lewis says none of this is painful to the child.

Adenosis and the other "iffy" DES conditions do not interest Lewis much. He is after the real thing, the big C, cancer. "Look," he argues, "adenosis or benign changes in the vagina and cervix are present in 90 percent of the daughters exposed. So you're not really looking for that. The problem is to diagnose the *cancer*." Lewis biopsies areas that feel or look abnormal, but he does not routinely use a colposcope.

Treatment

Should adenosis and the other benign abnormalities be treated? Sometimes they are, with hormones such as progesterone or "locally destructive measures" such as cauterization, cryosurgery, or excision. Some doctors have been quick to perform vaginectomies (removal of the vagina) and skin grafts, just for adenosis.

It seems excessive. The large majority of DES daughters may never get cancer at all, for in spite of having been exposed, prenatally, to the powerful carcinogen, they themselves may be genetically resistant, like some strains of mice. Herbst does not favor routine surgical excision of adenosis. He believes that "careful follow-up appears to be the most prudent approach to DES-exposed subjects without carcinoma at present."

Unfortunately, because the condition is so new and the outcome so uncertain, what constitutes "careful follow-up" has not been fully settled. The safest route for a DES-exposed person is to place herself in the care of a real DES specialist, whether he or she pursues a Herbst type of colposcopic examination or the Lewis approach.

There are other approaches too—and debates among the most knowledgeable specialists. Dr. Albrecht Schmidt of the Medical College of Pennsylvania, moderator of a symposium on Management of the DES Syndrome that appeared in the June 1976 issue of the *Journal of Reproductive Medicine*, explained that he prefers to cauterize abnormal areas of the cervix and the vagina. This, he said, "has a tremendous positive psychological effect on the patient and mother." Schmidt's procedure, in which all abnormal areas are burned off, requires a two-day hospitalization.

Several others at the panel, all reputable specialists, also believed in "doing something" to lesions that might be precancerous. Some apply acidifying creams to the abnormal areas. Others choose laser treatment. One doctor said that he regularly weeds the vaginas of his DES patients "as one would weed a garden." Either in the operating room using general anesthesia, or in his office with local, he uses a small biopsy instrument to pluck out all the areas that have abnormal cells, a procedure called "multiple-punch biopsy." When such areas are extensive, he does this in gradual stages so that adhesions and scarring will not form.

There were nine symposium participants, and while their approaches differed, *none* advocated hysterectomy, vaginectomy, or other extreme measures. The doctors who take radical approaches, *when there is no cancer,* are viewed by most colleagues as quite out of line. The DES daughter and mother should be warned: The doctor who wishes to use cautery, ointments, or other moderate measures reflects a respectable school of thought. The doctor who advocates major surgery to *prevent* cancer may be a charlatan.

New Light on Birth Control for the DES Daughter

Dr. Louis Burke of Harvard had a fascinating finding: When DES daughters select the diaphragm for contraception, the jellies used with it seem to have a *healing effect* on their adenosis because they help acidify the vagina. In addition, the annoying problem of mucus discharge, which 15 percent of DES daughters suffer from, also responds favorably to the spermicidal jellies used with diaphragms.

DES specialists are starting to counsel their patients toward the diaphragm. When this is not feasible, they prescribe products such as Aci-Jel—or sometimes the very contraceptive jellies sold for use with the diaphragm—to be applied nightly over a six-month period.

The DES daughter must inform herself on birth control because her doctor may not be as aware as he should be of the drawbacks or benefits of the different methods. For example, the pill or an IUD could cause harm in the chronically inflamed cervix many DES daughters have.

Anger and Guilt

The symposium participants were understandably concerned about the anguish DES has brought its victims. Dr. Burke remarked: "An extremely important part of the management of these patients is the necessity for psychological counseling of both the patient and her mother. Many of the young women are very hostile and resentful. . . . The mothers' guilt feelings must also be assuaged. Both tasks are accomplished by pointing out the fact that it was considered good medical practice to use diethylstilbestrol at the time."

Burke's concern is genuine, but his information is not strictly accurate outside of Harvard and Boston, where he works. Once the New Orleans and Chicago studies were published—in 1953—many doctors viewed DES as chancy and ineffective. Because of its Harvard origins, though, some of the best-trained and brightest doctors did continue to use it.

The symposium brought some good news for DES daughters, and other news that was not so heartening.

The good news is that adenosis may diminish with maturity after peaking in the teens. As time passes, many cases seem to heal themselves—all the more so if they get some extra help from the diaphragm and jelly. One doctor went out on a limb and predicted that 98 percent of adenosis may gradually mature into normal tissues, while only 2 percent will change toward malignancy.

If he is right, these are very good odds for the DES daughter who has regular checkups. They mean that 49 out of 50 may ultimately be dismissed with a clean bill of health. The remaining 1 in 50, who might develop cancer, at least will have it diagnosed before it spreads. Some specialists see their DES patients every four months. Dr. Joan Celebre of the Hospital of the University of Pennsylvania in Philadelphia is observing 600 patients, aged 18 to 25, of whom 80 percent sought consultation because of the news media.

The less heartening news concerned possible infertility and a different kind of cancer (different, that is, from the rare and fast-spreading adenocarcinoma Herbst first detected).

DES daughters need not panic on the score of infertility—a number have already borne normal children, and most appear in good reproductive shape. But there does seem to be a higher incidence of infertility among DES-exposed women than in the population at large. And in a Miami study of 70 patients, "an inordinate number" of menstrual irregularities, such as scanty or shortened menstruation, were observed.

As for the cancer, Adolf Stafl of Milwaukee emphasized the absolute necessity of tracking and early detection. Stafl is now following 280 young DES daughters of whom 5 have already developed a condition called carcinoma *in situ*, which is a localized and highly curable form of early cancer, while 5 others have developed dysplasia, a form of abnormal tissue that either regresses with time or matures slowly into cancer. Stafl surveyed 386 doctors who are interested in colposcopy and who use that technique to examine DES daughters. Among them, they reported having seen 20 patients with carcinoma *in situ* of the vagina, 48 with carcinoma *in situ* of the cervix, 52 patients with marked vaginal dysplasia, and 117 with marked cervical dysplasia.

Some of these colposcopists had many DES patients, and some had only a few. Stafl was not able to calculate how many patients they were seeing in all, so he could get no clear notion of frequency from his survey. Still, it now appears to Stafl and many other DES investigators that *other forms of cancer*, more manageable and more common than Herbst's clear-cell carcinoma, should be watched for very closely in the DES daughter. The cervix especially should be monitored, for it seems most vulnerable.

Dysplasia and carcinoma *in situ* are common enough among women generally—but not in women quite so young as most DES daughters.

Dr. Joseph Scott of the University of Miami School of Medicine is more worried about Stafl's thesis than is Stafl himself. Of Scott's 70 DES patients, 47 percent had conditions he deems as precancerous. One had cancer itself. These patients ranged in age from 10 to 26.

Scott is a rare figure on the DES landscape, more extraordinary than he seems to recognize. We salute him. His 70 daughters *are babies he delivered, the children of women to whom he prescribed DES*.

As far as we know, Joseph Scott is the only doctor who became active and prominent in DES detection by looking after his own mistakes. Here is Scott speaking, and may his tribe increase:

"When the dramatic work of Herbst and his associates was published, I felt it incumbent upon me, as one who had used DES extensively in high-risk patients, to locate these patients. This monumental task required 1,500 hours by a medical secretary, with my personal reviews of all suspect charts. I then mailed a letter with a DES information packet, advising these patients that their daughters should be examined by a gynecologist of their choice."

Some of Scott's patients are very young because, as he explains, "arbitrarily I selected the age of 7 years for the first examination, since that is the youngest age at which carcinoma has been reported."

When Scott was prescribing DES, right up until the first Herbst publications, he should have known better. But he knows better now, and he is doing his utmost to save these little girls.

The Treatment of Cancer

The DES daughter must learn to look cancer in the face. If her doctor says she has it, she must ask him what kind.

Carcinoma *in situ* is not an emergency and should not be confused with Herbst's clear-cell adenocarcinoma. Carcinoma *in situ* can usually be cured with minor surgery. Clear-cell adenocarcinoma, on the other hand, is very serious indeed. Fortunately it is also rare.

Our most tentative calculations suggest the following:

• Of each 250 DES daughters, 1, at the maximum, may develop adenocarcinoma by age 30. This, we believe and hope, is a *high* estimate. Possibly the number is as low as 1 in 1,000.

• The chances of DES daughters developing the less virulent cancers described by Stafl look now as if they could be ten times as high as that. One in 25 DES daughters may have carcinoma *in situ* by age 30. Many more will have dysplasia and other changes that should be attended to. It is possible that up to half of DES daughters may need minor surgery before they leave their twenties. Carcinoma *in situ* of the cervix is usually treated by cryosurgery (freezing) or by conization—the coring out of the afflicted portion of the cervix, leaving reproduction intact.

The Treatment of Adenocarcinoma

The management of adenocarcinoma, a far more treacherous problem, is much more debatable. Surgical excision and radiation each produce a 75 percent cure rate, at least for the time being. Because this iatrogenic illness is new, we do not yet have a lengthy follow-up. Surgery is currently in favor, but advocates of radiation, including Dr. J. Taylor Wharton at the M.D. Anderson Hospital and Tumor Institute in Houston, Texas, present a good case.

Wharton and his associates favor *local* radiation therapy whenever feasible, for external radiation, like surgery, may leave the patient with a "nonfunctioning vagina," unable to have intercourse. Wharton argues: "The concept that radical therapy designed to treat the entire vagina and pelvic nodes is needed to cure patients with early cancers should be questioned on the basis of results of less radical treatment."

Wharton's group has treated 5 adenocarcinoma patients, aged 15 to 23, with local radiation, usually after the cancer itself—but not the surrounding tissue—had been surgically removed. Three received a "transvaginal cone" of one to four and a half centimeters, and 2 had "interstitial irradiation" involving radium needles. One of the latter, a 19-year-old, suffered a pulmonary embolus following removal of the radium needles and died. The other 4 are living and well, two to eight years after completion of the therapy. The most remarkable case is that of the second "needle" patient, who was twenty weeks pregnant. She delivered an apparently normal child by caesarean section and has since had two more.

Wharton admits that he, like all DES therapists, is charting the unknown. Despite his success with a pregnant patient, he is concerned about genetic damage from irradiated ovaries. He summarizes the speculative state of our knowledge when he says:

The use of local therapy for patients with small lesions seems to be adequate from the results of this small series of patients. When local irradiation therapy is chosen for lesions up to 2 to 3 cm, it should be anticipated that some patients' cancers have spread beyond the vagina, and, therefore, in a large series with longer follow-up time, a few failures would undoubtedly appear. Would it be justified to strive for 100 percent cure rate in such situations by employing such radical therapy that all of the patients would lose the function of their ovaries, uterus, and vagina, or is it not better to accept a few failures and allow the survivors to enjoy a normally functioning genital tract? If the incidence of regional metastases proves to be high as additional data accumulate, then more comprehensive management will be indicated.

Favoring surgery, however, is Howard Ulfelder, Herbst's colleague and the doctor who operated on the first known patient with DES-related cancer. In Philadelphia in 1975, he reviewed the question of treatment at a National Cancer Institute conference. In the course of his talk, Ulfelder emphasized that whatever tracking method may be used thereafter, he believes it is essential for every DES teen-age daughter to have at least one thorough and complete examination that includes cytologic tests, iodine staining, colposcopy, and biopsies.

Ulfelder has performed extensive surgery on 17 young women with adenocarcinoma. He acknowledges that such treatment has a serious emotional overlay, but he adds that the results were "satisfactory technically, and the women were able to have sexual intercourse." As a surgeon, Ulfelder is less keen than Wharton on radiation treatment. He feels that, even if the disease is controlled, the patient's life expectancy—almost fifty years—is more than enough time for the patient to develop and suffer every possible negative consequence of therapeutic radiation.

Advice to DES Daughters and Mothers

If you are a DES daughter, what can you do for yourself— or, if you are the mother of a daughter who was exposed to DES *in utero*, what can you do for her?

1. Obtain the pertinent medical records if they exist. Do not allow the doctor to be evasive. If he or she won't reply to phone calls or written inquiries, enlist the help of another doctor, or a lawyer if necessary. If DES or other hormones were administered before the eighth week, you will probably show effects, but these may not be of a serious nature. Don't panic, but do investigate.

If hormones were administered between the 8th and 18th week, vaginal abnormalities are likely, but not inevitable. After the 18th week, the syndrome of hidden birth defects which constitute the DES vagina are extremely rare, and *no case of adenocarcinoma has been reported*.

Do not, however, be lulled by false assurances that "the dosage was low" or the duration of administration too short to create problems. Adenocarcinomas have occurred in young women whose mothers received only minuscule doses for a matter of only days in early pregnancy. The essential issue then appears to be *timing*, not duration or dosage.

2. Go to a DES specialist for a thorough checkup. One way to find a specialist is to contact the DES registry in your area of the country. Dr. Samuel Behrman, professor of obstetrics and gynecology at the University of Michigan Medical Center, has written: ". . . we owe patients at risk *constant surveillance* during their teenage and early reproductive years."

3. *If you are a DES mother* exposed before the 18th week of pregnancy, you should start your daughter's checkups by age 14, at the latest. If you prefer to start sooner, find a super-specialist, like John Lewis, who has developed techniques for examining young girls. There is a small risk of cancer in waiting, and a larger risk of emotional distress in starting too early. But if the examination is handled with gentleness and tact, possibly the psychological effects can be minimized. We know two prepubescent DES daughters who are checked out regularly, and seem to take it in stride.

4. Be wary of further exposure to hormones. Herbst points out that oral contraceptives "introduce another hormonal variable into a complex situation, and we have usually discouraged their usage until more information is available." Therefore many doctors advise DES patients against the pill. Certainly it would seem injudicious for the DES daughter to take more DES as a "morning-after" contraceptive (see chap. 5), or to use replacement estrogens as she gets older.

The DES residues in meat pose a thorny problem. Dr. Frank Rauscher, head of the National Cancer Institute, has testified that if he were a pregnant woman, he would not eat liver. The DES daughter might also wish to avoid it, and perhaps, if she is very cautious, all DES-fed meat (see chap. 6).

5. The best specialists do *not* recommend "preventive surgery" for adenosis. Widely practiced in some cities, such as Detroit, it occasionally leaves the recipient with a "dysfunctional" vagina. Why be a guinea pig twice? If you are a DES daughter who is cancer-free, but your doctor proposes vaginectomy, be sure to get further opinions—from other doctors as well as from patients who have had such surgery.

6. Join with other DES victims for emotional support and up-to-date information. (Addresses of DES action groups are provided in the back of the book.) Through organizing, victims of rape and other crimes have obtained sweeping changes. If DES daughters and parents succeed in bringing the makers and promoters to accept responsibility they will set a precedent that may bring about a more cautious approach to all prescription drugs.

7. As of 1978, there is preliminary evidence that DES mothers may be developing breast cancer, as well as cancers of the other female organs, at a higher than normal rate. Mothers are urged to learn self-examination and to be scrupulous in checking themselves. Further exposure to estrogens, including menopausal treatments, is probably inadvisable for any woman who took DES during pregnancy, including those who did not carry to term. For up-to-date information on breast cancer screening in DES mothers, write to: Diane J. Fink, M.D., Director, Division of Cancer Control and Rehabilitation, National Cancer Institute, Blair Building, Room 732, 8300 Colesville Road, Silver Spring, Maryland 20910.

Dr. Fink is chair of the DES Task Force which was convened by the Department of Health, Education and Welfare in 1978.

There is yet no concrete evidence that breast cancer occurs at higher rates in DES daughters. There are, however, anecdotal reports that daughters who have now reached their thirties (i.e., those whose mothers were among the first to receive DES in the 1940s), may also be especially susceptible to breast cancer. Few DES daughters in their thirties are presently under study; but, as a precaution, and until the matter is settled, regular self-examination of the breasts would seem advisable for daughters, too.

According to attorney Paul Rheingold, over two hundred American companies were making DES in its prime, some of them locally, for sale in their own areas. The principal manufacturer was Eli Lilly, which, with five or six other companies, supplied 90 percent of the market.

DES lawsuits are pending in almost every state, and Lilly lawyers are coordinating the defense nationally. The Smiths, for example, have turned over all their records to Lilly.

What Rheingold had hoped to achieve, with his class-action case, was to shift some of the financial burden from patient to manufacturer. The manufacturers, he feels, could pool their resources and share the damages. Thus, if Eli Lilly has held 60 percent of the DES market, it should contribute 60 percent of the cost of aftercare. Squibb and the others would contribute proportional amounts.

And what of the "constant surveillance" that obstetrician Samuel Behrman and the officials of the AMA and ACOG say we "owe" the DES daughters? How can they be "surveyed" if they are not identified? Rheingold thinks the drug companies should be made to run newspaper ads, telling women about DES.

Paul Rheingold's class action was thrown out of federal court in New York. A similar suit in Michigan, brought by 129 women, is still pending, and another has been filed in Manhattan Supreme Court by attorney Aaron Broder. Broder's three clients, residents of Nassau County, range in age from 15 to 23. All claim that they have developed cancer, and are seeking personal and punitive damages, as well as a $500 million "class" fund for treatment and research. DES is providing a lot of work for lawyers. It has no precise legal or medical precedent.

Doctors, even the good ones, are wary of the situation, and reluctant to entangle any colleagues in lawsuits. Time after time, physicians reporting successful treatment of early DES cancers explain, in their scientific papers, that the patients have been alerted by the newspapers to come in for examination. And yet, almost in the same breath, many of these doctors minimize the value of publicity. "The problem is," insisted one doctor, "that the people writing these articles don't understand the subtleties."

"The problem is," said a second doctor, "the people affected by DES have been 'victimized' by a bad press."

Isn't the problem, rather, that doctors—albeit with good intentions—unwisely prescribed DES to pregnant women in the first place?

CHAPTER 4

Of Mice and Men

> [Doctors] *were giving the drug without any good*
> *reason. We're ashamed to say it, but it's the truth.*
> *We're afraid to say it because of lawsuits.*
> Dr. Marluce Bibbo, 1976

Virginia Apgar, the pioneering anesthesiologist and inventor of the "Apgar Score" to assess the condition of newborn babies, used to observe: "It's easy for a woman to succeed in medicine—provided she's twice as smart as a man and works twice as hard."

Marluce Bibbo, M.D., Sc.D., FIAC, of the University of Chicago has a touch of an exotic accent, but she minces no words. She is the only American DES researcher who says right out that the early studies were done on "perfectly normal" pregnant women. This is a matter of record, easily confirmed at any medical library, unless Duane Townsend's mysterious fires have destroyed all the old obstetrics journals as well as the private records of so many prescribing doctors.

But today the shocking facts are nowhere mentioned in print, and few doctors, reporters, or DES victims seem to be aware of them: *DES was tried out on large numbers of normal women, without their informed consent.*

The Mini–Mop-up

Let us hop now to Washington, where Dr. Philip ("He's too young to be an administrator") Corfman, another medical "son" of the Smiths, presides as director of the Center for Population Research at the National Institute of Child Health and Human Development. In this capacity, he has been dispensing contracts for DES research, and has so far awarded $730,000 to Marluce Bibbo's group in Chicago.

A different government agency, the National Cancer Institute, is also laying out over $2.5 million, through the Mayo Clinic and the three other regional DES registries, to locate and examine 4,000 DES daughters. These efforts are commendable, but limited. They reach only a tiny fraction of the women exposed. Since the drug companies and medical societies have not as yet agreed to contribute anything to aftercare, we, as taxpayers, are financing the current mini–mop-up.

Bibbo's Study

Marluce Bibbo, in her follow-up study of Dieckmann's work, used a tracing agency to find patients who had moved. She discovered that 70 percent have adenosis. However, she prefers the cautious approach to adenosis, and believes the treatment for it at some centers is "much too aggressive."

Bibbo, like Herbst (who has moved from Harvard to chair the department at Chicago) favors careful monitoring of DES daughters "as soon as they start to menstruate," with colposcopic observation every six months. She is hopeful that natural healing of adenosis may occur.

By 1975, Bibbo and some dozen associates reported on 84 DES daughters whom they compared to 43 controls. All were around 22 at the time they were examined. The exposed and nonexposed had started menstruating at about the same time, at an average age of 12. However, in frequency of menstruation, duration of flow, regularity of the cycle, and ability to become pregnant there were minor but worrisome differences. Some of the DES daughters were having trouble conceiving, but it is too soon to say whether DES daughters will have substantially more fertility problems than other women. However, more of the DES daughters had also been given *hormones* to regulate their menstrual cycle. We suggest that no DES daughter accept such treatment without getting at least a second opinion from a cancer specialist or endocrinologist.

DES Sons

But Bibbo's bombshell was not her tentative finding of menstrual irregularity in DES daughters. The big news concerned DES sons. In the turmoil over daughters, examination of boys born to women who had taken DES had been neglected. Four years after the Herbst report there was no thorough data on sons. Bibbo, who is professor of pathology as well as obstetrics and gynecology, and her Chicago colleagues began to perform urologic examinations on the male children of DES mothers.

Remember that in the late 1930s, when Shimkin and Grady fed sesame oil laced with DES to male strain C_3H mice, the animals developed "serious abnormalities of the spleen and sex organs" as well as breast cancer. No one seemed interested in this finding. Then, in 1963, other researchers specifically reported *cysts of the epididymis* (the epididymis is a part of the sperm transport mechanism) in newborn male mice injected with DES.

Bibbo *was* interested and worried. She and her research team looked for such cysts in the sons in the early 1950s Dieckmann study and regretfully found *they were there*. Of the first 42 DES sons who were examined and compared to other young men of the same age, *10* had genital abnormalities, including undersized penises (2 cases), varicocele (or enlargement of a vein on the testicle) (1 case), abnormally small testes (2 cases), testicular mass (1 case), and *the same cysts of the epididymis that had long since been demonstrated in mice*. By contrast, only 1 genital abnormality, a varicocele, was observed in any of the 37 controls.

The Chicagoans have now completed studies of 100 DES sons and 100 controls. Cysts are still being found at the rate of 10 percent in the DES sons. Bibbo comments: "Our patients are all still single. The cysts might be of no importance, or they might cause some fertility problems. The proof will come after they are married."

In the meantime, close on the heels of Bibbo's first published reports, further mouse work appeared in *Science*. Dr. John A. McLachlan of the National Institute of Environmental Health Sciences gave DES to pregnant mice. Sixty percent of the sons were sterile, and on autopsy showed many reproductive abnormalities, including intra-abdominal testes attached to their kidneys, and the all-too-familiar epididymal cysts.

McLachlan commented: "In light of these results in rodents . . . boys whose mothers had been treated with DES during gestation . . . should be evaluated for latent alterations in the genital tract. . . . These findings raise the possibility that the disturbance of genital tract development following prenatal exposure to DES may be . . . in the male as well as the female fetus."

Few DES sons are receiving special checkups, perhaps because infertility seems less ominous than cancer. But, in 1978, occasional cases of cancer of the testicles started to be reported. Besides a detailed physical and urologic exam, laboratory studies, which include urine and prostatic fluid cytology, radioimmunoassays of pituitary hormone and testosterone levels, and semen analyses should be performed.

McLachlan and other colleagues have also found that the female offspring of mice treated with DES reveal vaginal changes comparable to those changes observed in human DES daughters. If the females of both species respond alike, it's not surprising that the males do also.

Strange as it may seem, the DES sons are well-advised to learn self-examination of the breast. It's possible that in later life, some of them, like DES-exposed male C_3H mice, may also develop breast cancer.

Some DES sons have already fathered children, according to Arthur Herbst. Among mice, "only" 3 in 5 males are sterile; according to figures released by the National Institutes of Health in April 1976, it looks as if the figure among human males will be smaller—closer perhaps to 1 in 3.

If DES damage is high, concern for it in the medical establishment is low, even among those who are taking in our tax money for the mini–mop-up. Duane Townsend, gynecological oncologist and head of the DES registry in Los Angeles, for example, is skeptical. He said to *Medical*

World News: "What you have is one mouse study [sic] with a small number of mice, and one clinical study in Chicago with a small number of men. . . . They found two undersized penises. What do you compare them with?"

Should we tell him?

CHAPTER 5

After the Morning After

Edward Kennedy, U.S. Senator: "What would you say to the young women of the country who are using [DES] indiscriminately?" Grace M., DES mother: "Stay away from it, as far away as you can get."

Senate hearings on DES, 1975

Despite the bulletin to physicians warning against the use of DES in pregnancy, which Congressman Fountain had wrested out of FDA in November 1971, DES sales *rose* by 4 percent in the next nine months! Now that DES had proved carcinogenic in humans, doctors were prescribing it more than ever. The DES market had been salvaged in the nick of time by a new application, the morning-after pill.

It's worth recalling that in 1949, when the Smiths presented their claims that DES could "make a normal pregnancy more normal," Dr. Willard Allen expressed doubt because in his experiments with rabbits "the administration of estrogen is very deleterious to the fetus. In early pregnancy, estrogen will *prevent* implantation or produce abortion. . . ."

In those days, before Gregory Pincus and John Rock led the way with the oral contraceptive, it was unthinkable to interfere with the *human* ovary just for birth control.

How flexible population ethics are. In the 1940s and 1950s, it was all right to give women a potentially dangerous drug *in the hope of preserving their pregnancies*, but not for birth control. In those days it was a woman's duty, her purpose in life, to reproduce. By the 1960s and 1970s, when the world, in the opinion of its Western political leaders, was sufficiently filled up, the posture of population ethics duly shifted. A dangerous drug was not to be used to preserve a pregnancy, but was acceptable for contraception.

By the 1960s, it was all right to apply Willard Allen's discoveries about DES and rabbits to human subjects— women. This time Yale, not Harvard, led the way. New Haven researchers Drs. J. McLean Morris and G. Van Wagenen were first to publish their trials of oral DES as a morning-after contraceptive. Others followed suit, including Dr. Joseph Massey of the University of Pennsylvania, who reported 4 pregnancies in 500 exposed patients who took the new pill.

The morning-after dose of DES is 25 mg twice daily initiated within seventy-two hours following mid-cycle exposure, and continued for five days. There is a difference of opinion on the effectiveness of this treatment, since pregnancy cannot be diagnosed so early. The DES contraceptive, or "interceptive" as it is sometimes called (because it may work, *if* it works, by preventing implantation), had never been studied in a carefully controlled manner, in which women receiving it after mid-cycle exposure were compared with women who did not take it.

Dr. Christopher Tietze, the statistical wizard of modern contraception, calculates that a woman's chances of getting pregnant from a single unprotected exposure range from 1 in 25 to 1 in 50.

Thus, the Health Research Group states the dilemma like this:

"Estimates are that $\frac{1}{25}$ to $\frac{1}{50}$ of women given the morning-after pill are actually pregnant. Thus, if 4 pregnancies occur in a group of 500 given the pills, the failure rate is much higher than it might seem. Of the 500, only 10 [using the 1 out of 50 figure] would become pregnant without the pill. If 4 get pregnant with the pill the effectiveness is only 60 percent."

Then in 1976 Vicki Jones of our National Center for Disease Control (CDC) in Atlanta presented further evidence that DES is an unreliable contraceptive. Out of several hundred rape victims treated with DES at Grady Memorial Hospital, 5 sustained pregnancies anyway. In fact, the proportion who got pregnant seemed to be about the same as among *untreated* women.

The Michigan Health Service

In the late 1960s, the morning-after pill was being prescribed tentatively by some physicians. But by 1972, an official at the National Institutes of Health announced: "Most university health services are giving the morning-after pill."

How did this happen, and why? What persuaded so many doctors to give their patients, *who might or might not be pregnant*, high dosages of a known carcinogen?

Some of the credit must go to the health service at the University of Michigan. On October 25, 1970, just two weeks before the FDA took action *against* DES as a pregnancy booster, *JAMA* published a report on 1,000 women in and around the university who had used it as a morning-after contraceptive. "No pregnancies resulted," according to the author, "and there were no serious adverse reactions"—an amazing statistic, considering the fact that no contraceptive, *not even sterilization*, has ever been 100 percent effective in a population of 1,000 people.

"The problem of requests for postcoital help by the female patient when she has been exposed to unprotected sexual intercourse for whatever reasons—rape, neglect to use prophylaxis, or failure of prophylaxis, such as condom breakage—is familiar and challenging to most practicing physicians. Formerly in this clinic, we had only told the patient to wait for her next menses—not very consoling advice to a woman who does not want to be pregnant."

The report was like a green light to thousands of health-service doctors, and also to a small Franklinville, New Jersey, drug company called Tablicaps, which merchandised its 25-mg DES tablets called "DESMa" as ". . . the optimum contraceptive since it does not compromise the spontaneity of the sex act."

The Cowan Study

But something embarrassing happened. Local women in Ann Arbor, who were patients at the student health service, chanced upon the *JAMA* report. They didn't believe it. It didn't fit the facts.

First of all, a few women who had been given the

morning-after pill were pregnant, although they acknowledged it could have been from exposure earlier in the cycle. (DES does not work "interceptively" unless it is started within seventy-two hours of the latest exposure and preferably within twenty-four hours after conception. No claims are made that it interrupts an earlier conception.)

Other pregnant women treated at the health service had not had *any* earlier exposure, but were unable to finish the five-day course because the DES pills made them vomit.

Then there was a third group: Women who had not had earlier exposure, were not too nauseated to swallow their medication, but were nonetheless . . . pregnant.

Whatever the scientific explanation, those among the pregnant women who did not believe in abortion were in a bad situation, carrying to term babies who had been exposed to DES early in pregnancy and might get cancer. The morning-after DES dose of 50 mg a day is several dozen times higher than the minimum of 1.5 mg which has been associated with adenocarcinoma.

But how could the student health service know of these pregnancies when in fact it had *never followed up most of the DES patients?*

The investigation took place in 1971, when the notion that patients might check up on their doctors was only beginning to take hold. The Ann Arbor DES patients were pioneers because, as disbelievers, they performed their own surveys. The first survey, of 69 DES patients, revealed that only 1 in 4 had been contacted by the health service doctors *after* the morning-after pill was administered.

Local Ann Arbor women continued to monitor the effects of DES, and repeatedly found facts that contradicted those in the *JAMA* report. On February 27, 1975, Belita Cowan, a health instructor, testified at Senator Kennedy's hearings (the Senator broke precedent for congressional health hearings by seeking opinions from *patients* and consumer advocates, as well as physicians and scientists):

"Last summer, I conducted a survey of over two hundred women, ages 18 to 31, who had taken DES as a morning-after pill in Ann Arbor, Michigan, between 1968

and August of 1974. Twenty-nine percent of my sample
stated that they had taken the morning-after pill at least
twice within a year's time.

"The study showed that DES is being prescribed with
carelessness and casualness. Forty-five percent were not
given pelvic or breast exams. Fifty-six percent stated that
the doctor did not take a personal and family medical history. Eight women said that they got the morning-after pill
not for themselves but for a friend or roommate. Only 26
percent were followed up to see if they were pregnant.

"The study also revealed that DES is being given to
women for whom estrogens are contraindicated. Women
who cannot take birth control pills are being given the
morning-after pill. They are not aware, nor are they informed, that the morning-after pill is estrogen.

"Fifty-seven percent of the sample were unaware that
the morning-after pill did not have FDA approval and that
it had not been proven safe and effective.

"Further, the study revealed that many women are not
being told of the possible cancerous effects to the fetus if
the woman is [already] pregnant. I could not find a single
case where a pregnancy test was given prior to and after
the DES regimen.

"Six percent of those in the survey stated that they
themselves were DES daughters; that is, their mothers took
stilbestrol when they were pregnant in the early 1950s. Of
all the doctors I interviewed, only one expressed hesitation
about giving the morning-after pill to DES daughters. Dr.
Ann Pfrender of the University of Michigan Health
Service stated that, 'We don't know the effects of the morning-after pill on DES daughters, so I don't give it to them.'

"The most interesting finding of the study is that 24
percent of the women stated that they did not take all 10
pills in the series. As one woman put it, 'I got so sick from
the first pill that I never took the rest. I couldn't stand to
be that ill.' And not surprisingly, 65 percent stated that if
they had been fully informed about DES, they would not
have taken it [the morning-after pill] in the first place."

Second Thoughts About the Morning-After Pill

The AMA's medico-legal expert, Don Harper Mills, has warned that in ten to twenty years there may be lawsuits arising from misuse of the morning-after pill. "Whereas physicians today have little or no real exposure to liability for the occurrence of vaginal cancer from DES prescriptions in years gone by, their liability potential henceforth is completely reversed. They, rather than the manufacturers, will have the major defense burden for malignant complications from the contraceptive use of DES."

The drug companies themselves are patently uneasy about morning-after DES. As FDA commissioner Alexander Schmidt admitted in 1975: "DES is a generic drug and is made by many manufacturers, none of whom came forward with data to support the use of DES as a postcoital contraceptive."

They didn't come forward—they backed off! On December 10, 1974, 230,000 United States physicians and 55,000 pharmacists received an unusual letter from DES's most faithful manufacturer, Eli Lilly. The letter said in part:

> Although postcoital contraception is recognized by some authorities as an indication for diethylstilbestrol, Eli Lilly and Company has neither conducted nor supported laboratory or clinical investigations to establish efficacy and safety of its product for this indication. Therefore, diethylstilbestrol supplied by Eli Lilly and Company is not recommended for postcoital contraception, and we are deleting from our product line the 25-milligram dosage forms. We continue to endorse diethylstilbestrol for the indications included in our current literature.
>
> Although diethylstilbestrol is supplied by many manufacturers, Eli Lilly and Company believes it important to acquaint the medical profession with this information.

Profits notwithstanding, Lilly wanted out and still wants out of the morning-after pill—or so it claims. It is instructive to look at page 951 of the *Physicians' Desk Reference*, 1977 edition. The *PDR*, as it is called, is a basic source book wherein the major drug manufacturers supply information about their principal products. Lilly's thousand-word description of its diethylstilbestrol tablets starts out with a warning in oversized capital letters: "THIS DRUG PRODUCT SHOULD NOT BE USED AS A POSTCOITAL CONTRACEPTIVE."

The Kennedy Committee Hearings

And yet according to Morton Mintz, a top-notch investigative reporter for the *Washington Post*, Eli Lilly supplies DES to Tablicaps—the company that markets morning-after pills "that don't compromise the spontaneity of the sex act." Eli Lilly is one of its two DES suppliers. If that is true, what is going on? Can Lilly be talking out of both sides of its mouth?

At this writing, the University of Michigan is still using the DES pill, and so are thousands of other health services and private doctors. The situation is almost without precedent. Doctors, the guardians of health, are prescribing a product for a purpose which its major manufacturer, a frankly profit-making concern, is publicly warning against.

And what of our government guardian, the FDA? Its posture on all DES matters is simply unfathomable—even, as we shall see, to some of its own employees. Commissioner Edwards left the FDA in 1973 and was replaced by Alexander Schmidt, a cardiologist and dean from the University of Illinois Abraham Lincoln School of Medicine. Schmidt testified at the 1975 Kennedy hearings that he was very concerned about "this widespread use of an approved drug for nonapproved use." He added that the FDA was about to approve DES as a morning-after contraceptive *in order that it could be better regulated.*

The logic of this seemed obscure to most observers. The AMA had cautioned doctors against any use of DES in pregnancy while the Michigan Health Service's influential study concerning efficacy had been discredited, or at least severely challenged, by local Ann Arbor patients. The premier DES manufacturer, Lilly, had gone out of its way to inform doctors that neither efficacy nor safety have been established.

Why didn't the FDA just forget it? Why didn't it warn doctors—and women—to stop using the morning-after pill? Why was it approving it now?

Approving it *now?* The reporters at the Kennedy hearings did a double-take. Hadn't the FDA approved DES as a morning-after contraceptive almost two years earlier? Yes, it had, or so most people thought. In May 1973, the FDA mailed a drug bulletin to physicians stating that DES was effective in preventing pregnancy and was approved under restricted conditions. The following September, a similar press release went to reporters.

No one doubted that the FDA had approved morning-after DES. If it really hadn't, this was surely a well-kept secret.

Even the scrupulously careful *Medical Letter*, the *Consumer Reports* of prescription drugs, had stated in its issue of July 16, 1973: "Diethylstilbestrol (DES), a nonsteroidal synthetic estrogen that has been in clinical use for many years, has recently been approved as a 'morning-after' contraceptive. Although the exact mechanism of action is unknown, it probably interferes with implantation of the fertilized ovum."

Like others in the hearing room, Senator Richard Schweiker was confused. If FDA hadn't approved the morning-after pill in 1973, the bulletin to physicians and the press release to reporters must have been a mistake.

Senator Schweiker: "Well, how could a bulletin that erroneously indicated FDA approval for two years not be withdrawn. . . . How do you account for two years nonwithdrawal?"

Commissioner Schmidt: "All the drug bulletin did is specify the conditions under which it would be marketed as a postcoital contraceptive. None of this has taken place yet."

None of this has taken place? Hundreds of thousands of young women, including DES daughters, were getting more DES at student health services, while a new generation of DES children was being born out of what *Medical Letter* had called the "treatment failures."

Why wouldn't the FDA put a stop to it?

Two courageous FDA employees, Dr. Marvin Seife, director of the Generic Drug Division, and Dr. Vincent Karusaitis, an obstetrician and gynecologist, testified that they were puzzled and shocked at their agency's behavior:

Dr. Karusaitis: "I could not understand that we would approve this in a simplistic manner. . . ."

Dr. Seife: "In all my years with the FDA, this is the first time in my experience that a drug has been published for a new use in the Federal Register without any study, without any investigative new drug application for a totally new indication."

Senator Kennedy: "Was that the correct thing to do?"

Dr. Seife: "No."

Senator Kennedy: "Who made the decision to do it?"

Dr. Seife: "I have no idea."

And so in 1973 we have the FDA telling doctors and reporters it was approving the morning-after pill, and then in 1975, because it had no evidence on which to approve it, and because none of the major manufacturers wanted it approved, we have the FDA denying that it had taken this action. Still, the bulletin and press release existed and were there for all to see—just as the 1971 "analyses" of the Herbst and Greenwald data did not exist.

DES as a Milk Suppressant

"For twenty to thirty years, almost every American woman who chose not to breast-feed her baby was given DES, often for several days after birth, to relieve breast engorgement and to dry up her breast milk," Doris Haire, president of the American Foundation of Maternal and Child Health, has stated.

The use of hormones to suppress lactation had been steadily increasing in the United States as breast feeding declines. In 1946, according to pediatrician Herman Meyer of Northwestern University, only 35 percent of newborn babies were bottle-fed exclusively when they left the hospital; by 1966 the figure had jumped to 73 percent. The trend continued through the early 1970s, at which point it was estimated only 5 to 10 percent of newborns were breast-fed. (But today a turnabout is occurring, a spokesman for an infant formula company explained. Breast-feeding has sufficiently increased, so that the company in changing its ad campaign. Instead of promoting its formula as the ideal nourishment for newborns, the ads will suggest that formula is better than cows' milk later, after the infant is weaned.)

American women are rarely told that if they decline

to breast-feed, it is not necessary to use hormones to dry up their milk. Indeed, many do not know that they are getting hormones for this purpose. Medication is merely brought to them, and they are not expected to ask questions. Besides DES, other hormone products commonly used for lactation suppression are the pill, Tace, and Deladumone. Tace, made by the Merrell Company, is a synthetic estrogen employed for most of the same indications as DES, and known to have many of the same side effects. Deladumone, made by Squibb, combines estrogen and a form of testosterone, given in a long-acting slow-release injection. It has the usual estrogen dangers also. DES and Tace are administered for from two to six days, depending on the size of the dosage. Deladumone is given in a single shot.

What do they look like? It's a good idea to know if you had them—and also you'll want to recognize them if you are offered them in the future. In the 12-mg dose, Tace is a large, soft green gelatin capsule. The 25-mg dose is a hard, two-tone green capsule, and a whopping 72 mg can be found in a green and yellow soft gelatin capsule. The Amfre-Grant Company's Dicorvin, another diethylstilbestrol pill, is a yellow scored tablet. Lilly's diethylstilbestrol line is extensive: Red-coated tablets and off-white scored tablets come in dosages from .1 to 5 mg. Tylosterone, a combination of methyltestosterone and diethylstilbestrol, is also an off-white scored tablet.

Why are hormones especially dangerous after childbirth? A major cause of maternal illness and death is blood clotting in the period just after delivery. Hormone administration substantially increases the risk of developing post-partum clotting. Deladumone, the long-acting injectable, seems particularly treacherous in this regard because, should blood clots develop, the overload of hormones cannot be halted. Most doctors advise their patients to stop taking the pill or other estrogens some weeks before going into the hospital for elective surgery. This is specifically to avoid the extra blood-clotting risk.

All new mothers take risks when they accept hormones to dry up their breast milk. We would especially urge DES daughters to avoid hormonal lactation suppressants, whether the product is specifically DES or its chemical cousins, such as Tace, Deladumone, or the pill. Some of these medications may also produce other startling and undesirable side effects such as the growth of facial hair.

Doris Haire, in observing childbirth practices worldwide, notes that "in Sweden almost all women nurse their babies while they're in the hospital, and then taper off if they plan to bottle-feed at home. It is much safer to dry up a mother's milk gradually over a week's time than the way we do it here." Beth Gall, a pediatric nurse practitioner in Ann Arbor, concurs: "It only takes a few days for milk to dry up. A woman who nursed for a week or so could remain comfortable and then gradually taper off and wean the baby to the bottle. This method would not require the use of lactation suppressant." Hormones do not always dry up milk—they may only delay lactation until the woman gets home from the hospital. So many new mothers complain of this "post-hospital rebound" that obstetricians can hardly be unaware of it. Symptoms include swelling and breast engorgement, as well as severe pain, which is usually treated with breast-binding and ice packs. Of course, once the patient returns home it is *her* problem, no longer a nuisance to hospital personnel.

In contrast to hormone therapy, the Swedish method of tapering off offers health benefits to mother and baby. The infant's sucking contracts the mother's uterus, helps it return to normal size, and may prevent uterine hemorrhages. And for the baby, even temporary nursing, especially in the first few days, is thought to convey immunity to some illnesses.

Most recently, doctors in Greece and England have started to substitute 200-mg dosages of vitamin B_6 for post-partum estrogen. Newly dubbed "the sleeping giant of nutrition," the vitamin relieves breast engorgement in 90 percent of women. It works in half the time of the hormone (ten to twelve hours instead of twenty-four) with no danger of blood clots, and less rebound effect. B_6 is usually administered for 5 days.

In 1978, the FDA's Advisory Committee on Obstetrics and Gynecology reviewed the evidence and recommended that approval of hormones to suppress lactation be withdrawn.

DES and Other Types of Cancer

Today DES is still used interchangeably with Premarin and other brands of replacement estrogen for menopause, while Premarin is offered as a morning-after contraceptive at some health centers where DES has a bad reputation, including Barnard College. Some of the women who have suffered cancer of the endometrium (the lining of the uterus) as a result of menopause therapy were, specifically, users of DES.

Why then do doctors continue to prescribe it?

Some of them do not realize that its association with cancer is firmly proved. They believe that DES was administered *only to women who were having problem pregnancies*, and that when daughters born to DES users develop cancer, it may be due to a natural weakness in the fetus, or maternal environment.

But as we now know, DES was given to many healthy pregnant women in the 1940s and early '50s in the hopes of making "normal pregnancies more normal." When that practice was abandoned, doctors still gave it to patients who merely had a previous history of miscarriage—even when there was not the slightest hint of present trouble.

Another defense we've heard from DES-prescribing doctors is that it has been proved carcinogenic only in fetuses but not adults. Once again this in incorrect. *Adult males treated with DES in medical experiments have developed breast cancer as a consequence.*

Concerning adult women, on September 28, 1972, a report appeared in the *New England Journal of Medicine* which should have received as much attention as the Herbst study but did not. Since it, too, came from Massachusetts General Hospital, it was like the dropping of a fateful second shoe. The doctors who made the later study observed a series of young women who, due to a condition called ovarian dysgenesis (congenitally defective or absent ovaries), were under treatment with DES for five years or longer. Several patients had developed cancer of the endometrium or precancerous changes. All told, pathological specimens from five women with ovarian dysgenesis who got endometrial cancer in association with estrogen therapy were carefully evaluated. Three of the five were of a most unusual mixed or adenosquamous type, *reminiscent of the adenocarcinomas found in the vaginas and cervices of women exposed to DES prenatally*. The average age of these 5 endometrial cancer patients was 31.

Thus, by 1972, DES had proven carcinogenic in adult women as well as in fetuses, causing cancer of the uterus rather than the vagina and cervix.

Detail men (drug company salesmen) are very, very nice to doctors. Some are pharmacists or scientists by training, but most are hired for their likability and charm. They entertain doctors—at least, those who'll let them—and provide free drugs and vitamins for their personal use, and even more elaborate gifts, including office equipment and trips. A detail man's commissions rest on the number of prescriptions that the doctors in his territory write for his products. When a doctor writes a prescription for DES, he could be returning a favor or helping out a friend.

Cancer is good for the economy too. There is a grim joke that "more people live off cancer than die from it." The total care of a terminal cancer patient averages $20,000. Cancer provides lots of jobs for medical workers and morticians.

CHAPTER 6

Fed Up with DES

Every consideration favors removing DES from cattle feed. Every other country in the world has banned DES. United States exported meat is rejected in a number of countries because we continue to use it.

Dr. Jean Mayer, 1976

Olive and George Smith may have failed to grow bigger and better "stilbestrol babies," but others who took a similar notion—veterinary scientists—had more success.

A free and mentally competent adult U.S. citizen is not permitted to medicate herself or himself with hormones or antibiotics. Such powerful chemicals are available by prescription only—in drugstores. In feedstores, however, hormones and antibiotics are sold *without prescription—by the carload.* The veterinary market for some of these products is much larger than the human market.

Eighty to 85 percent of our livestock is raised on DES. Residues remain in the animals after slaughter and are served up with our meat. The consumer gets it, wanted or not, on the dinner table.

Additives to packaged foods must at least be listed on the label, but the hormones, arsenic, and antibiotics that lace our meat are, like pesticides, totally invisible and silent.

The U.S. Department of Agriculture (USDA) claims that DES saves the average American $3.85 a year on his or her meat bills. It fattens up livestock so that animals can be brought to slaughter sooner, cutting feed costs by 10 percent.

The raising of cattle, sheep, and poultry on DES has been popular since the end of World War II. The Animal

Health Institute, an industry association that represents major manufacturers of animal health and nutrition products—drugs, biologicals, and feed additives, among others —maintains that progress in animal health and nutrition and in veterinary medicine, including the use of DES, has helped the American farmer to produce 88 percent more meat and poultry today (1976) than he did in 1950.

DES-Fed Animals and the Consumer

Natural food advocates reply that any economic benefits from DES are not, in truth, passed along to the meat shopper. M.E. Royce, a physician from El Centro, California, compares the fattening of animals with DES to certain practices that were "hanging offenses" in years gone by: "If the figures supplied me are anywhere near correct," he writes, "the increased weight [of DES-fed cattle] represents a less than 2 percent increase in protein, about 25 percent increase in fat, with the balance of the increase representing retained salt and water. The meat animal on DES retains salt and water in its tissues, even as the lady on birth control pills retains salt and water in her tissues. The old-time farmer knew not to slaughter a female animal 'in heat' because of the excess salt and water in her tissues at that time. . . . All the retained salt and water does for the consumer is to cause the meat to splatter in the pan while frying, making it necessary to clean the top of the stove more often. . . .

"In days gone by, some unscrupulous farmers gave their cows salt, followed by water, just before taking them to market. The stockyard operators soon learned to wait a couple of days until the cattle had excreted the salt and water before weighing the animals and paying for them. This process of salting and watering the stock, if discovered, was a hanging offense in some areas of the country. Now, however, accomplishing the same result on a longer-term basis by using DES is thought of (by some) as good farming practice and scientific animal husbandry. There is the further 'advantage' that if retained by the action of DES, the salt and water will not leave the animal's body in only a day or two in the stockpen.

"I can find no justifiable reason on a human nutritional basis for adding DES to animals, either in the feed or by implant. If it is in order to sell salt and water at high prices, there is only one excuse for so doing—greed."

Beatrice Trum Hunter, the natural foods writer, agrees: "Stilbestrol yields poorer meat because it produces weight that is watery fat, but not protein. . . . From the consumer's viewpoint, this is not only undesirable but an economic fraud."

FDA and the Pellets

In 1938, the U.S. Congress attempted to extend consumer protection afforded by the original 1906 legislation through an amended Food, Drug, and Cosmetics Act that defined any food as "adulterated" if it contained substances that might be injurious to health. The act also gave the FDA authority to proceed against food products that contained harmful residues.

Then in May 1945 the FDA received an application to use stilbestrol pellets in the necks of chickens to produce a feminized male bird called a "caponette."

The capon, like candied sweet potatoes or mince pie, was a popular novelty item for holidays and special occasions. In her book *Consumer Beware!*, Ms. Hunter explains why poultry farmers found DES pellets useful: "It was easier and faster than the old castration process. Poultrymen without special training necessary for caponizing could 'castrate' with the hormones."

Soon DES was widely used in the poultry industry, for, Ms. Hunter reveals, it could also "put weight on birds quickly, and could even give old birds the appearance of youth, with plumper, more attractive flesh. There are greater cooking losses in hormonized birds—in some cases 20 percent more—than in untreated ones."

Men exposed to large amounts of estrogens sometimes grow breasts; indeed they need not even take it internally, for antibaldness scalp treatments containing estrogen produce this effect in 1 user out of 50. It is not surprising that prodigious consumers of chicken necks—such as restaurant workers who were free to snack on the portions of the bird not served to customers—were reported to be showing this effect. The first such case occurred in New

York City, and was duly noted by the health department, which registered concern about the new caponizing practices.

Yet, in the course of the next decade, FDA sanctioned the addition of DES to the feed of poultry, cattle, and sheep, as well as pellet implants in the necks of poultry and the ears of cattle and sheep. Their rationale was that residues of DES would not appear in any *edible tissue*. The stilbestrol implants, in theory, would all have dissolved, and stilbestrol-laced feed was to be withdrawn twenty-four hours before slaughter.

Ranchers and poultrymen like to produce a wholesome product, and they were wary at first. But DES gave the breeders who used it a competitive advantage, so reluctantly a majority went along. As late as August 1955, *Farm Journal* carried an editorial called "Stilbestrol-fed Cattle: How They're Selling Now" which advised: "If you feed stilbestrol to your cattle, better not say anything about it when you send them to market. You might end up getting less money. One packer has this to say: 'Stilbestrol cattle just don't cut out a carcass that's as good as they look on the hoof.' . . . The beef we're seeing today does not measure up to the old corn-fed beef. It looks plump and good on the outside, but when you cut it open, the quality isn't there. Can buyers tell by looking at cattle whether they've been fed stilbestrol? Generally not. So while it's hard to nail down anything concrete at those markets, one fact stands out: If you feed stilbestrol, better keep mum about it."

But one group of animal breeders—mink ranchers—could not "keep mum" about stilbestrol, not when they discovered that the poultry implants were sterilizing their minks!

If you have a pet in your household, look at the labels on some of the canned products you probably keep for them in your cupboard. You will see that they contain mysterious ingredients such as "digest of chicken by-products and chicken parts." Chicken by-products—portions of the chicken (and other animals) that do not command a large human market—are normally recycled for other carnivores, including minks. Minks like the head and neck of chicken, which happens to contain (contrary to FDA and stilbestrol-industry assurances) the remains of the DES pellets that had been implanted in chicken necks and had not dissolved. And as we discussed earlier, the side effects of DES include not only cancer but *sterility and feminization in males*—which is what happened to many ranch-raised minks. This discovery by the mink ranchers was proof of DES residue and should have caused DES treatment of food animals to be discontinued at once. But though the FDA did ban DES in poultry in 1959, pellet implants in cattle were allowed to continue.

When DES pellets were ordered out of chicken necks, poultrymen were stuck with a surplus of 12 million pounds of stilbestrol chicken. With the blessing and connivance of the USDA, it was legally converted into canned, boned-meat chicken products. Thus, while minks were protected from stilbestrol-implanted chickens, we and our household pets were not.

The Delaney Amendment

FDA also took sides against consumer protection by opposing the 1958 Delaney Amendment to the Food, Drug, and Cosmetic Law. This amendment stated that *"No [food] additive shall be deemed safe if it is found to induce cancer when ingested by man or animal. . . ."* George Larrick, then commissioner, fought it. (When he retired, Larrick accepted a job as consultant to Dow Chemical.)

FDA successfully subverted the Delaney Amendment in 1962 by persuading Congress to *permit the use in animal feeds of drugs found to promote cancer, provided such use did not result in detectable residues of the drug in edible tissues.* FDA assured Congress that the DES in meat would be gone by the time it reached our tables.

However, in the late 1960s a scientist at Eli Lilly & Company devised an improved method for measuring DES residues in what Congress and the FDA called "edible tissues." Using this method, the Agriculture Department began to report residues of DES in beef liver, and in the kidneys and the musculature of beef and lamb. From then on, through 1971, DES residues were consistently found in the livers of .5 to 1 percent of all beef cattle examined. Pressure to take action mounted on the FDA.

This was a clear violation of the Delaney Amendment, even as modified in 1962. Detectable residues of a carcinogen were *not* gone from the meat we were eating. At the Fountain Committee hearing on DES, conducted in 1971 and '72, Commissioner Edwards resisted . . . and resisted. Flanked by attorney Peter Barton Hutt, Bureau of Drugs Director Henry Simmons, and C. D. Van Houweling, D.V.M., director of FDA's Bureau of Veterinary Medicine, the commissioner dug in his heels. Defending his decision to overlook the residues, Edwards made as many excuses as the chap who "had never borrowed his neighbor's lawn mower, in the first place, claimed it was broken when he borrowed it, and avowed that he returned it in perfect condition."

Edwards argued that the new, improved method of finding DES residues, informally used by the Agriculture Department, didn't really count because it had not yet been officially approved.

He insisted that low-level residues, if they existed, were "safe," contrary to the animal research that showed that levels of 6.26 parts per billion—much less than those found in beef liver—were carcinogenic in mice.

In April 1970 a committee formed by the United States Surgeon General consisting of cancer experts from the National Cancer Institute, the National Institute of Environmental Health Sciences, and the academic community had submitted a report entitled "Evaluation of Environmental Carcinogens," which stated flatly that "no level of exposure to a chemical carcinogen should be considered toxicologically insignificant for man. For carcinogenic agents, a safe level for man cannot be established from our present knowledge." (Curiously, this report was *not* publicized by the Surgeon General until Morton Mintz of the *Washington Post* got hold of it a year and a half later.)

The Surgeon General, along with the FDA commissioner, is an officer of the Department of Health, Education, and Welfare, so the environmental carcinogens report was presumably made available to FDA also. One can only conclude that FDA ignores the advice of its own blue-ribbon scientific experts. Even FDA's special cancer adviser Roy Hertz had stated that "any amount [of DES] in any foods to be ingested by human subjects, and for that matter even pets around the house, constitutes a substantial hazard which we would all be better off without." Yet Commissioner Edwards stated publicly, "I do not think Dr. Hertz has had a great deal of experience with . . . some of our regulatory and compliance problems. . . . I do not question his scientific knowledge at all, but I question his regulatory knowledge."

"In terms of environmental carcinogens," Edwards declared, "we must be pragmatic."

No Ultra-ban from FDA

Under pressure from Fountain, Edwards took the lesser action of requiring that DES be withdrawn from the feed of meat animals *seven* days before slaughter, instead of two. Not only did residues fail to decline—they were found even more frequently. By June 1972, the Agriculture Department was reporting DES residues in 2 percent of the livers sampled, up from 1 percent in earlier years.

FDA was plagued not only by Fountain and his tenacious staff, but also by consumer groups such as DOOM (Drugs Out of Meat), Federation of Homemakers, Health Research Group, and the Nader organizations.

Finally, on August 4, 1972, FDA revoked approval of DES in animal feed, to become effective in January 1973. Implants (still permitted in the ears of cattle) were to be terminated on April 25, 1973.

But Edwards was still playing games with the consumer, appeasing us while giving industry an out. He declined to invoke the Delaney Amendment, which would have left the manufacturers without further recourse. Jean Mayer, the Tufts University nutritionist, tells the story: "The law gives the FDA two ways to deal with a carcinogenic substance. The first is to apply the Delaney Amendment, which forbids the use, in food or feed, of any substance that in any concentration causes malignancies in any animal species. When this law is involked, there is no legal appeal.

"The FDA has seldom applied the Delaney Amendment, preferring to use the alternative course, which is simply to declare that a substance has not been shown to be safe and for this reason should be withdrawn.

"The FDA chose this second method of banning DES, and as a result, FDA hearings first had to be held. Then appeals and counterappeals . . . [were] . . . heard in the federal courts. The FDA attempted to institute the ban on DES; they were then challenged in court by the feedlot operators on the grounds that hearings had not been held, as the law requires.

"The feedlot operators were upheld, and there the matter has rested legally. . . ."

In the midst of all this delaying litigation, Dr. Alexander MacKay Schmidt from the University of Illinois took over the reins at FDA in 1973 and now the pressure was on him. Nearly two years passed, during which Schmidt did nothing, even though he has claimed, as a cardiologist, to be concerned about the effect of estrogens on the cardiovascular system. Yet, when the feedlot operators won their case and the courts overturned the DES ban in January 1974, Schmidt took no immediate action.

In December 1975 the Health Research Group issued a letter to the Secretary of HEW demanding that DES be banned in animal feed, and the Senate passed a bill (S. 963) prohibiting such use. Supporting congressional intervention—made necessary only because of FDA's refusal to invoke the Delaney Amendment—was Congressman (now Senator) John Melcher from Montana.

Melcher said: "For the cattleman, the question is not just an economic one. It is also a question of consumer confidence. As a veterinarian and former feedlot operator, I have used DES as a growth stimulant and understand its beneficial aspect as such. It does promote growth, it does save on feed costs, and it does help to get our product to market faster. That there are economic advantages, when seen on paper, cannot be disputed.

"But," said cattleman Melcher, "DES is a proven carcinogen. It causes cancer. . . . The United States public is in some danger. . . . There is a much more important matter at stake than the economics of raising cattle. That, of course, is the consumers' fear of eating meat from animals fed a known carcinogen. . . . The use of DES in the feedlot ration is a poor policy . . . consumer confidence in the wholesomeness of the product will be jolted.

"I believe DES should be unconditionally banned in livestock feeds. . . ."

Once again, however, FDA failed to name DES a carcinogen and invoke the Delaney Clause. It simply "proposed to withdraw approval for the use of DES as a growth promotant."

This means that, at this writing, DES is *not* out of our meat. Hearings and legal hassles will go on for years. DES manufacturers, unlike consumers, have endless funds to finance their battle. In our corner, theoretically, is FDA, but—with one or two exceptions—its officials lack conviction.

"Safe Levels"

Some scientists maintain that there are probably "safe levels" of human exposure to carcinogens. One who has argued such a position in *JAMA* (the *Journal of the American Medical Association*) is Dr. Thomas H. Jukes, a biochemist and nutritionist, who worked for Lederle Laboratories for almost twenty years. Jukes has stated: "Apprehensions about [estrogen] residues in food are widespread among the American middle class, who are able to afford the higher prices that will result from the extra costs of producing and processing food without chemical technology. The world's problem is that the higher prices will [affect the] less well-to-do and that no actual benefit to public health will result from banning the technology in any case."

Jukes believes that the addition of DES to cattle feed at most yields a risk of "one case of cancer per 2,500 woman years in the United States population." He says, "It seems likely that there must be a threshold level for cancer caused by estrogens, for these are present in all human beings, and not all human beings develop cancer."

Curiously, most of the pertinent officials at FDA and the Agriculture Department share Jukes's optimism. One has stated: "If DES were present in liver at 2 parts per billion, you would have to eat 500 pounds of that liver to get an amount of estrogen equivalent to the daily estrogen production in premenopausal women."

Maybe the FDA's and the chemical industry's typical spokesmen are right. Maybe DES is not dangerous in our meat, and does help poor people get more protein. But maybe cancer specialists like Hertz and many others and the natural-food advocates are right. *They* say that there are no safe levels of DES exposure, nor any economic savings to speak of, for the extra weight of DES-fed livestock is mostly water.

Can we afford to take chances with such a powerful drug?

Piecemeal Legislation

. . . or with *any* powerful drug? Alexander MacKay Schmidt, FDA Commissioner through November 1976, comes from an academic background, not from industry. The excuses he had given for inaction on DES do make some scientific and moral sense.

Schmidt is opposed to "piecemeal legislation" governing DES on the legitimate grounds that all estrogen products are equally dangerous. On January 21, 1976, he explained to Senator Kennedy at the estrogen hearing: "We have no reason to suspect that DES is unique among estrogens in its ability to harm the fetus. It was simply the first synthetic, inexpensive estrogen to be marketed in the United States and is, therefore, an estrogen which has been commonly [used] for many years."

Schmidt has also expressed concern about the male hormone, testosterone. "Interestingly," he commented, ". . . testosterone can also produce tumors in rodents if tested under similar conditions."

Does it make sense to ban only DES in cattle feed when nine other hormones are permitted? Does it make sense to ban it as a morning-after pill when student health services are already substituting Premarin, megadoses of the birth control pill, and other hormone products for the same purpose?

Schmidt acted indecisively (products should be *out*, not *in*, until proven safe), but his administration did, for the first time, acknowledge the crucial damages and similarities of *all* hormone products. He may go down in history as the well-intentioned Hamlet of our modern FDA commissioners.

On the face of it, Schmidt's dilemma seems legitimate, for if DES is banned, he argued, why not Premarin and the pill?

For starters, FDA might distinguish between the *hidden* and *overt* uses of hormones. When DES or other hormones are used medically, consumers (patients) usually have some choice in the matter, if not always an *informed* choice. When such drugs are used "nutritionally" we have no choice at all. To feed us a known carcinogen without our knowledge or approval might be considered a violation of the Bill of Rights, a kind of chemical assault on our persons. On this basis, hormones and other dangerous chemicals could surely be banned from cattle feed, whether or not they are still retained in medicine.

Later in 1976 an HEW committee chaired by Dr. Carl Schultz acknowledged that Schmidt's dilemma was legitimate. The committee was formed to consider what might be done to help DES families. Soon it recognized that many pressing questions remained unanswered. How *much* would it harm DES daughters to use the pill, take hormone lactation suppressants, or eat estrogen-laced meat? Hoping to issue guidelines quite quickly (the committee, in fact, had planned to set up a telephone hot line to answer consumer questions), Schultz and his group are now bogged down in intricate studies.

For Appearance's Sake

At Albert Einstein's Department of Social Medicine, Dr. Ernest Drucker has suggested—only half in jest—that the very word FOOD be dropped from the FDA's title. "Why not just call it the Drug and Cosmetic Administration?" he suggests, since food, as we used to know it, hardly exists anymore.

Drucker is right. Most of us know about the dyes and sequestrants used, for cosmetic purposes only, in our packaged foods, but few are aware that hormones and other chemicals in our unlabeled animal feed have also been approved, in many cases, just for appearance's sake. They serve no value as growth promotants or preservatives, and are officially sanctioned just to seduce or tempt the buyer, like a lady of the night.

In poultry, for example, certain hormones and arsenic are permitted just to "improve finish," "improve pigmentation," and "enhance bloom."

Among the animal-maintenance products to which Americans are still exposed, and which many other nations have banned along with DES, are nine additional hormones:

• Chlormadinone acetate, permitted in feed for beef heifers and beef cows for synchronization of estrus (heat).

• Progesterone, permitted for subcutaneous implantation in lambs and steers for growth promotion and feed efficiency.

• Dienestrol diacetate, permitted in feed for broilers, fryers, and roasting chickens for the promotion of fat distribution and for tenderness and bloom.

• Estradiol benzoate, used in combination with progesterone and testosterone.

• Estradiol monopalmitate, permitted for injection under skin at base of skull of roasting chickens to produce more uniform fat distribution and improve finish.

• Testosterone, permitted for subcutaneous ear injection in beef cattle to stimulate growth.

• Testosterone proprionate, permitted for subcutaneous ear implantation in heifers to promote growth and increase feed efficiency.

• Medroxyprogesterone acetate, permitted in feed for breeding cattle and ewes for the synchronization of estrus and ovulation.

• Melengestrol acetate, permitted in feed for heifers for growth stimulation, improved feed utilization, and suppression of estrus.

The liver and, to some extent, the kidney are the body's filters in which drug residues are most apt to collect. Until such time as FDA bans all drugs from meat, it seems judicious to avoid these two organs—for your pets as well as yourself and your family. (Organic desiccated liver tablets can supply the proper nutrients you should be getting from fresh liver. See chap. 35 for additional information.)

Senator Melcher's fears that our trust in the wholesomeness of meat has been "jolted" seem warranted. Many people who can afford meat are eating less of it. A vegetarian diet can be nutritious and healthy, but should not be embarked upon lightly. Sources of instruction for vegetarian eating are listed in the appendix.

Your economic weapon is your meat dollar, while your political weapon is consumer action. A list of consumer groups whose literature you might wish to send for is also included.

Some ranchers and breeders, usually the smaller ones, have taken it on themselves to avoid unnecessary drugs. Perhaps 15 percent of the meat and poultry raised in the United States remains free of chemicals. Unmedicated cattle and poultry are more expensive at present, partly because they are raised with more care, and partly because the weight gain in medicated livestock, legitimate or not, gives breeders who use DES a competitive advantage. Wherever it's possible to buy meat of unmedicated animals, consumers would do well to consider it.

Oral Contraceptives: From the
Wonderful Folks Who
Brought You
the Pill

In 1967 a delegation of Western journalists was granted an interview with Boris Petrovski, the Soviet minister of health. When the writers asked why the pill was not being used in Russia, Dr. Petrovski replied: "We do not want our children born with deformed hands and feet."

The journalists were confused. Had Dr. Petrovski confused the pill with thalidomide? There was then no hint, in the annals of Western medicine, that the pill might be associated with any such birth defects.

Some years later, in 1973 and '74, studies by researchers in the United States confirmed that a thalidomide-like syndrome, involving limb defects, does occur in a small number of the offspring, especially males, of mothers exposed to hormones during the early weeks of pregnancy. In some cases this exposure is due to hormonal "pregnancy tests," while in others it is associated with "breakthrough" pregnancies that occur to women on the pill. (These are less rare than we think. While the pill is near-perfect in theory, in practice *6 percent of pill users get pregnant during the first year* and most continue taking these hormones until the pregnancy is diagnosed—which may not be for months.)

If the Russians knew so long ago that the pill can cause birth defects, why weren't we informed? Whenever a new and alarming side effect of the pill is uncovered, why do some doctors and population controllers hasten to minimize its importance? It's bad to *frighten* women, according to this doctrine, but all right to *kill* and *maim* them. And some doctors who won't hear a word said against the pill have personal or professional ties with drug companies. For example, Dr. Robert Kistner, author of a book and many articles defending the pill, has performed research for the following pharmaceutical houses: Wm. S. Merrell, Mead Johnson, Cutter, Squibb, Searle, Parke, Davis, Upjohn, Wyeth, Lilly, and Organon. In his writings, he is identified merely as a Harvard professor, not by his other connections.

In 1975 we were notified, as if out of the blue, that the pill is associated with a much-increased risk of heart attacks. *Users in their thirties, we learned, are three times as likely to have heart attacks as nonusers.* Users in their forties are five to six times as likely. A woman in her early forties who does not take the pill stands an annual risk of 1 in 5,000 of suffering a heart attack; if she is a pill user, her risk increases to 1 in 1,000.

These heart attack studies were performed in England. Upon learning of them, our FDA commissioner urged American doctors to stop prescribing the pill to women past 40. The FDA appears to be on its toes, and yet . . . in 1969, when we were preparing a book called *The Doctors' Case Against the Pill*, we called on Dr. John Schrogie, who was then the FDA's principal expert on the subject. Dr. Schrogie admitted he was extremely worried about the possibility of heart attacks in pill users.

Did the FDA warn American women in 1969 that, theoretically, the pill was apt to be dangerous to their hearts? No. Did the FDA order the pertinent studies to be done? No. Instead it was left to the British, who have fewer pill users than we and a lower budget for this type of research, to clarify the issue six years later. In the meantime, women died, women who might have chosen not to take the pill if they had understood the risks.

Today, in spite of the formidable mass of accumulated evidence that the birth control pill can and does cause fatal or disabling blood clots, fatal liver disease, cancer, depression, birth defects, and a wide spectrum of less serious but nevertheless disabling or discomfiting symptoms, it is still widely prescribed. Some birth control organizations continue to offer it as the choice method to women who come to their clinics. They present the spurious argument that the pill is safer than childbirth—as though there were no other options available. (What is the logic in comparing a method of contraception with *birth*? Doesn't it rather make sense to compare one contraceptive with *another*?)

Schrogie, like so many FDA officials, left his government post some years ago to become an executive with a drug company.

CHAPTER 7

How the Pill Happened

We may be condoning the use of an entirely elective drug by young, healthy women without adequate evidence of its thrombogenicity. This is a sobering responsibility—particularly if this drug can contribute to deaths from pulmonary embolism in some ancillary way that is not currently appreciated.

Dr. Stanford Wessler, assistant professor of medicine at Harvard Medical School, September 1962

The pill was a brainchild of Margaret Sanger, founder of Planned Parenthood, popularizer of the diaphragm, and an indomitable fighter for women's rights. Surviving jail, ridicule, and decades of harassment, she, more than anyone, made birth control respectable. In 1950 or 1951, when she was about 88, Ms. Sanger was introduced to Gregory Pincus, a reproductive scientist from Massachusetts. She raised some $150,000—mainly from her friend Katharine McCormick, heiress to a farm-machinery fortune—to get Pincus started on research toward a "universal" contraceptive.

It's regrettable to note that Margaret Sanger, for all her great works, was a bit of an elitist. In a fund-raising letter to Katharine McCormick, she stated: "I consider that the world and almost our civilization for the next twenty-five years is going to depend upon a simple, cheap, safe contraceptive to be used in poverty-stricken slums and jungles, and among the most ignorant people. . . . I believe that now, immediately, there should be national sterilization for certain dysgenic types of our population who are being encouraged to breed and would die out were the government not feeding them."

Pincus, Chang, and Rock

By the 1930s, animal researchers knew that hormones could prevent ovulation in rabbits and other species. Some observers claim that Hitler's scientists used crude hormonal birth control methods in concentration camps.

Outside of the Third Reich, most doctors were wary of trying any such experiments on humans. First there was the fact that the physiology of female reproduction depends on a delicate, imperfectly understood "feedback" system. If you introduce extra ovarian hormones in contraception, you interrupt the normal oscillating signals that trigger pituitary hormones which, in turn, seem to mediate most of our metabolic functions. You are throwing a monkey wrench into the entire body system.

Second, estrogens, at least, were known to be cancer-producing. By the year 1940, hundreds of studies had been published with titles such as "Estrogens in Carcinogenesis" and "The Significance of Hormones in the Origin of Cancer."

Even so, Pincus and his research colleague, Dr. Min Cheuh Chang, had the tantalizing notion that perhaps some form of progesterone, the second ovarian hormone, might be used more safely for birth control. It did not, at least, have a long-established connection with cancer.

Pincus and Chang began to experiment with progestins (artificial progesterones) which in the early 1950s were just becoming available in a form to be taken orally. They discussed their efforts with Dr. John Rock, a Harvard gynecologist, who, as an infertility specialist, was also doing experiments with ovarian hormones. Soon they joined forces—Rock from Harvard and Pincus at his nearby private establishment, the Worcester Foundation for Experimental Biology. Pincus and Chang were giving hormones to rabbits and rats, while Rock gave them on a short-term basis to women with complex fertility problems. They pooled information.

By the mid-1950s they were ready to move into the next stage of their work—testing a *contraceptive* pill on humans. The first volunteers, some 60 women, included medical students and a group of chronic mental patients at a hospital near Worcester. Pincus wondered if his pill would make men as well as women infertile. It did! Among the very first patients were a group of male psychotics at the same state hospital. Thus, before the pill ever became available to women, Pincus established from sperm samples that it worked on men as well. (See chap. 21.)

Syntex, Searle, and Progestin

Our primitive ancestors, we are told, had knowledge of medicinal plants. They presumably used them as diuretics, astringents, emetics, stimulants, and pain relievers. Throughout human history, until chemists learned to synthesize drugs, people relied upon plants and animals entirely for their medicines.

For a time in the 20th century, medicinal plants were neglected by all but a few believing scientists. One such, in the 1930s and '40s, was an organic chemist named Russell Marker who taught at Pennsylvania State College. Marker was interested in the chemistry of steroids, including sex hormones. His research led him to conclude that plants of the sarsaparilla family might be a good source of steroids. From time to time, Marker would go into the steamy jungles of Mexico on plant-hunting expeditions. He discovered that a certain species of wild yam produced a high progesterone yield. In 1944 he and some associates from Mexico City started a small pharmaceutical supply house, called Syntex. The demand for progesterone was going up—mostly to treat menstrual problems—and Syntex hormones found a ready market. However, production was still expensive and painstaking, and the new plant derivative was not sufficiently potent to work when taken by mouth. A Syntex chemist, Carl Djerassi, tackled the problem of creating an oral compound. By 1951 he was successful, and Syntex patented the first oral progestin, norethindrone.

Meantime, in Chicago, G. D. Searle & Co. was also becoming interested in hormones and occasionally hired Gregory Pincus as a consultant. Searle had been founded in the 1880s by an Indiana pharmacist, Gideon Daniel Searle, and was still managed by the family. However, it had grown to be a good-sized company, manufacturing opticals, medical instruments, and lab products as well as drugs. Today Searle has subsidiaries or branches in forty-one countries.

Shortly after Djerassi's research was published, Searle applied for a patent on a remarkably similar progestin. Surprisingly, no suit for patent infringement was ever filed by Syntex, although one still hears rumors that it was contemplated. Unlike Syntex, the Searle scientists had no long history of pertinent discoveries and publications or original research. Marker and Djerassi were highly esteemed and innovative chemists, while the Searle personnel investigating progestins were not of comparable stature.

Pincus and his associates used both Searle and Syntex products for their tests at first, but then switched to Searle's progestin exclusively. By 1956, when widespread trials of the compound were initiated in Puerto Rico, Syntex was out of the picture, and Pincus had a well-cemented connection with the Searle company.

But now a curious error was discovered. It was found that the compound being tested was not, after all, pure progestin; tiny fractions of estrogen had somehow intruded. Production methods were hurriedly revised to get rid of the estrogen, but the purer pill didn't work as well. Many women were getting breakthrough bleeding (i.e., bleeding between periods), and it appeared doubtful that ovulation was entirely suppressed. So now the estrogen was *returned to the pill,* for progestin alone, it was concluded, was not an adequate contraceptive after all. (Years later, progestin-only pills were reintroduced. Known as the mini-pills, they are still considered safer but far less effective than pills that combine both hormones.)

Thus, the original concept of the pill was to *avoid using estrogen,* and the first reports described it as an all-progestin product. But by the time that Searle's Enovid was patented and the Puerto Rican trials were under way, the pill, as it came to be known, was admittedly a combination product.

The So-called Tests

When Enovid was approved as a contraceptive, in 1960, we were led to believe it had been tested on thousands of women in Puerto Rico. In truth, as a Senate investigation revealed in 1963, the FDA's decision to approve Enovid was based on clinical studies of only 132 women who had taken it continuously for a year or longer. Most of the other original subjects drifted in and out of the testing program and were lost to follow-up. Three young women died but were not even autopsied. The person at the FDA who got behind Enovid was a Dr. William Kessenich, then the director of the Bureau of Medicine. He apparently had persuaded FDA Commissioner George Larrick that the evidence concerning Enovid's safety was far more substantial than it really was. Then, in 1964, FDA's top physician, J. F. Sadusk, left to become vice-president of Parke Davis, a maker of oral contraceptives.

Today we hear arguments that any drug must be in widespread use before all the possible side effects can be tallied. These arguments have merit, but the pill was a special case, for several reasons.

• The ancient cornerstone of medicine is the motto "First, Do No Harm." Powerful drugs are, ordinarily, prescribed for the treatment of powerful diseases. The doctor and, ideally, the patient also—after a thorough discussion —weigh the *benefits* against the *risks*. With the contraceptive pill—for the first time in pharmaceutical history—a powerful drug was being recommended *for normal healthy women*. Wishing to prevent pregnancy is hardly the same as being seriously ill, and there were many safer alternatives to the pill, including the diaphragm, which, if fitted and used properly, is almost as effective.

• The pill was for continuous, long-term use, not just for a few days or weeks, like most such potent medicines.

• Estrogen was known to be carcinogenic, and therefore the original pill, as planned by Pincus, Chang, and Rock, did not contain it. Their 1950s discussions and papers all referred to the *progestin* pill. When the pill makers decided to add estrogen, the issue of carcinogenicity was suddenly dropped.

• The question of pituitary suppression was of grave concern to reproductive scientists. In 1955, on hearing of Pincus's plans for the pill at an International Planned Parenthood meeting in Japan, Sir Solly Zuckerman, the pioneering British anatomist, commented: "The fact that you could suppress an ovary by means of estrogen or progesterone . . . had been known for years and years. We need better evidence about the occurrence of side effects in human beings; there is an urgent need for prolonged observation before we draw any firm conclusions."

A few years later, when the pill was marketed, Sir Charles Dodds, who had made the first synthetic hormone in 1938, said: "The women who have continuous treatment with the contraceptive pill have an entirely different hormonal background due to the pituitary inhibition. One cannot help wonder what will happen if this state of affairs is allowed to continue."

Thus, of all new drugs, this should have been *more* thoroughly pretested than others, but it was not. So crude were the initial trials that appropriate dosage was not even established. It was discovered only after millions of women had taken Enovid that the amount of estrogen in the pills was *ten times as high* as is usually necessary for contraception. The dosages today are a great deal lower, a fraction of what they were.

The Curious News Blackout

It is puzzling now that such brilliant reproductive scientists as Pincus and Rock felt impelled to minimize the pill's side effects. Throughout the sixties, however, the pill enjoyed a sort of diplomatic immunity, and all those who attacked it publicly were accused of being puritans or scaremongers.

Rock particularly denied that the pill was associated with blood clots or any serious side effects, and argued in his 1963 book, *The Time Has Come*, that the product was "natural," "physiologic," and therefore safe.

He further avowed that ". . . the pills, when properly taken, are not at all likely to disturb menstruation, nor do they mutilate any organ of the body, nor damage any natural process."

Many of Rock's colleagues were pleased by his explanation, but gynecologist Robert Hall of Columbia University, reviewing *The Time Has Come* for the *New York Times Book Review*, was not: "I would like to dismiss this theory as a harmless euphemism; as a doctor, I must aver it is medical fantasy."

The First Pill Conference

In 1962, when the pill had been on the market for a little over a year, Searle had a file of *132* reports of thrombosis and embolism among the pill users, including 11 deaths, and there was talk that the government might withdraw the pill for general contraceptive use. At this point, Searle called the first major conference to discuss the safety of the pill.

It was held at the Chicago headquarters of the American Medical Association in September, and chaired by heart surgeon Dr. Michael De Bakey.

Almost all the pill scholars were at the conference, including Pincus and Rock. Pincus informed the conference that some pill users had shown a reduction in blood-clotting time, but it was generally felt that this was nothing to be alarmed about. Nor, evidently, was anything else that came up at the conference, the transcript reveals.

There was even merriment about some of the deaths said to be associated with the pill. One death, someone suggested, was caused by a "tight girdle," another by a "long trip." The verbatim record shows laughter at these disclosures.

By midafternoon, Chairman De Bakey said, "I would like to try to get everyone out of here by 4:30," and proposed a resolution stating that up to that time there was no evidence suggesting a causal relationship between the pill and clotting disorders. Only one doctor, Dr. Stanford Wessler, assistant professor of medicine at Harvard Medical School, spoke up against the resolution.

Chairman De Bakey: "You are not in favor of the resolution. Will you tell us why you are not?"

Dr. Wessler: "The point at issue that disturbs me is that a decision is being reached on a statistical basis, yet the pertinent statistics are not available."

De Bakey: "You do not think we have enough statistics?"

Wessler: "I am not referring to the quantity of the statistics. I am referring to their pertinence. . . . My concern—and I have no evidence to support the view that Enovid is harmful—is that we may be condoning the use of an entirely elective drug by young, healthy women without adequate evidence of its lack of thrombogenicity. This is a sobering responsibility—particularly if this drug can contribute to deaths from pulmonary embolism in some ancillary way that is not currently appreciated."

De Bakey: "It seems to me that you have got to be realistic and accept whatever evidence is available and make reasoning on that in light of past experience."

The conference also discussed a resolution urging more research. Dr. Rock objected. "Would this give anyone the impression that we thought there was still a relationship between Enovid and thrombophlebitis which we have not yet been able to dig out, but if we keep on digging we think we will get to it?" he worried.

As it turned out, a statement endorsing "the need for continuing study" was unanimously adopted. The meeting adjourned at 4:15 P.M., and the resulting reports gave the public reason to believe the doctors had pronounced the pill safe.

The serious studies of the pill, the *pertinent* statistics Dr. Wessler had called for, were a long way off. In 1963, the FDA assembled a group of consultants, known as the Wright Committee, which once again could reach no concrete conclusions. In 1965, the World Health Organization convened a meeting of experts in Geneva to study the pill. It was like a popularity contest, with the doctors divided almost equally for and against. As one member of the task force later admitted to a reporter: "The people who were concerned about population problems had already decided that we were going to deliver a whitewash."

Not until 1968 did the British Dunlop Committee on the Safety of Drugs firmly establish that there was a cause-and-effect connection between the pill and (sometimes fatal) thromboembolic or clotting disorders. It is still a puzzle why this tiny little committee, with a permanent staff of only twenty-five people and a budget of less than $200,000 a year, had succeeded where all the other committees and agencies, American and international, had failed.

Metabolic Effects of the Pill

Relatively few women (and, we fear, doctors) are fully acquainted with the metabolic effects of the pill. Research in this area is time-consuming and costly. Most of it is not performed by gynecologists and does not appear in their journals. But there is one essential book that every pill-prescribing doctor should have: *Metabolic Effects of Gonadal Hormones and Contraceptive Steroids* contains the proceedings of a scholarly international conference held at Harvard in December 1968. At that conference some fifty-five metabolism researchers presented their findings, and they were grim.

As the introduction by Drs. Hilton Salhanick, David Kipnis, and Raymond Vande Wiele states: "These accumulated data and others suggest that no tissue or organ system is free from a biological, functional, and/or morphological effect of contraceptive steroids. Many of these changes appear to be reversible after short periods of treatment, but it is impossible to form judgments on the reversibility of some of the changes resulting from prolonged administration. This question becomes more important *daily* for the many patients who already have had long-term contraceptive steroid treatment."

As one young Englishman told us afterward, many of the assembled scientists had been inclined to think that the particular organ or system on which each was personally working might be the only one affected by the pill. "It was a shock to sit there for five days and listen to all those papers. I wasn't the only one who called home long distance and advised my wife to stop the pill at once."

A most worrisome metabolic effect is diabetes. Dr. William Spellacy of the University of Florida College of Medicine, in Gainesville, has been investigating diabetic-type changes in the metabolism of pill users since 1962. He and other researchers report that a majority of long-term users show some abnormalities, and a smaller group, some 5 to 15 percent, have rather pronounced reactions. In the winter of 1970, Spellacy testified at Senator Gaylord

Nelson's hearings on the pill. He was asked whether he feared that the pill users with grossly abnormal glucose tolerance might be headed toward diabetes. "Yes," he answered.

Recently, we checked with Dr. Spellacy again. Some of the women in the susceptible group *have* become diabetic. And Spellacy has lost his federal funding. He has had to decrease his contraceptive studies.

Perplexed, we checked with Dr. John Schrogie, who, as mentioned, now works for a drug company but had been in charge of pill research at the FDA when that agency was funding Spellacy. "Spellacy's work is of such importance to women," we pointed out, "and he's been following some of the patients for such a long time. Everyone's always insisting that we won't have any final answers on the pill unless large numbers of long-term users are carefully tested. How could the FDA let Spellacy's decade of careful work go down the drain? How will we know which women—and how many—are getting diabetes from the pill?"

"It was somebody else's turn for funding," was all Schrogie would say.

Then we contacted Dr. Myron Melamed, a pathologist at Memorial Sloan-Kettering Cancer Center, who, in 1965, had begun a study of early developing cervical cancers in pill users as compared to diaphragm users. About that time, Dr. Louis Hellman, who was chairman of the FDA's Advisory Committee on Obstetrics and Gynecology and later the HEW assistant secretary for population, had commented: "It's quite obvious that something is going on in the cervix [of pill users] but what it is we don't know." After three years, Melamed found that the earliest-developing cancers are more prevalent in pill users, but he was unwilling to conclude that there was any cause-and-effect relationship, since there are too many other factors that may have bearing. (If cervical cancer is associated with a virus, for example, the diaphragm may provide a barrier.) Melamed attempted to publish his study in the *Journal of the American Medical Association*, but refused to accept suggested editorial changes. After considerable delay, the report was sent instead to the prestigious *British Medical Journal* and published there. At the time, in 1969, Melamed felt that a lot more work was required. Now he, too, has lost his funding and has given up pill research altogether.

In contrast to Drs. Spellacy and Melamed, consider the case of Dr. Joseph Goldzieher of San Antonio, a consistent devotee and defender of the pill.

In 1971, *Medical World News* reported that the San Antonio researcher had given placebos to 76 women—all poor, Mexican-American, and with many children—who had come to his clinic seeking oral contraception. They were not told they were getting dummy pills, but were only advised to use vaginal cream as added protection. Goldzieher wanted to find out if, as he believed, some women were not imagining side effects such as nausea, bloating, and fatigue. Indeed these symptoms did occur in 11 women receiving dummy pills; they got pregnant.

The report set off a small furor. Some gynecologists speaking off the record scored the Goldzieher research as "totally unethical." Protests were heard at meetings of women's groups. Eventually the FDA notified Goldzieher and the drug companies that sponsored him that they would no longer accept his research on human subjects because it was improper.

As a result, Goldzieher lost his drug company support —drug companies find it fruitless to sponsor research that the FDA won't accept. But our government's Agency for International Development is not so fussy. It awarded Goldzieher's Southwest Foundation for Research and Education more than a million dollars for further contraception studies!

And that's not all. In addition to his AID money, Goldzieher had also been granted $93,290 in 1973 by the National Institutes of Health's Center for Population Research. His contract was renewed in subsequent years. So now, having lost his drug-company support, he is funded by us, out of our taxes. Officials at both AID and NIH informed us that Goldzieher was conducting metabolic studies. Ruth Crozier of the Center for Population Research noted that Dr. Goldzieher would be working with *baboons and beagles. "This contract does not support any human investigations,"* she pointed out.

So well is Goldzieher supplied with grants that by 1976 FDA itself—which avowed his research on humans to be unacceptable—awarded him $112,352 for a one-year study of estrogen effects on cattle. The purpose of the study is to see whether other estrogen products, in cattle feed, might be less carcinogenic than DES. Also in 1976, the World Health Organization gave him $12,800 for additional research on baboons.

CHAPTER 8

Where the Pill Is Now

> *Dr. Huddleston Hargrave, the tough Federal Drug*
> *Administrator who was responsible for the recall*
> *of Whizzadrine, made by the Plowboy Drug Co.,*
> *has resigned to become vice-president in charge of*
> *public affairs for Plowboy at $150,000 a year. His*
> *last act before leaving the FDA was to rescind his*
> *recall of Whizzadrine, which he admitted was a*
> *"terrible" mistake.*
>
> Art Buchwald, *Washington Post*,
> June 1976

The year 1975 was a bad one for the drug industry, a turning point, especially for manufacturers of tranquilizers and antibiotics. For the first time in twenty-five years, the number of prescriptions written in the United States declined. The era of naïve faith in the notion that if one pill is good for you (or your patient), two must be twice as good was drawing to a close.

Some companies were harder hit than others. G.D. Searle, for one, was still flourishing. In 1975 Searle achieved record sales and earnings for its ninth consecutive year, and its stockholders received dividends.

Yet, as the company's annual report to its shareholders states tactfully: "For G.D. Searle, 1975 can best be summarized as a year of marked contrasts." Outside, business went on as usual, but within Searle's offices, a blue-ribbon team of twenty FDA inspectors, including Dr. Frances Kelsey, who had blown the whistle on thalidomide, were performing a relentless audit of Searle's research procedures. At issue, according to the FDA, was the finding that Searle had consistently faked results in drug safety tests, cutting out tumors from animals and then restoring the animals to the study, or switching sick animals from the group receiving drugs to the unmedicated control group. The FDA auditors' formal memorandum, completed in March 1976, is a frightening document that should be read by any patient who places trust in any Searle product, including, of course the pill.

Searle was also in trouble on the business side, specifically with the Securities and Exchange Commission, for paying bribes to foreign governments in return for favors.

The Pandora's Box of Adrian Gross

The scientific audit began in 1972, when FDA evaluator Adrian Gross was charged with reviewing Searle's material on a drug called Flagyl, used to treat vaginal infections. Gross had made himself an expert on carcinogenesis, and was also spearheading a kind of palace revolution within the FDA to ban DES in cattle-feed.

Independent studies had convinced Gross that Flagyl was a potent animal carcinogen, yet Searle's reports to the FDA did not reflect this danger. Puzzled by the discrepancies, Gross demanded more data from Searle. The data indicated either fraudulent or extremely careless research practices. Unannounced, Gross called on the company and asked to see further documentation of their animal tests. The company scientists said they had mislaid the material. Undaunted, Gross whipped into his rather original technique for wresting information out of Searle. Here is how he describes it:

"I go to a desk, open a drawer, and throw its contents up in the air. 'Not here,' I say. Then I repeat the procedure at the next desk. After about three minutes of this, they usually find what I've asked for."

Convinced now that Searle was concealing negative data, Gross filed his report to the commissioner. Nothing happened at the FDA for a year, even though *Medical Letter* issued a strong warning against Flagyl, and Sidney Wolfe, the consumer-minded doctor and associate of Ralph Nader's, formally asked the FDA to ban it.

Finally, in the all-too-familiar pattern, Senator Kennedy applied pressure on the FDA, as Congressman Fountain had in the case of DES, and Senator Nelson with the pill. Only then did the commissioner order a large task force to conduct a three-month inspection of Searle.

Gross's original findings were amply confirmed, and FDA Commissioner Alexander Schmidt seemed shaken and stunned. He admitted that the Searle evidence cast doubts on the believability of *all* drug safety tests, from *any* pharmaceutical house. He called for sweeping reforms in drug testing, and FDA supervisory powers.

The Searle products ultimately included in the investigation were: Flagyl; Aldactone, an antihypertensive; the Ovulen oral contraceptive; the Cu-7 intrauterine device; Aspartame, an artificial sweetener that is not yet marketed; Norpace, and experimental heart drug; and a birth control product for animals called Syncro-Mate.

Concerning Ovulen specifically, it was learned that a fibroadenoma of the abdomen (a benign tumor containing glandular tissue) has been surreptitiously removed from a test dog who was then restored to the study, and that only the vaguer and more favorable company analyses by different scientists had been submitted to the FDA; others had been withheld.

In the spring of 1976, the FDA called for a grand jury investigation and possible criminal action against the executives of Searle. Incredibly, the suspect products were selling as well as or better than ever, and Searle continued to issue stockholder dividends. A company spokesman told us that sometimes adverse publicity *increases* prescriptions, perhaps because it reminds doctors to try a product they had forgotten. "Then too," the Searle publicist said thoughtfully, "a lot of doctors are on our side. They don't like the FDA any better than we do. They know what's good for their patients."

Following the FDA's lead in December 1976, Gloria G. and her husband, Mortimer, filed a $7 million suit against both Searle and Mrs. G.'s doctor, alleging that the Searle product prescribed for her hypertension was "carelessly and negligently manufactured and tested." The cancer Mrs. G. subsequently suffered has led to a double mastectomy. Her case is still pending.

Searle is not in any danger of going bankrupt, although some of its executives and scientists face a threat of being indicted. Searle seems especially worried about the future of Aspartame, which is not approved for marketing, and for which the company holds high commercial hopes. Searle, like Ayerst, has an aggressive public relations approach. It used to maintain a pill-pushing "information center," much like Ayerst's Information Center on the Mature Woman. (See chap. 23.) In 1969, by which time the pill had been proved to cause fatal blood clots, Searle attempted to prevent three books on the subject from being reviewed. At the same time Syntex tried to cash in on the alarm about conventional oral contraceptives by hiring J. Walter Thompson to help push its new all-progestin, or mini-pill.

While prescription drug companies do not directly advertise in the mass media, they still have clout with it, for many drug companies are parts of large conglomerates which do such media advertising.

Exaggerated Credit Given the Pill

More than twenty years have passed since Gregory Pincus announced his daring pill experiments to a somewhat appalled audience at an International Planned Parenthood Meeting in Japan. At that point John Rock was still uncertain of the ethics of giving healthy women such a powerful drug—and fearful of the questions his colleagues might raise; he declined Katharine McCormick's offer to pay his fare and expenses to the meeting.

More than twenty years have passed, but the same debates continue undiminished among scientists and unrevealed to many pill users.

It is widely believed that our declining birth rate, the increasing liberation of women, and other socially desirable fallout can be attributed to the pill. The pill is, of course, one factor, but it is less central than many people think.

First, the main acceptors of the pill have been middle- and upper-class women in developed countries. These women were the daughters of successful diaphragm and/or condom users, and now, in fact, in the third generation, *their* daughters are returning to the old-fashioned but harmless barrier methods. The pill has had some acceptance among the starving hordes for whom Margaret Sanger envisioned it—it is very popular in China especially—but by and large it has succeeded with the middle class. The IUD and sterilization have had greater acceptance in the "third world" than the pill, although a revolt against these methods, sterilization in particular, is rapidly developing.

Other social measures have had *more influence* on declining birth rate than the pill. These include improvements in child health (when parents know that most of their children will live to maturity, they usually want to limit family size), the opening up of jobs for women, and legal abortion.

Also, very few women stay on the pill for most of their reproductive life span because no more than 15 percent stay totally free of symptoms. Some believe the symptoms are worth enduring, but many others do not.

Through most of the 1960s, supporters of the pill maintained that side effects were imaginary or extremely rare. Now they admit their existence, but still minimize their seriousness, exaggerating the risks of not taking the pill, as if the only choice were to take it—or be pregnant.

The Good News

The pill remains attractive to women for two important reasons.

Except for the word "no" it *is* the most effective and convenient reversible contraceptive ever devised. No wonder Margaret Sanger lusted for it, and no wonder other liberated women have agreed with Clare Boothe Luce that with the pill, "modern woman is at last free, as a man is free, to dispose of her own body, to earn her living, to pursue the improvement of her mind, to try a successful career."

In addition, menstrual distress plagues many women, and in perhaps 1 case in 20 (especially during adolescence and menopause), it is so severe as to be incapacitating for days at a time. The pill can cure such problems for, in point of fact, it eliminates menstruation. Women who take the pill with estrogen in it neither ovulate nor menstruate, but, due to the artificial manipulation of hormones, have something called "withdrawal bleeding," which resembles menstruation. (A few pill users experience an *increase* in cramps or irregularity, but relief is much more the rule.)

These benefits notwithstanding, a thoughtful woman may want to consider the risks she is taking, before she decides in favor of the pill.

By 1969 and '70, the evidence against the pill had grown so weighty that two successive FDA commissioners, Dr. Herbert Ley and Dr. Charles Edwards, as well as the HEW secretary, Robert Finch, all affirmed that every pill-using woman had the right to be informed about what she was getting. Detailed consumer labeling was devised by the FDA, and it was announced that this labeling would be included in every pill package. The American Medical Association objected on the grounds that it could needlessly frighten many women, as well as interfere with the doctor-patient relationship. A compromise was reached. Only the briefest labeling was included in the packages, but a pamphlet called "What You Should Know About the Pill" was printed up and sent to doctors to give their patients.

Few women have had the opportunity to read "What You Should Know About the Pill." The AMA has distributed only *6 million* copies (and most of these apparently have gone into doctors' wastebaskets), even though *100 million* pill prescriptions have been written in the United States since 1970. Once again, women have been protected from the frightening knowledge that they are taking a dangerous drug.

Types of Pill

Until recently there were three basic types of pill available: the *combined*, which provides progestins and estrogens simultaneously; the *sequential*, designed to provide these ingredients in a sequence more reflective of the normal menstrual cycle; and the newer, *progestin-only* varieties.

Brand names in the combined category include: Demulen, Brevicon, Enovid, Loestrin, Lo/Ovral, Modicon, Norinyl, Norlestrin, Ortho-Novum, Ovral, Ovulen, and Zorane.

In 1976, three major drug companies announced that they would stop marketing sequential pills. The withdrawn products were Oracon, made by Mead Johnson;

Ortho-Novum SQ made by Ortho; and Norquen made by Syntex. However, supplies currently on the market were not recalled, and women taking these pills were advised to finish their present cycles before selecting an alternative.

Progestin-only contraceptives (mini-pills) include Micronor—Nor-Q.D.—and Ovrette.

The combined pills are the most reliable. Taken according to directions, with no skipped pills, they are said to be 99.5 percent effective. As noted, however, their actual "use" effectiveness is as low as 94 percent. In some populations it is lower yet, for one must be motivated to make the pills work. It is not enough to have them—one must *take* them.

The sequential pills, which used to comprise about 10 percent of the U.S. oral contraceptive market, were less reliable and more dangerous than the combined. There was some indication that sequential users might have a higher risk of clotting disease than that found in users of the combined formulations. There was also a suggestion in two recent studies that sequential pills, containing what is called "unopposed estrogen," may be associated with cancer of the endometrium.

The progestin-only pills are the least reliable, quite possibly less reliable than, say, a good brand of fresh condom. They also produce frequent bleeding irregularities, leading to a high dropout rate. On the other hand, they may be less apt to produce clotting disorders or high blood pressure than pills containing estrogen.

As this is written, the FDA is in the process of revising its labeling on the pill. Cancer is a particularly thorny issue, for one important study suggests a tentative association between the pill and breast cancer, while others do not. There is also new evidence linking various pills with cancer of the liver. Pill users have also been shown in some studies to have higher rates of early-stage cancer of the cervix, but this evidence is still considered tentative.

The FDA has again promised to order the manufacturers to include in pill packages full information about side effects. We shall see. There is sure to be industry and medical lobbying against such a move, for a great many women refuse to take the pill when they are fully informed about it.

The Bad News

For women who take the pill—or are considering it—here is a simplified summary of the contraindications and side effects presently acknowledged by the FDA:

• You should not take the pill if you have *ever had* clotting disorders, cerebral vascular disease (stroke), or coronary occlusion (heart attack). You should not take it if you presently have impaired liver function (as in hepatitis), tumors, known or suspected breast cancer, or undiagnosed vaginal bleeding. You should not take the pill if there is any chance you might be pregnant.

• Pill use increases your risk of developing blood clots four- to eleven-fold. It doubles your risk of stroke. It increases your risk of heart attack three- to six-fold.

• If you are aged 20 to 44, and do not use oral contraceptives, your annual risk of being hospitalized with a blood-clotting disorder is 5 in 100,000. If you use oral contraceptives, your risk increases nine-fold—to 45 in 100,000. There is some evidence that products containing 100 micrograms or more of estrogen cause a higher risk of clotting disorders than those containing lower amounts.

• If you are going to have surgery, you should discontinue the pill at least two weeks before, and not resume until at least two weeks afterward. Pill use increases your risk of postsurgical clotting disorders.

• You should stop taking the pill and call your doctor immediately if you develop severe leg or chest pains, cough up blood, experience sudden and severe headaches, or cannot see clearly.

• The pill may cause liver tumors, involving serious or fatal hemorrhage, and may also be linked to cancer of the liver.

• The pill should be avoided for a period of time (up to three months) and another method of birth control used before deliberate conception.

• The pill doubles the risk of gall-bladder disease, decreases glucose tolerance, and increases certain blood fats.

• Small but significant numbers of women develop high blood pressure on the pill. It is usually reversible.

Women who had high blood pressure during pregnancy may be more likely to suffer this effect.

• Breakthrough bleeding, spotting, and absence of menstruation are frequent side effects. If you have any of these, you should get a checkup. Doubling of pills (as some doctors advise when patients miss a day or two) or changing to brands with a higher estrogen content may increase the risk of blood clots.

• Women with a history of irregular or scanty menstruation may not regain their ovulation or periods after stopping the pill. Women with such a menstrual history should be encouraged to use other contraceptives.

• Oral contraceptives are more effective in preventing normal pregnancies than ectopic (or tubal) ones. Hence the ratio of ectopic to uterine pregnancies is higher in pill users. Every patient who becomes pregnant while using the pill should be evaluated carefully to determine whether the pregnancy *is* ectopic.

• A small residue of hormones from the pill has been identified in the milk of nursing mothers who take it. The long-range effects to the infant have not been determined.

• Endocrine and liver function tests may be affected by the pill. Fibroid tumors may increase in size. Conditions influenced by fluid retention—such as epilepsy, migraine, asthma, or kidney dysfunction—may be affected by the pill. If you have a history of depression, you should discontinue the pill if depression recurs. If jaundice develops, the pill should be discontinued. The pill may cause a deficiency of certain vitamins, such as pyridoxine (B_6) and folic acid.

The following adverse reactions are known to occur in patients receiving oral contraceptives: nausea, vomiting, birth defects, abdominal cramps and bloating, breakthrough bleeding, spotting, change in menstrual flow, cessation of menstruation during and after use, fluid retention, skin discoloration (possibly permanent), breast tenderness, enlargement and secretion, weight increase or decrease, change in cervical erosion and secretion, reduction in breast milk when used after childbirth, jaundice, growth of uterine fibroid tumors, rash, mental depression, reduced tolerance to carbohydrates. (This last may ultimately produce diabetic or hypoglycemic symptoms.)

The following adverse reactions have been reported in users of oral contraceptives, but research is incomplete: infertility after discontinuance of use . . . premenstrual-like syndrome . . . intolerance to contact lenses . . . change in corneal curvature . . . cataracts . . . changes in sex drive . . . occurrence of involuntary jerking movements . . . changes in appetite . . . cystitis-like syndrome . . . headache . . . nervousness . . . dizziness . . . fatigue . . . backache . . . hirsutism (excessive hair growth in the wrong places) . . . loss of scalp hair . . . skin disease . . . skin hemorrhages . . . itching . . . vaginitis . . . and metabolic disease.

Should any pill user have laboratory tests, she should be sure to tell her doctor she is taking oral contraceptives. The following common laboratory tests are among those that may be altered by its use: liver function, blood clotting, thyroid function, glucose tolerance test, serum lipid values, serum folate values.

Here is a final, little-known fact about the pill: It changes the acid-alkaline balance of the vagina, making the user more susceptible to VD, as well as to other annoying infections. If a woman who uses *no* method of birth control has sex relations with a gonorrhea-infected man, she is thought to have a one-third chance of contracting his infection. If condoms and/or foam are used, her chances are considerably lower. If, however, she is on the pill, her chances of contracting it from one exposure jump to more than 90 percent.

Former Pill Users

What about the health of *former* pill users? Although, as we have noted, some 10 million U.S. women may take the pill at any given time, this is an ever-changing population. Two users out of three stop within five years because of side effects. Some of these return to the pill later.

Apparently, most of the problems associated with the pill are reversible, *although some,* such as skin discolorations, *usually are not.* Some women undergo a period of adjustment after stopping the pill, while waiting for their own pituitary and ovarian hormones to reassert themselves.

During this interim, women may notice changes in their skin, hair, and figure, as well as the absence of menstruation and ovulation. In the book *Lunaception*, author Louise Lacey claims that, at the suggestion of a nutritionist friend, she got her "in-house" glandular system working again by priming it with extra doses of vitamins B and E.

Over the years we have obtained the histories of more than 6,000 current or former pill users, or their survivors. We are especially apt to hear from women (or their survivors) who were familiar with our earlier writings but who didn't believe them until disaster struck. Many people have asked us why, when it was known and reported in the 1960s that the pill causes heart disease, liver disorders, and birth defects—to name only three side effects—the FDA failed to acknowledge these conditions until 1975.

The FDA as Consumer Adviser

The FDA has an advisory committee on obstetrics and gynecology which has no consumer members, and few if any specialists from medical disciplines other than obstetrics and gynecology. The lack of outside specialists is more significant than it may seem. When a pill user gets into serious trouble, she is usually treated by a doctor *other* than her gynecologist. If she has a stroke, she is cared for by a neurologist; in depression, by a psychiatrist; for retinal vein thrombosis, by an ophthalmologist, and so on. Many gynecologists say, quite honestly, that they have observed few serious complications in their patients. The catchword here is *observe*. Like all doctors, gynecologists *should worry more* about their patients who don't come back. Most women who have a serious pill side effect are so outraged that they never wish to see the prescribing doctor again. (This is more true with the pill than with other drugs, for these women were *healthy* when they started. They feel justifiably betrayed.) We encourage such women—with mixed success—to notify their doctors by letter, at least. When we made this suggestion to one patient, who was in the hospital following a pulmonary embolism, she said, "Listen, if my doctor were to walk into this room, I would leap out of my bed and strangle him."

One cannot help but notice that within FDA many officials charged with responsibility for monitoring the pill go on, as we have shown, to lucrative drug company positions when they leave the agency. The FDA advisory panel, which rotates, has had more than its proportion of members who have ties to the population control movement, drug industry, or both. (Dr. Elizabeth Connell, for example, who is presently Associate Director for Health Sciences at the Rockefeller Foundation, and Chairman of the National Medical Committee, Planned Parenthood World Population, also has had commercial connections with the following firms: Eli Lilly & Co.; Syntex Laboratories; Mead Johnson Laboratories; Organon, Inc.; Ortho Pharmaceutical Corporation; and G.D. Searle & Co.

Many intelligent and honest doctors have helped to monitor the pill, both within the FDA and on its advisory committees but they do not have the advantage of official input from patients or patient advocates, or from specialists who deal with pill catastrophes. The mix at FDA is disadvantageous to the consumer. It ranges from members who are neutral to committed pill defenders, with few if any critics or skeptics ever permitted a voice.

When the FDA "concedes" a side effect, you can be sure that it has ample reason. Side effects usually have appeared in the medical literature for six to seven years, or longer, before the FDA takes formal cognizance of them.

Dr. J. Richard Crout, director of the FDA's Bureau of Drugs, stated in a recent interview:

"The decision on what contraceptive to use ought to be made basically by the patient and not her physician. She ought to ask of her physician information and advice, but not ask him to make such an important decision for her. . . . She should know that the standard old diaphragm, followed by an abortion in the event of failure, is probably the single safest approach to birth control." Crout went on to comment that while the relationship between the pill and breast cancer is still unsettled, every patient should be thoroughly and accurately informed about the fifty-plus side effects of the pill—as well as the unanswered questions concerning cancer—before deciding whether to take such risks. He admits that the information presently given out with the pill is "obsolete," as well as much too short. He admits that many women have been falsely led to believe the pill is safe.

In January 1976, at Senate hearings, Crout swore that FDA would see to it that users of estrogen products, including the pill, would have detailed warnings within three months. Then, women would be free to make up their own minds.

The AMA and drug companies are not happy about such patient warnings. They argue that women don't read them anyway. But since 1970, the FDA has been experimenting with various brief warnings that are included in the pill packages. And a national survey, made in 1975 by the FDA itself, showed that almost all users read the scraps of information offered with the pill, and eight out of ten recognize that this information is inadequate. Specifically, users want much more information, *full* information, about side effects.

Early in September 1976, eight months after Crout's public promise, the new labeling to go on the pill and ERT packages was still not published in the *Federal Register*, a preliminary step, much less being anywhere near the point of inclusion in the packages for women to read. We asked Crout why. He said the delay was because the warnings for other estrogen products were turning out to be "more complex than expected." The agency, he explains, "wants to make sure that all estrogen labeling is consistent. . . . Great pains are being taken to get considerable input from the public and advisory committees on what the labeling should say."

The labeling for menopausal estrogens was finally published in the *Federal Register* at the end of September, and the pill labeling not until December 7, almost a full year after Crout's Senate testimony. Consumer advocates were, once again, dismayed with the whitewash in the proposed insert for patients. Rose Kushner, a breast-cancer victim and author of an investigative book on the subject, has joined with Marlene Manes, wife of the borough president of Queens, New York, in a suit against the FDA for hedging on cancer risks.

By April 1978, all estrogen products and birth control pills were supposed to contain a long user warning, dispensed by the pharmacist at the point of sale. Spot checks in various regions indicated that some pharmacists were failing to comply. Earlier, the Pharmaceutical Manufacturers Association, supported by both the AMA and the gynecologists' organizations, attempted to bring injunctions barring these patient package inserts. It was disillusioning to many health consumers and to some enlightened doctors when organized medicine chose to side with the drug industry against the patients.

The FDA's wishy-washy defense of the labeling was dismissed in Delaware's First U.S. District Court. Luckily, Margaret Kohn, Marcia Greenberger and other attorneys at the Center for Law and Social Policy had filed a more convincing brief on behalf of several feminist and consumer groups. The judge was persuaded and ruled that the inserts be dispensed after all.

If you know of a pharmacist who is not complying, please notify Dr. Donald Kennedy, Commissioner, Food and Drug Administration, 5600 Fishers Lane, Rockville, Maryland 20852.

Send a copy of your letter to the National Women's Health Network, Suite 203, 1302 18th Street, N.W., Washington, D.C. 20036.

The Weakness of the FDA

The FDA's reliance on outside advisory committees is illegal, according to a unanimous report released in 1976 by the House Committee on Government Operations. Congress charged that FDA uses such committees as "window dressing" and to "dilute its responsibility for effective regulation of the drug industry." FDA has also "disregarded statutory requirements that advisory committee meetings be open to the public [we have personally been ejected from at least two] and has grossly understated the cost of maintaining its advisory committees in reports to the President."

Other events give further pause about the FDA. In 1974, fourteen current and former FDA employees—sincere people, evidently, who believed their job was to protect the consumer—brought charges that due to industry pressure they were suddenly and improperly transferred, reassigned, or removed from positions where they were either holding up drug approvals or preparing warnings and cautionary labeling. Some were suddenly moved to departments where they had no knowledge or expertise, and were thus rendered ineffectual. One FDA dissident, Alice Ling, charged that her superior beat and kicked her when she tried to copy incriminating documents.

Almost everyone, from FDA commissioners, through Consumers Union, through the American Civil Liberties Union, through the National Organization of Women, has agreed in principle that consumers and patients should see the full prescription labeling on drugs. A former FDA commissioner, Dr. James Goddard, has written:

"An American buying prescription drugs is like no other American at any other counter at any other store in the country. . . . Although he is the consumer, he is not the shopper; he buys (on faith) what the doctor has prescribed. He is like a child who goes to the store with his mother's shopping list, which he cannot even read. He is totally unsophisticated as to the workings of the $5,000,-000,000 industry to which he is contributing and which his tax money is already helping to support. The consumer of drugs pays up and takes his medicine, and the Drug Establishment, about which he knows nothing, scores again."

Goddard was one of our more outspoken FDA chiefs. Today he is president of the Ormont Drug and Chemical Company, a small manufacturer developing skin tests for cancer.

Goddard's immediate successor, Dr. Herbert Ley, was almost equally forthright. "The thing that bugs me," he said, "is that the people think the FDA is protecting them—it isn't. What the FDA is doing and what the public thinks it's doing are as different as night and day."

Since his retirement from the FDA, Ley has worked as "a consultant to the food and drug industry," according to his listing in *Who's Who*.

But you don't have to be an ex-commissioner to better your position when opportunity knocks. Within weeks after FDA turned its case against Searle over to a grand jury, a man named Owen Lamb, who was compliance chief for FDA's Chicago District—Searle territory—resigned his job to go to work for the pill company.

Some months later, Searle also appointed James Phelps its new vice-president and general counsel. Phelps is a former trial attorney with the FDA.

CHAPTER 9

Side Effects—Are They Rare?

There is no cell in the body that is not affected by oral contraceptives.

Dr. Victor Wynn

In 1974 the British Royal College of General Practitioners released a five-year interim report on the side effects of the pill. It was a very large study, based on 46,000 women patients, half of them pill users. The well-publicized conclusion of the report—which was partially financed by six pill manufacturers—was this: ". . . it seems that the estimated risk at the present time of using the pill is one that a properly informed woman would be happy to take."

Later, Dr. William Inman, head of Britain's Committee on the Safety of Drugs, was skeptical in his evaluation of the study, saying that many of the morbidity and mortality statistics were too low.

Dr. Philip Corfman, director of the U.S. Center for Population Research at HEW, deemed the study valuable, "even though it doesn't prove what it says it proves, because it provides evidence of *hitherto-unknown side effects.*" Dr. Valerie Beral of the London School of Hygiene and Tropical Medicine noted in a letter to the British medical journal *Lancet*, that *if one looks closely at the study, it reveals that users and ex-users of the pill have a combined mortality from all causes that is 39 percent higher than the mortality rate of the control group.*

Vascular disease and suicide, Dr. Beral calculated, appear to be the main contributors to the excess mortality of pill users. "The 39 percent excess mortality among users and ex-users of oral contraceptives, who previously were healthier than the controls, is a cause for some concern . . .

the . . . risk . . . may not be one that a properly informed woman would be happy to take." (Note: Many of the control group women had used other methods *because of pre-existing conditions*, such as diabetes, tumors, or high blood pressure, which made them poor candidates for the pill. This is what Beral refers to when she says the pill users were "previously healthier.")

Over the next several years, Beral collected World Health Organization data from twenty-one different countries, confirming that pill users everywhere demonstrate a much increased susceptibility to heart disease and stroke. Her analysis, published in *Lancet* in November 1976, also showed that the low-dose pills (those containing no more than 50 micrograms of estrogen) are not reducing these problems as much as had been hoped.

The pill can cause almost any symptom you might name. Dr. Louis Hellman, the obstetrician who for many years was chairman of the FDA advisory committee on the pill, says that when a patient asks if a certain problem might be caused by this medication, he can never say for sure that it is not.

Dr. Elizabeth Connell, looking on the bright side, has stated: "I think the most amazing thing . . . is the side effect of having less ear wax! It's great to point out that there are rather nice things that go on when one uses the pill."

Blood Clots

Two major factors in blood clotting are affected by the pill: It causes the walls of the veins to dilate, thus slowing the flow of blood; it affects clotting characteristics of the blood itself, increasing the adhesiveness and aggregation qualities of the platelets, causing cells to stick together.

Since surgery can sometimes lead to blood clots, the FDA now cautions women to stop the pill for a cycle or longer before an elective procedure. It does *not* caution them that their chances of succumbing to post-partum blood clots, a leading cause of maternal deaths, increase threefold when they take hormones to suppress breast milk.

Clotting factors in the blood are extremely complex; the more scientists discover the less they know. An astute student of the subject is Dr. Stanford Wessler, the only scientist who spoke out against the crowd at the 1962 Searle conference. Six years later he was proven correct.

By the 1970s Wessler had moved from Harvard to the New York University School of Medicine, where he continued his work on the pill and blood clots. With several colleagues, Wessler discovered that a normally occurring factor called antithrombin III, which plays an important role in maintaining the fluidity of blood, is adversely affected in 16 percent of women on the pill. Wessler has developed an assay to identify those pill users who are at increased risk of thrombosis. The test would cost about fifteen to twenty-five dollars, and could be performed at most laboratories. Wessler also suggests that low-dose heparin (anticoagulant) regimens might be administered preventively to pill users who require emergency surgery or have accidents.

In a massive collaborative study, performed by scientists in the United States, Sweden, and the United Kingdom, it was found that women with Type O blood are less likely to develop clots than those in the A, B, or AB groups. This was true in general, but especially striking where the clots occurred in connection with either pill use or childbirth.

Another finding that may be connected is that patients of blood group O are *more likely* to develop bleeding as a complication of peptic ulcer than are those of groups A, B, or AB.

Scientists like Wessler, or Hershel Jick, who headed the international blood-type study, are trying to diminish the clotting risks in pill users. If a patient is carefully selected—if she has Type O blood, and if her antithrombin III factors are checked before and after going on the pill—her risks of future illness might be substantially diminished.

And of course there are other issues, too. Dr. William Spellacy, an expert on the metabolic effects of the pill and a strong proponent of tracking the sugar and fat metabolism of users, says that he is perplexed and disappointed when he raises such matters at FDA and other official bodies where he sits on several councils.

"We have the medical technology to do it," he explains, "—to eliminate a lot of the high-risk patients—but the argument I get against it is that less developed countries don't have the means. They say it could make us look bad abroad to require tests on our women when they can't test theirs."

Blood clots usually form in the veins of the legs, feet, or pelvic region, where they can permanently impair the circulation, often necessitating surgery—or, in some cases, amputation of the affected limb, as happened to Susan.

A young, once-active woman, Susan had been on the pill for only a month when she was admitted as an emergency hospital patient because of a painful swelling in her left leg. A large number of clots were found, but efforts to remove or reduce them proved futile. Circulation in her leg came to a complete halt and gangrene developed. First, her leg below the knee was amputated, then, when that proved insufficient, the upper part of her leg was also removed. Two years later, Susan was still struggling to adapt to an artificial limb, for her a lifelong reminder of the pill.

While some women lose their limbs, others lose their lives because of pill-caused blood clots. If a clot breaks loose from the vein where it originated, it can travel to the lungs or elsewhere—with fatal results. Pulmonary emboli —clots that have traveled to the lung—cause more officially recognized deaths than any other pill side effect. When the arteries in the lungs are blocked by a clot, the blood supply is cut off, and part or all of the lung becomes necrotic. The FDA acknowledges that a minimum of 300 to 500 otherwise healthy young women die each year in the United States from pill-associated pulmonary embolism. This figure *does not include* pill deaths from clotting disorders in other vital organs of the body, nor does it include the deaths from other causes such as cancer—or depression leading to suicide, which may claim many more victims than pulmonary embolism.

If a clot travels to the brain, or originates there, it can cause a stroke—a cerebrovascular accident (CVA)— that can kill or cripple. Before the pill era, strokes in young, premenopausal women were extremely rare. When they did occur, they were usually connected with some pre-existing disease—diabetes or high blood pressure (more about the pill's connection with these later). Soon after the pill became available, neurologists began reporting a steady increase in the incidence of strokes "from no apparent cause" in healthy young women. The reports had one common denominator: All the women were taking oral contraceptives.

The following case, reported in the *Canadian Medical Journal* in 1974, vividly describes the rapid progression of clot formation to CVA to death:

A 22-year-old single woman was well until June 3, 1973, when she developed a severe, generalized headache. . . . Three weeks earlier her family doctor had given her a prescription for a low-dose birth control pill. . . . Owing to the severity of the headache, she was referred to a neurologist whose examination yielded normal findings. . . . She was sent home on analgesics, but the headache did not subside and she also began to vomit. On June 6 she was admitted to the Women's College Hospital. Physical examination, including a detailed neurologic assessment, yielded no abnormal findings apart from fever. The next day she had a generalized convulsion, followed by paralysis of the right side which persisted. A detailed neurologic examination on June 10 revealed partial blindness, weakness, and loss of sensation of the right side of the body, difficulty in expressing her thoughts and evidence of increased pressure in the head.

The patient was transferred to the neurosurgical department at The Wellesley Hospital. During examination in the emergency department, she suddenly complained of increasing headache, became restless, screamed, and then stopped breathing and became comatose. She was sent immediately to the operating room. Extensive thrombosis of the superficial cerebral veins was observed. Postoperative treatment was ineffective. The patient died on June 11, 1973, eight days after the onset of the headache.

The young woman's physicians concluded: "Our patient died from the sequelae of extensive cerebral venous thrombosis. Except for the intake of oral contraceptives, none of the numerous predisposing factors . . . was present. Therefore, we believe that in this case the oral contraceptives were the cause of the venous thrombosis."

While it was originally hoped that the lower-estrogen pills would decrease the incidence of blood clotting, evidence has proved inconclusive, and pill-caused blood clots are not necessarily dose-related. The drug company propaganda that low-dose pills are "safe" is somewhat misleading, although it's usually advisable to take the lowest effective quantity of *any* medication.

Women who take oral contraceptives should be alerted to the warning signs of blood clots in the limbs, lungs, or brain; these signs include: pain and swelling; increased temperature of the affected areas; visual disturbances; headaches; chest pains; numbness or tingling in the limbs, and shortness of breath. In about one-quarter of the cases of stroke there seems to be no warning. In the rest there is a preceding period characterized by recurring headache and also by vomiting, convulsions, drowsiness, impaired or blurred vision, and an increase in body temperature.

Other Neurologic and Eye Disturbances

Strokes are not the only neurological damage caused by the pill. In the early 1960s, Dr. Frank Walsh, an ophthalmologist at Johns Hopkins Hospital, identified a wide range of visual disturbances in pill users.

A review of 5,000 patients with adverse reactions to the pill disclosed 112 cases of eye complications. Of these, 15 were cerebrovascular disturbances with ocular symptoms, such as blurred vision, temporary blindness, and loss of part of the field of vision. Other eye disturbances linked to the pill were inflammation of the optic nerve, swelling of the optic disc, double vision, blockage of the arteries or veins in the eye, retinal hemorrhage, contact lens intolerance, swelling of the eye membranes, inflammation of the cornea, inflammation of the iris.

Cataracts *may* be associated with the pill, but this is not established. Laboratory studies have proven that the pill can cause cataracts in animals, and cortisone, a chemical cousin to the pill, has definitely been linked to cataracts in humans. Retinal vein thrombosis, causing blindness, has also been reported in pill users.

A link between the pill and epilepsy has also been observed. Dr. Gilbert Ross, chairman of the Department of Neurology at Upstate Medical Center, State University of New York, has said: "I feel there is a definite risk in the use of the pill in the female patient with a convulsive disorder or migraine headaches."

Harriet J. had been on the pill for a little over three years when, without warning, she had four epileptic seizures in twenty-four hours.

"The first happened while I was asleep," she told us. "My husband and I were having coffee when he told me that I had wakened him the night before. He said the bed was shaking, I was shaking, and my whole body was rigid. I laughed and told him he must have been having a bad dream. I was laughing when my right arm suddenly became completely paralyzed."

She was hospitalized and given anticonvulsant medicine. She continued to take the pill along with her medicine until her doctor, chancing upon an article that mentioned a possible link between the pill and epilepsy, told her to stop taking it.

She is still an epileptic—in fact, the seizures have become worse. She says she's learned to live with it, but adds: "I can't even take a shower without my husband being in the bathroom. So many things could happen."

Another neurologic disturbance that has been reported in pill users is chorea—an uncontrolled twitching and jerking. Victims usually notice that they suddenly become clumsy—they drop things, fumble with keys in locks, and so on. Sometimes the symptoms become so severe that an afflicted woman finds it impossible to perform simple chores like zipping a zipper or brushing her teeth.

Liver Disease

In 1973 Dr. Janet Baum, a radiologist at the University of Michigan, noticed a connection between the pill and liver tumors. Such tumors were medical oddities, yet Dr. Baum reported finding 7 cases among pill takers in five years!

Shortly thereafter, physicians at the University of Louisville in Kentucky discovered 13 further cases, all in pill users. Four of the 13 women were found to have malignant tumors, and 3 died. But even "benign" tumors of the liver were causing fatal hemorrhages.

One of the Louisville physicians, Dr. William Mays,

tracked down almost 50 additional cases within a few months, convincing the FDA to add benign and malignant liver tumors to its list of pill side effects.

Other kinds of liver disease caused by the pill have been recognized since the early 1960s. Jaundice is usually an early symptom of liver complications, so any woman who becomes jaundiced while on the pill should stop at once. There is some evidence that women of Scandinavian stock may be more susceptible to liver complications than most.

Here a grieving father speaks: "It is six months to the day that I lost my dear daughter Janet to 'the pill.' Janet, a beautiful, strong, healthy young woman of 25 when the pill was prescribed by the doctors of the student health service at her university died of liver disease in Mount Sinai Hospital in New York City after an agonizing period of ten months during which she was in the hospital six times. Janet was assured by a sweet, fatherly, gentle doctor that 'the pill is perfectly safe.'

"He prescribed it for twelve months and told her to watch for redness or swelling in her legs. She was given a breast and pelvic examination and a Pap smear. No provisions were made for periodic examination. In twelve months the prescription was renewed with the same kind of examination. Three months or so later she started having pains in her midsection. She went to the university clinic several times, and they told her she was nervous, probably working on an ulcer. No mention was made of the pill. Not until she completed her master's degree and came home to New York in April did we get her to a doctor who recognized her dangerous situation by taking a blood test. He took her off the pill immediately—by that time it was *too late*. Is there anything we can do to stop this killing of our young women?"

High Blood Pressure

Once considered a "rare" side effect, high blood pressure (hypertension) is now acknowledged to be common. According to Dr. John Laragh, director of the hypertension and cardiovascular center at New York Hospital–Cornell Medical Center, 5 percent of pill users—1 in every 20—

develop high blood pressure; a far greater number of women show a rise in pressure, though still within the normal range.

Laragh, writing in the *American Journal of Obstetrics and Gynecology*, first observed the increased incidence of hypertension in pill users during the mid-1960s. Other clinics have since confirmed his discovery; some report an even higher frequency than 5 percent. Laragh points out that pill-induced high blood pressure usually can be checked and reversed if the woman stops the pill, but cautions that *women with a history of high blood pressure —or kidney disease, toxemia of pregnancy, excessive pre-menstrual weight gain and fluid retention*—or a family history of high blood pressure, should avoid use of this contraceptive. Obese women or women with a previous history of hypertension are more likely to experience high blood pressure while on the pill.

Cancer

As far back as 1940, scientists had demonstrated that estrogens, such as those in the pill, can *speed up* the progress of an already existing cancer. What was not known was whether the pill could actually *cause* it. As Dr. Roy Hertz, now of George Washington University, explains, when a carcinogenic agent is applied to a human subject, it usually requires about a decade before a cancerous tumor begins to grow. It can then take another ten years before the tumor manifests itself enough to cause symptoms. Back in 1969, Dr. Hertz predicted that the seventies could mark the beginning of a pill-caused cancer epidemic in American women.

A study of the pill's effect on benign or malignant breast disease was begun in 1970—a decade after the pill was first available. Two California researchers, Elfriede Fasal and Ralph Paffenberger, reported findings in the October 1975 issue of the *Journal of the National Cancer Institute*. A frightening six- to elevenfold cancer increase was discovered in long-term (six or more years) pill users with a prior history of benign breast disease.

Fasal and Paffenberger were careful to note that the pill had been available for "perhaps too short a period to induce or promote cancer, but sufficient to enhance the growth of pre-existing cancer." They recommended that since benign breast disease per se predisposes women to breast cancer, women who have evidenced it should use other contraceptives.

It is not surprising that the matter has not been settled. DES and menopause estrogens, first marketed about 1940, were not finally proved carcinogenic in humans until the 1970s—a thirty-year interval. The pill was not marketed until 1958 (for medical conditions) and 1960 (as a contraceptive). We think it will be remarkable if the pill, alone among estrogen products, fails to cause cancer in the same sites in humans as in animals.

(These organ sites in animals include the breast, endometrium, cervix, ovary, pituitary gland, testis, kidney, and bone. As *Medical Letter* observed of estrogens in its issue for May 21, 1976: "No other drug effect so readily reproducible in such a wide variety of test animals has been generally regarded as not potentially applicable to man.")

Research on a total of more than 65,000 women implicated the pill as a possible cause of cervical cancer. Pill users have a demonstrated increase in nonmalignant cervical polyps; blistered, "eroded" areas; and dysplasias (cellular changes which some doctors consider malignant or premalignant).

Other changes in the reproductive organs of pill users may include cystic ovaries and enlarged uteri. A Dutch gynecologist, Dr. W. P. Plate, who studied the ovarian tissue of 11 women who had been on the pill found that of the 6 who had taken it for a year or longer, 5 had ovaries that showed abnormalities—parts of their ovaries resembled scar tissue. The remaining 5 had taken the pill for less than a year, but 2 had already developed similar pathology.

Many cautious physicians urge that a woman with any prior history of tumors in the breast or reproductive organs, or with a family history of cancer, should not take the pill. But women who obtain birth control from impersonal clinics are usually not questioned about their family history.

Infertility

While the evidence connecting the pill with cancer slowly accumulates, the belief that once a woman stops taking the pill she becomes super-fertile has proven to be a myth. It turns out that just the opposite is true: Many women experience an "oversuppression syndrome"—that is, infertility.

Some women find they have irregular or scanty periods after they go off the pill; others have no periods at all. Either way the result is the same; such women are sterile. In most cases, but not all, the situation is reversible, although it may take years before a woman can conceive. We will return to this problem in chapter 11.

Diabetes

Some of the most potentially serious effects of the pill are the changes it brings about in carbohydrate (sugar) and lipid (fat) metabolism.

Women who take the pill show a significant change in glusose-tolerance levels as well as an increased output of growth hormone. Both of these changes can lead to diabetes, and in fact, according to Dr. Sheldon Segal of the Population Council, "the average woman who uses oral contraceptives is likely to test out as a diabetic or pre-diabetic." What this means is that their blood tests resemble those of diabetics, even though the symptoms of the disease have not yet developed.

Dr. Victor Wynn, the British endocrinologist, finds that 80 percent of women on the pill for a year or longer show a significant impairment of their glucose tolerance, and 13 percent have demonstrable chemical diabetes, which can be the precursor of the type of diabetes that may develop in middle age.

Women who are already diabetic probably should avoid the pill, for, as in the case with existing cancer, the pill can make diabetes worse. Dr. Spellacy has gone even further and said: "I think the pill is a real risk for any woman who has had abnormal blood sugar at any time—during pregnancy or surgery or severe infection."

Glenda R. is a diabetic who was put on the pill before its effect on blood-sugar metabolism was widely known. She went to her family doctor and announced that she was getting married. He warned her of the hazards of pregnancy for women with diabetes and suggested that she use an IUD or oral contraceptives. She decided on the pill, and her doctor recommended a gynecologist who would prescribe it. When she called the gynecologist's office for an appointment, the nurse told Glenda that since she only wanted birth control pills, it would not be necessary to have an examination and that she could come by any time and pick up the prescription.

Glenda felt nauseated from the time she first started taking the contraceptives, but didn't pay much attention since her friends had complained of the same thing as a routine side effect of the pill, which would disappear after a while. But she continued to feel queasy and then gradually lost her interest in sex. After six months of marriage and the pill, Glenda began having trouble with her eyes. She shuttled from doctor to doctor, and was eventually referred to the Mayo Clinic. No one bothered to ask if she was taking birth control pills, until it was too late, and Glenda was totally blind from the combination of her diabetes and the pill.

Dr. Spellacy and other metabolic experts have urged that any woman who shows even borderline glucose and insulin responses not be given oral contraceptives. Other high-risk groups who should not use birth control pills are women with a family history of diabetes, those who have given birth to very large infants (9 lb. or more), older women, obese women, and women who began menstruating early. He has also warned that women on the pill should watch for the development of monilia vaginitis—a signal of altered carbohydrate metabolism.

Dr. Spellacy believes that on "the basis of evidence already in hand, it seems reasonable that *all* women on oral contraceptives be tested for glucose tolerance at least once a year."

The changes in fat metabolism brought about by the pill have been connected to high blood pressure, blood clotting, and the associated risks of heart attack and stroke. What Spellacy sees as a most ominous change is the rise in triglycerides in the blood, which are associated with hardening of the arteries and, possibly, heart disease. The pill is depriving women of one advantage they have had over men—their ability to resist heart attacks.

Spellacy urges that women with a family history of stroke or coronary thrombosis should undergo a complete blood profile before taking oral contraceptives.

Another Pill Side Effect—Pregnancy

The interaction between oral contraceptives and other drugs is hardly understood at all, but some preparations increase the dangers of the pill, while others *reduce its effectiveness*, perhaps by causing the hormones to be metabolized too rapidly.

It's anyone's guess how many pill pregnancies are not —as is usually implied—due to user carelessness, but rather to the ingestion of a second drug that "canceled out" the pill.

There have been a number of reports of pill users who conceived while taking Rifampin, a drug used in the treatment of tuberculosis. Yet this has not deterred doctors from prescribing it along with the pill. In one recent case in Louisville, a woman conceived in 1974 while taking the pill and her TB medication. She denied missing any pill doses but, after an abortion, was placed back on the same pill and Rifampin regimen. Six months later she was pregnant again. This time she discontinued all medications, and carried the baby to term. Luckily—miraculously —the child appears to be healthy at age 2.

The doctors who prescribe the pill—gynecologists— often are not the same as those who prescribe competing medications. Thus, it is essential for the pill user herself to be familiar with all medications she is taking, and to raise the questions of interactions with any or all of her physicians.

A partial listing of other drugs that have been implicated in blocking the contraceptive action of the pill includes: antihistamines, barbiturates (Amytal, Nembutal, phenobarbital, Seconal), Butazolidin, Dilantin, Equanil, Miltown, Rifadin, Rimactane.

Sex Drive

Contrary to original expectations, the pill can cause women to lose their interest in sex. Studies carried out in this country, England, and Sweden have confirmed that a decrease in sex drive is more prevalent among pill users than an increase. Today, one of the first questions sex therapists ask a nonorgasmic woman is whether she is taking the pill. Dr. Michael Grounds of Australia reports that loss of sex drive is the main reason women in his country give up the method.

It would be naïve, however, to assume that all the sexual problems associated with the pill are entirely due to biochemistry. Dr. Roger Pluvinage, a Paris neuropsychiatrist, has studied women who develop migraine headaches on the pill. His patients confided a variety of secret fears that sometimes express themselves as headaches and migraine. (Note the word *sometimes*. At other times, remember, headaches can be warnings of a stroke.) The Pluvinage patients felt anxiety that the pill might cause birth defects in a pregnancy, and guilt feelings over what their friends or the priest might say. Often a wife felt repressed anger at her husband for allowing her to use a contraceptive that might be dangerous.

To complicate matters, mind and body are truly inseparable—especially when it comes to the endocrine system and hormones. Our emotions mediate the flow of hormones, and vice-versa.

The rhesus monkey appears to be the species with which we have most in common sexually. The female has a twenty-eight-day menstrual cycle, like ours. Her sex drive wanes and waxes, over the month, according to her natural hormone oscillations, but, even at her most receptive, any old male will not always do. She is selective and much more aroused by some males than others. Another area where rhesus sexual behavior parallels the human is female assertiveness. In many species, the females are indifferent to passive males. In the rhesus—and human—many females, but not all, will take an aggressive courting posture with males they fancy who are shy.

Animal researchers who study the sexual effects of the pill have therefore turned their sharpest spotlight on the rhesus. Their findings have not had the attention they deserve, for many of the parallels between the pill's behavioral effects on primates and humans are striking.

An early warning came from investigators at the Primate Research Center in Beckenham, England, who noted that rhesus couples became inhibited when the females were given oral contraceptives. Their male companions groomed them less (grooming, among apes and monkeys, is the equivalent of courting behavior and cuddling), mounted them less often, and generally worked much harder to attain fewer ejaculations. They didn't quite reject the females on the pill, but their enthusiasm and sexual vigor waned. The investigators concluded that possibly the synthetic steroids upset the normal olfactory (smell) signals between the sexes.

At Emory University, Dr. Richard Michael, professor of psychiatry and anatomy, has made enormous strides in clarifying the relations between sexual behavior and synthetic hormones. Michael works with rhesus monkeys and humans as well.

There are two aspects of feeling and behavior in both species that synthetic hormones alter. First is the question of receptivity, or interest, of the *female*. This is not by any means solely dependent on hormones, but there is no question that the hormones in the body affect sexual appetite in the brain. Under the influence of progesterones, like those in the pill, the female rhesus in Michael's study is much less inclined to tap a lever that admits a male into her cage as a reward. She's more apt to tap it if she is rewarded with a male she likes, but even so, progesterone has a *profoundly dampening effect*.

Progesterone is a most mysterious hormone, and its influence on sexual behavior could fill a textbook. Yet scientists remain uncertain whether to assign progesterone (the synthetic progesterone in the pill is usually called progestin) as a male or female hormone. Testosterone, a male hormone produced by both sexes, stimulates sex drive; estrogen, a female hormone produced by both, stimulates it under some conditions. Progesterone, a hormone chiefly connected with pregnancy or preparation for pregnancy in the female (although in some ways it has more in common chemically with testosterone than estrogen), often has an adverse effect on sex. Ordinarily in the female, progesterone levels are low for most of the monthly cycle. Pill users get an unremitting supply of artificial progestins.

Concerning the male response to the pill, Michael's research is illuminating and dramatic. No matter how receptive a female, the male must, of course, be "positively motivated." When the sexual scents of the female rhesus are altered, most males disdain her. When her scents are restored to normal, the interest of her male companions revives. What is the key to female sexual scent? It is *vaginal secretions*. Even though we may think we have no odor, the vaginal secretions from a healthy unmedicated female of various species, including the human, stimulate the male rhesus. When he is unresponsive to a certain female, the application to her of vaginal secretions from *other females* provokes his interest. Vaginal secretions, named *Copulins* by Dr. Michael, contain a half-dozen very specific short-chain aliphatic acids. Remarkably similar in a dozen different primate species, including humans, these chemicals have a marked stimulatory effect on the male. They are now considered to be major sex attractants. When synthesized in the laboratory they produce the same aphrodisiac effects.

The female on the pill, be she human, rhesus, or baboon, is robbed of her *Copulins*. The pill changes the underlying body chemistry, which, in turn, alters the action of lactobacillus (Doderlein's bacillus, specifically) in the vagina. Other drugs, including penicillin, also inhibit *Copulins*. In short, normal *Copulins* are produced by normal vaginal bacteria. Both hormones and antibiotics change the bacteria—and the *Copulins*. In 25 human females using the pill, vaginal acids and *Copulins* were lowered, and the normal cycle changes (in the vagina) disappeared.

We cannot claim that human males respond to smell as directly as do rhesus monkeys. This topic is considered so unpleasant that humans don't like to open it up for discussion. Still, on some level, we all know that smells do influence sexual attraction—very much. The male rhesus, at least, grows indifferent to pill-using females because of the way their normal vaginal secretions are altered. We do not know enough yet to say for sure that on this profound chemical level human females who take the pill are less attractive to human males. However, we can say that vaginal processes take place which might inhibit the male —especially since studies of intercourse frequency in human married couples suggest that it often declines when the wife goes on the pill.

The other insight gleaned from rhesus monkey research is that the progestins in the pill inhibit sexual interest on the part of the female. This is a function of brain chemistry, not *Copulins*.

On the other hand, a female whose vagina has abnormal secretions caused by the pill can suffer from vaginitis, and therefore feel less sexual.

One young woman, who had been married for three years, told us what happened to her when she began taking the pill: "I became totally apathetic toward sex— in fact, I was repulsed by the thought of it. Many times, when I'd go to take a pill, I'd think, 'Oh, God, I only have two pills left, and we haven't done it all month.' Then I'd take the pill and out of a sense of guilt go jump in bed with my husband. It got so bad that my husband, who is a very virile man, became impotent several times. He thought it was him. Even after I stopped taking the pill, it took a long time before I was back to normal."

Other women—1 to 2 percent of pill users—find the pill *increases* their sex drive. Still others complain that intercourse becomes painful or impossible because of dryness of the vagina.

All in all, the pill has not been the great sexual liberator that it originally was made out to be. Of course it has improved the sex life of some women by removing the fear of pregnancy. But the diaphragm and other methods can accomplish that without placing them in a state of chemical castration.

Depression

The pill can create havoc with the emotions and the mind. By 1969, British researchers had established that 1 pill user in every 3 studied showed depressive personality changes, and that 3 out of 50 became suicidal.

It is difficult to know just how many suicide attempts are caused by pill-connected depression. The British Royal College study stated that "Data on attempted suicides are available, but they have not yet been analyzed . . . it would be misleading to quote them." The figures they have for *successful* suicides show that twice as many pill users took their lives as nonusers. The same ratio applies to women who died from accidents.

Many pill users who suffer depression describe themselves as "hysterical" or "on the verge of a nervous breakdown." They feel helpless, hopeless, enervated, guilty, ashamed, worthless. Some lose their appetite; others eat compulsively. Many complain that when they try to read through something they have no idea of what they've read. Decisions, even simple ones like what to prepare for dinner, become impossible. They often feel overwhelmed, anxious, terrified.

Once the pill is discontinued, the depressive symptoms often disappear. But for some women, psychiatric help, including antidepressant drugs and sometimes shock treatment, is necessary. In the same way that the pill affects existing cancer or diabetes, it can add fuel to a depression that has been smoldering for a while.

Some researchers have suggested that pill-induced depression is a result of subtle alterations in brain chemistry associated with abnormal metabolism of various amino acids, and have connected depression in pill takers to decreased levels of vitamin B_6. Some women have been shown to improve with vitamin therapy. There is some evidence that pill brands containing relatively more progestin in proportion to estrogen have more unsettling personality effects. Nonetheless, a woman who responds badly to one formulation may respond *worse* to another. It is suspected, though not yet proven, that clots and strokes may occur with higher frequency after a brand switch. Of course the opposite can happen also—some patients do feel better. But brand switching is taking a chance.

Danger also lies in prescribing tranquilizers and antidepressants to counteract pill-caused psychiatric symptoms. Research indicates that the pill taken in conjunction with some mood-altering drugs can produce a number of side effects, including tremor and rigidity, as in Parkinson's disease, hyperactivity, twisting of the body so it is bent like a bow, tremendous weight gain beyond what the pill alone can cause, and increased interference with sugar metabolism.

Many women report that their personalities undergo a complete change—often for the worse—when they begin taking the pill. The change most often reported is increased irritability. One woman told us: "I hardly ever got off the couch except to slap one of the kids. I was always irritable and tired—I'd nap all the time. Getting dinner was a real effort. I wanted to stick it out to see if it got better, but my husband said that it looked to him as if I was never going to get beyond the first trimester. That's what it was like—like perpetual early pregnancy. So I stopped taking the pill."

Sometimes the psychiatric changes wrought by the pill build up slowly from cycle to cycle. The woman herself is hardly aware of them, but her close associates are. Many pill users have been urged to give it up by observant husbands or roommates. Many have only recognized later how much the pill had affected them. Lorraine P. stated, typically: "I was never a clumsy person, or what you might call *tense*. During my year on the pill I went through two complete sets of china—broke 'em accidentally. Finally my roommate delivered an ultimatum. 'Lorry,' she said, 'either you're giving up those pills or we're switching to plastic dishes.'"

Newly Acknowledged Side Effects

One of the most recently established side effects is an increased risk of gall-bladder disease. A study reported in the *New England Journal of Medicine,* early in 1976, documented that pill use causes higher levels of cholesterol saturation in the bile, which increases the risk of gallstones. According to Dr. Donald Small of the Boston University School of Medicine: "Patients who persistently have supersaturated gall-bladder bile—that is, bile more than 100 percent saturated with cholesterol—have an early chemical stage of gallstone disease, and many of them will go on to form stones."

Other studies have documented that the risk of developing gallstones is two to two-and-a-half times as great for pill users as for comparable women.

Pill users have a decreased resistance to many viral infections, but their loss of immunity to chicken pox is particularly startling. It may be related to the severe B-complex deficiencies that afflict so many women on the pill. (B-deficiency is a factor in many herpes conditions, and chicken pox virus is a member of the herpes family.)

Rebounding bladder and kidney infections are almost garden variety side effects. Some urologists think that these occur because the pill's hormones cause the tubes connecting kidney and bladder ureters to dilate, providing a "red carpet" for bugs. Hundreds of women have remarked to us that when they stopped the pill their persistent urinary problems evaporated. Forty percent of pill users have bacteria in their urine, as compared to about 15 percent of normal controls.

Arthritis-like symptoms, including pain and swelling in the joints, occur in a substantial number of users. Often these symptoms are minimal and are only noticed by pianists, professional seamstresses, artists, designers, or others who depend on their fingers for a living.

The leaders in this highly specialized area of pill research, such as Dr. Giles Boles at the University of Michigan's Rackham Arthritis Unit, think that these joint changes may reflect underlying—and potentially very dangerous—changes in immune responses caused by the pill. By now, many doctors know better than to give the pill to a woman with pre-existing arthritis, but few of them connect the pill with a healthy patient's complaints that her joints are becoming swollen and painful.

Alice J. is a serious pianist who practices four hours a day at a minimum, and much more when a concert is scheduled. Her fingers get a lot of action, or stress. When her joints started swelling she consulted *everyone*, her internist, gynecologist, orthopedist, and even her husband's allergist, as well as all of her music teachers and colleagues.

We asked if she were taking the pill, and when she answered affirmatively we suggested that she try a short vacation from it. Alice was otherwise happy with the pill and considered our comments to be (she admitted after) "off the wall." All of her doctors agreed that the connection was far-fetched—they weren't familiar with Boles's research, which appears in highly specialized journals. But Alice's piano coach, an 84-year-old European gentleman who was once a musical director at the Metropolitan Opera, agreed with us. He said: "Oh, my dear, of course you must stop with those terrible chemicals. You are an *artist*. I had no idea you were doing such experiments on your body and your hands."

So Alice vacationed from the pill, and six weeks later her fingers were fine. Now she advises other pianists *never* to take it.

The pill is also associated with gum inflammation and bleeding, similar to, but more persistent than, the gingivitis of pregnancy. A New York periodontist claims that when she performs gum surgery on a pill user it takes the patient six times as long as average to heal. A nutritionally minded dentist, she speculates that this may be related to the vitamin C and C-complex deficiencies in pill users.

Another serious condition that can be worsened or occasionally caused by the pill is colitis. Symptoms include acute abdominal pain, nausea, vomiting, and bloody diarrhea. The actual cause may be tiny blood clots in the digestive apparatus. If the damage does not progress too far, simply stopping the pill produces healing within a few months. The pain and bloody diarrhea may cease immediately. If however, sections of the bowel have turned gangrenous, surgery may be necessary.

Years ago, women started to tell us that they thought they were allergic to the pill. About one to three months after starting it—but sometimes sooner—they either developed hives or a chronic runny nose and sneezing. They stopped and the symptoms went away. They started again, and the symptoms recurred. There were no reports of any such allergies in the medical literature, and what is more, women with asthma sometimes noted that the pill made it better.

Once again, patients were way ahead of their doctors and should have been heeded. Now allergies to the pill are formally recognized. At the Allergy and Asthma Clinic in Denver, Colorado, Dr. Constantine J. Falliers decided to track such associations. In twenty-seven months, Falliers collected 14 cases—3 of women with chronic asthma who improved on the pill (1 also improved during a subsequent pregnancy)—and 11 of women *with no past history of allergic disease* who developed rhinitis or hives soon after starting it. Three of the patients with rhinitis got asthma as well.

Some of the women had endured their symptoms through *years* of pill taking. Five suspected a relationship, but it was ridiculed by their doctors. One blamed her own emotional problems with her husband. The remaining 5 "seemed startled" when the chronological connection was pointed out.

Women who wish to remain on the pill may be content to control their minor allergies with appropriate medication. On changing contraceptives, some improve immediately but others show no response. They have been "sensitized" for life.

Reporting these findings, Dr. Falliers has observed, in *Lancet:* ". . . it must . . . be remembered that in clinical medicine, once the fire is lit, removal of the match (in this case, the oral contraceptive) does not necessarily extinguish the flames."

Birth Defects

The potential danger of the chemicals in the pill to unborn fetuses is yet another serious consideration. It happens, more often than people realize, that even conscientious pill takers sometimes become pregnant. Not only are *their* fetuses at risk—so are the unborn babies of women who stop the pill and conceive very soon afterward.

As early as 1960, a report in the *Journal of the American Medical Association* demonstrated that progestins, when taken during pregnancy, can cause masculinization of a female fetus.

But even before that, back in 1955, when Pincus and Rock were just starting human trials of the modern pill, a professor at New York City's Baruch College, psychologist Jean Jofen, was beginning to investigate a chilling theory. Professor Jofen had been giving routine IQ tests to 5-year-old students at a Hebrew parochial school in New York.

She noted that a large subgroup of these children had below-normal scores. She discovered that in each of these cases the mother had been imprisoned at a specific concentration camp during World War II—Auschwitz. Further research revealed that inmates at Auschwitz—men and women—had been fed daily doses of liquid estrogen in their soup. (The women stopped menstruating, and the men lost their sex drive, just as the Nazi scientists expected.)

As their estrogen source, the Nazis had first used a plant that comes from Brazil. In time they switched to synthetic estrogens, similar to those found in the current pill. "They just poured it in the soup," Jofen explains. "There was no dosage." In a paper presented at the Fifth World Congress of Jewish Studies in Jerusalem, Jofen reported that after testing hundreds and hundreds of young children, "the Auschwitz sample had the lowest range." Only 2.7 percent of the Auschwitz children had IQs over 115, while in comparable groups of youngsters, including those whose mothers had been interned at other Nazi concentration camps *where estrogen had not been added to the diet*, one-third or more had IQs over 115.

Does estrogen also have a long-range effect on the children of men who were given it? This is a most important question for families considering the male pill. Here Jofen's findings are reassuring: "Those children whose *fathers only* were interned in Auschwitz, but whose mothers belonged to the other groups, fell into the normal range of IQ," she reported.

Jofen has also found that the younger the mother had been when she was first introduced to the drug, the lower the IQ of the child.

"Not all facets of intelligence are affected equally," the psychologist explains. "I am not saying these children are retarded. . . . Intelligence is made up of many things, logical thinking, auditory memory, visual memory, motor coordination. . . . If a child has very poor coordination with hand and eye movements, this will depress the whole intelligence score."

Jofen states flatly that she believes: "Among women who have taken the pill, we will find a larger number of lower IQ children than among mothers who have not taken the pill." Although the FDA acknowledges (and only after all these years of widespread use) that birth defects increase if a woman takes hormones *during pregnancy*, or *just before*, neither it nor any other official health organization is seriously considering Jofen's finding, i.e., "that the estrogen administered to the mothers in Auschwitz had an effect on the intelligence of their offspring born many years later."

Jofen's research, ongoing now for twenty years and conducted over the opposition of most concerned parties, does not conclusively indict the pill. There are many reasons why the children of concentration camp survivors might have some minimal brain damage or other subtle medical and social handicaps. The poor nutrition the parents suffered could be one factor. Overprotectiveness could be another. It is eminently understandable why concentration camp survivors tend to coddle their children, but modern research does tell us that overprotection lowers IQ. On the other hand, the children of female survivors who received *no estrogen* do not have a comparable IQ deficit.

One further study, from Puerto Rico, has lent what may be tentative confirmation to Jofen's research. Younger children in Puerto Rican families usually have higher IQs than older ones. When the mother took the pill in the period between births, the younger children were still as bright as, or brighter than, their old siblings, but the difference was less marked than usual.

Jofen's research also lends weight to the hypothesis that hormones given to men are less apt to cause long-range handicaps in their children. (See chap. 21.) While her studies and the Puerto Rican report do not prove that pill users' children will have lowered IQs, they are certainly grounds (one would think) for further investigation.

By 1969 there was more data suggestive of birth defects. Dr. David Carr of McMaster University, in Canada, found a striking increase in a rare type of chromosomal defect known as triploidy among the babies of women who conceived within months after going off the pill. Most of the babies with this defect die in the womb or at birth. Moreover, a study performed at Andrews Air Force Base, in Washington, D.C., revealed the following: Women who had taken the pill for two years or longer and then conceived within one month had double the miscarriage rate of women who had never used the pill, or who, after using it, had waited longer to conceive. There were also more major birth defects among the infants born to the group who conceived very soon after going off the pill.

Women who take the pill have been shown to be deficient in certain vitamins and minerals, among them the B-complex group (including folic acid), zinc, and magnesium. Since folic acid is essential for a normal pregnancy because it promotes growth and helps develop healthy red blood cells, some researchers have pointed to this as a possible cause of increased miscarriages and birth defects among pill users.

Dr. Dwight Janerich, testifying before a Senate subcommittee on health in early 1976, described his own study showing that women who were exposed to synthetic hormones had five times as great a chance of bearing a child with defective limbs—missing parts of arms or legs—as women who had not taken the hormones.

A further report from the Hadassah Medical School in Israel showed a 25 percent increase in major birth defects and a 33 percent increase of minor birth defects in infants of women taking hormones.

Admittedly, not all of these abnormalities were caused by oral contraceptives. Some occurred in babies whose mothers underwent hormone pregnancy tests which the FDA has now banned, and others occurred in women who were taking hormones for other reasons. But the products are similar to the contraceptives, and, as Dr. Janerich testified, "there is some concern in the scientific community that even the use of these hormones just before pregnancy may pose some risk to the developing fetus." The evidence now indicates that women who stop the pill in order to get pregnant should wait for several normal periods to pass before conceiving.

Neither should a nursing mother take the pill. Hormones travel in her breast milk, and no one knows what the long-range effects on the baby might be.

Francine P. chose to breast-feed her infant daughter, Katy. When she went to her gynecologist for a six-week checkup, he put her back on the pill but cautioned that it might diminish her milk supply. At Katy's next checkup, the pediatrician asked Francine if she was still nursing. "Yes," Francine replied, adding that she had been on the pill for six weeks without any lessening of her milk.

The pediatrician became livid and called Francine's gynecologist. "Don't you ever read a medical journal?" she shouted into the phone. "Don't you know the hormones in the pill get into the milk, and no one knows what effect that could have on an infant? Giving the pill to nursing mothers is monstrous! You may be Francine's physician, but I'm Katy's, and as such I'm ordering Francine to stop the pill immediately."

Pill defenders claim that serious side effects are "rare." We disagree. At present "only" one out of several hundred users must be hospitalized annually with emergency complications such as blood clots, stroke, heart attacks, or liver tumors.

But these figures will probably go up, for long-term use increases risk. Consider heart attack, the rate of which climbs so dramatically in pill users over 40. Is this a reflection of their age only, or their length of use as well? We put the question to Dr. Christopher Tietze, the pill's leading statistician, and he admitted he didn't know. This factor, length of use, had not even been examined in connection with heart attacks. But few women start the pill suddenly at 40, so presumably most of these victims were on it a long time.

The relationship between the pill and breast or cervical cancer will not be settled for years. For now, women who get cancer are not listed as pill casualties (except for cancer of the liver, and endometrial cancer in former users of sequential brands), but in time they may well be. The risks of diabetes (or conditions akin to it), hypertension, and infertility *are* being quantified, and they are much higher than was formerly thought.

But these conditions, serious as they are—and they can leave a women's health or psyche in ruins—do not usually warrant emergency hospitalization. Thus, they tend not to be tallied with annual casualties.

Neither is suicide. Some doctors, in specialties other than psychiatry, don't really think of depression as a "life-threatening" illness. Psychiatrists do! Suicide is among the leading causes of death in several age groups, and, as noted, pill users commit it at least twice as often as comparable women.

During the sixties, some open-minded psychiatrists hedged on this matter. Perhaps, they suggested, the suicides were not directly caused by the pill but merely coincidental to it. For example, they said, these unfortunate women might be casualties of the sexual revolution; perhaps the pill made it hard for them to say "no" in situations where they would have liked to.

Such excuses are no longer defensible, for—while there are often secondary factors—we now know too much about the pharmacology of *both* the pill and depression. As we shall see in the next chapter, certain cases of pill-caused depression can be promptly cured with a vitamin! The women who get such depressions are suffering from a severe metabolic disturbance, like those who get gall-bladder conditions from the pill. Such depressions must now be viewed as a major *medical* side effect.

Let's just total the figures for four of the complications we've mentioned:

—5 percent of pill users get high blood pressure
—13 percent get chemical diabetes
—30 percent get mild to severe depression
—5 percent are infertile—and sometimes permanently sterile—when they stop

Thus, even allowing for some overlap (a given woman may get more than one), about half wind up with one of these four conditions, none of which is "trivial."

A recent ad, from a pill manufacturer, pokes fun at the personal testimonials of women and appeals to the most authoritarian (and sexist) instincts of the doctors who read the journal in which it appeared.

The ad shows a quartet of women playing bridge and gossiping. The copy informs the doctor how to "reassure" his patient when "her medical society" (i.e. her bridge club) scares her about the pill.

And yet, from the beginning, most of the now established complications were suspected, and reported, by intelligent users. They were dismissed by some doctors because the scientific evidence hadn't been compiled. (Other doctors did learn from their patients.) In the late 1960s a woman's magazine carried an article that mentioned all the FDA's officially recognized side effects of the pill, a list that has doubled in length in the ensuing years. The magazine was inundated with mail. A comment that kept recurring, in too many letters, was: *"I felt as though I was up against a stone [or brick] wall. My doctor kept saying that it [fill in any symptom] couldn't be from the pill—it was all in my head. Your article is the first I've heard that this is a recognized side effect."*

Since 1969, when Dr. Herbert Ley was FDA Commissioner, the agency has promised full disclosure to pill users (a complete lay-language warning in every dispensed packet) but has still not delivered. Each successive commissioner supported *the idea* of such a warning.

Thus, if a woman's doctor dismisses her questions or complaints, she has only her friends to consult. Unless the doctor is female (only 3 percent of U.S. gynecologists *are*, and the figure is declining) her friends can speak from personal experience, while her doctor cannot.

CHAPTER 10

Recovering from the Pill

Many women taking oral contraceptives show biochemical evidence of a multifactor hypovitaminosis. . . .

Drs. Michael and Maxine Briggs

One of the best-kept secrets about estrogen is that it wreaks havoc with nutrition—both vitamins and minerals. The same seems to be true of progestin.

As Dr. J. E. Jelinek of New York University Medical School stated: "While some . . . effects are seen in patients taking either estrogen alone or progesterone alone, the combination of the two agents seems to produce a unique clinical array of side effects."

And as the Australian researchers Michael and Maxine Briggs (see chap. 21) recently wrote in a medical journal: "Many women taking oral contraceptives show biochemical evidence of a multifactor hypovitaminosis [vitamin deficiency] involving vitamin C, riboflavin, thiamine, vitamin B_6, vitamin B_{12} and E. Clinical signs should be detectable. These would be expected to involve a general malaise and depression together with increased susceptibility to infections. Skin signs should be common. . . ."

Folic acid is seriously deficient in many pill users, as are B_6, E, and essential trace metals, such as zinc and magnesium. Conversely, other nutrients are mysteriously *increased*—to levels considered dangerous by some researchers. Of special concern are marked increases in plasma vitamin A and copper which, in excess, may be associated with birth defects, emotional disturbance, and hair loss. Moreover, pill users need less niacin and possibly less iron as well.

All told, vitamins D, K, pantothenate, and biotin *may be the only major nutrients left unaltered by the pill.*

Should pill users take supplementary vitamins to compensate? One who thinks so is Dr. Richard Theuer, a nutrition researcher. In January 1972, an article by Theuer—"Effects of Oral Contraceptive Agents on Vitamin and Mineral Needs: A Review"—appeared in *The Journal of Reproductive Medicine.* This was the first that many gynecologists had heard of the pill's effects on nutrition, for most of Theuer's 90 references came from obscure biochemistry or nutrition journals that busy practitioners rarely have time to read.

Theuer stated firmly: "Biochemical and clinical findings point to an increased need for vitamin B_6. . . . The absorption of the major food form of folic acid is substantially impaired. . . . The pill also appears to increase the requirement for vitamin C and perhaps for vitamin B_2 (riboflavin) and zinc. . . ."

Theuer, as it happens, is an industrial scientist—employed by the Department of Nutrition Research at Mead Johnson. A heavy advertiser in *The Journal of Reproductive Medicine,* Mead Johnson is also the manufacturer of Feminins, "a unique vitamin-mineral supplement for the special needs of women taking oral contraceptives."

Nonetheless, and despite subsequent research which challenges the precise ingredients in Feminins (in particular the inclusion of vitamin A), Theuer's article was a landmark.

There is no question that vitamins can reverse certain pill symptoms, including some cases of severe depression and disturbed sugar metabolism (relieved by B_6), or anemia and reproductive organ disturbances (relieved by folic acid). On the other hand, many scientists caution against using vitamins to (as they put it) "mask" the disturbances of the pill. *What they—and we—tend to advocate is stopping the pill and taking carefully selected vitamins afterward to speed your return to normal.*

But it's not that simple for many women. Some must stay on hormones because of serious medical conditions that the hormones control. They may feel terrible while they are using such medications—and worse when they stop.

Robin H. took her first Enovid tablet in 1958, the year it came out. She has been on and off Enovid ever since, for it is the only treatment that controls her endometriosis. (See chap. 29.) Without Enovid, Robin has much more pep and energy, and her chronic mild depression lifts. Her husband puts it like this: "When Robin is taking Enovid, I have to walk with her slowly, like an old man. When she's off it, I have to run to keep up."

But when Robin gives up Enovid her endometriosis recurs. She walks faster—to hospital emergency rooms.

Others, like Irene L., say they have no peace of mind with any other method. "I have excruciating vaginal infections when I take the pill. No matter what brand I use they always come back. But when I don't take the pill I get pregnant. I've been pregnant on the IUD, the diaphragm, and the *combination* of condoms and foam."

Although many symptomatic women feel relief as soon as they stop the pill (Irene's infections clear up within days), others take a long time to revive, and still others *get worse symptoms than they had while using it.* It's a "post-pill syndrome" or "adjustment period" that's well known, but far too little discussed.

Women frequently return to the pill (or other hormones) in a desperate effort to alleviate such symptoms.

For example, Corinne K. complained, "When I went off the pill, I just couldn't have intercourse. My vaginal secretions were *gone.* Something funny happened to my eyesight, too, and my voice changed. I was able to hit high notes better—I sing in the chorus of a Gilbert and Sullivan light opera group—but my speaking voice got squeaky. I felt real close to my 15-year-old nephew; it was as if both of our bodies were out of control. Our chats were comical, if you could have heard them."

A West Coast physician, Leah G., said: "It's such a familiar syndrome—it's happened to so many of my friends and patients. But in my case the symptoms are worse. I've been on and off the pill for ten lousy years on account of them. They develop over several months. My hair starts coming out in patches. I bruise if you touch me. My breasts and stomach get ugly stretch marks. I get chest pains and backaches. Worst of all is the depression. No, maybe the worst thing is the skin. Once I kept off the pill for half a year; my skin got worse and worse until I had severe acne. I never had it as a teen-ager—no more than a bump or two before my periods."

Rita P. told us: "I just didn't get my periods back. I went back on the pill because I don't believe in abortion. The irony is I'm probably sterile, but as long as I don't menstruate, how can I tell if I'm pregnant?"

Gynecologist Marcia Storch sums it all up this way: "When a woman comes off the pill, before her own hormones function again she is not protected . . . either by her own or the pill's hormones."

The purpose of this chapter, then, is twofold: to help women who are determined to take their chances with the pill compensate for some of its nutritional ravages, and to help women who wish to go off the pill—or who have recently done so—to hasten recovery and avoid the post-pill syndrome. Sample regimens are offered at the end of the chapter.

VITAMIN B$_6$ (PYRIDOXINE)

> 5 to 10 mg daily needed preventively by 7 out of 8 pill users
>
> 30 to 50 mg daily for pill users suffering depression
>
> Up to 100 mg daily to relieve hypoglycemia, or chemical diabetes

Victor Wynn is an esteemed metabolic researcher in England. In his laboratory, Dr. P. Adams and other co-workers studied 39 women who had developed depression while on the pill. Nineteen had severe B$_6$ deficiency, and improved significantly when treated with 40 mg daily of the vitamin. This important research has led many psychiatrists to treat pill-associated depression with B$_6$. Such deficiency is not the *only* cause of pill depressions, but seems to be implicated about half the time. The only women in the Adams study who did *not* improve on B$_6$ therapy were those who were not so notably deficient in the vitamin.

For the 5 to 15 percent of women who test out as "chemical diabetics" on the pill, even more B$_6$ is necessary. Doses as high as 50 or 100 mg a day are advocated.

B$_6$, or pyridoxine, is one of the most essential—

and underrated—vitamins. It affects our state of mind and nerves, as well as our skin, reproduction, sexuality, and hormones. The recommended allowance of 2 mg is too low for many people, since there are substantial inborn differences in our ability to utilize B_6. Some of us need a lot of it under the best of circumstances. Anyone afflicted with a metabolic disorder, including diabetes, hypoglycemia, celiac disease, or even water retention and overweight, should look to B_6 deficiency or malabsorption as a possible factor. A person suffering from depression or nervousness, severe premenstrual symptoms, skin problems or dental caries should look to it too. After C, B_6 might be the vitamin that does most to make all the others "work."

DIETARY SOURCES OF VITAMIN B_6

High:

    Liver (beef, calf, pork), herring, salmon

    Walnuts, peanuts, wheat germ, brown rice

    Yeast, blackstrap molasses

Medium:

    Bananas, avocados, grapes, pears

    Barley, cabbage, carrots, corn, oats, peas, potatoes, rye, kale, tomatoes, turnips, yams, brussels sprouts, cauliflower, spinach, soybeans, wheat

    Beef, lamb, pork, veal (heart, brains, kidney); cod, flounder, halibut, mackerel, whale, sardines, tuna

    Butter, eggs

Low:

    Apples, cantaloupes, grapefruit, lemons, oranges, peaches, raisins, strawberries, watermelons, cherries, currants (red)

    Asparagus, beans, beet greens, lettuce, onions

    Cheese, milk

Roger Williams, who in 1933 discovered and named pantothenic acid, one of the many B vitamins that work so intimately with B_6/pyridoxine, cautions that most vitamin supplements do not contain much B_6 because it is expensive to extract and synthesize. When babies do not get enough B_6—and some, like pill users, need many times the usual intake to maintain normal blood levels—they have convulsions, brain damage, and mental retardation.

The processing of many starches and sugars depletes their supply of vitamin B_6. Enriched white bread "returns" thiamin, riboflavin, and niacin, but not B_6 or E. (According to Carlton Fredericks, whole wheat is four times as rich in B_6 as white flour.)

Psychiatrist Carl Pfeiffer of the Brain Bio Center in Princeton, New Jersey, believes that ordinarily the nutrition-conscious individual should be able to derive sufficient B_6 from his or her diet. "When supplements are required," he cautions, "that is to be determined by individual need."

Nausea and lack of appetite in the morning are clues to B_6 deficiency, discovered at the Brain Bio Center. Also, deficient patients have trouble remembering dreams. The proper supplement corrects this, but too much B_6 (or too much at night) produces restlessly vivid dreams and insomnia. Pfeiffer himself relies on 50 mg of B_6 each morning in order to dream normally at night. But he says that if he uses the same dose on vacation—when he is less stressed— he dreams *excessively*. On vacation, he cuts his 50-mg tablet in half.

Pfeiffer and his colleagues at the Brain Bio Center urge their patients to give up the pill. High therapeutic doses of B_6 are chancy for a pill user, for *certain amino acids are already too low*. High doses of B_6 can *aggravate this deficit*. A pill user's B_6 deficiency symptoms improve, but her protein metabolism becomes more disturbed.

B_6 should never be used by patients with Parkinson's disease who are also receiving levadopa. However, we hope and trust that no one with Parkinson's disease is further assaulting her system with the pill!

VITAMIN C
500 to 750 mg (or more) daily (in two divided doses —morning and night)
Needed by many pill users to avoid bleeding gums, easy bruising, spider veins, cold intolerance, weakness, listlessness, rough skin, aching joints, slow healing of wounds, impaired maintenance of cartilage, bones, and teeth

The normal requirement of C is said to be 60 mg. Pill users need to take 500 mg, or more, routinely if they wish to avoid side effects. C deficiency impairs iron absorption, and interferes with metabolism of tryptophane, phenylalanine, and tyrosine. C is also required for normal hormone synthesis.

C "conserves" many of the body's vitamins, including most of the B's, E, and A. (Of course it may be inadvisable to conserve A in the pill user, since her levels are in some respects already too high.)

HIGH C PROBLEMS

Hidden complications can also occur when pill users take too much C. Mega-C is tricky in the first place, and not everyone can handle it. Side effects include diarrhea, abdominal pain, and kidney stones. The staff at the Brain Bio Center often places patients on large amounts of C (up to 3 or 4 grams daily in several divided doses), but they advise such patients to test their urine with dipsticks, available in drugstores. This way they can tell if they are taking too much.

The risk of kidney stones can be diminished in C users if calcium is avoided—a poor idea—or if magnesium is taken with the calcium, as in dolomite. Vitamin C has exceedingly complex interactions with aspirin. Two aspirin tablets inhibit the intake of C by the white blood cells. Thus, in theory, pill users who are also taking aspirin may need even more than 500 mg of C. On the other hand, doses of 3 to 5 g of aspirin daily—along with high C— have complicated and undesirable effects on the kidneys.

Very high C doses may adversely affect the cervical mucous lining. The cervix of a pill user is already in some trouble.

High doses of C (and B_6 also) create what is called "vitamin dependency." There may be symptoms upon withdrawal. Plasma levels may drop to well below pretreatment baselines for ten to fourteen days.

But the most serious drawback to mega-C for pill users concerns the "blood" vitamins, folic acid and B_{12}. These two are apparently not conserved by extra C, quite the opposite. Too much C increases urinary excretion of folic acid—washes it out—and simply destroys B_{12}. In one recent study it was found that 250 mg of C could destroy up to 81 percent of the B_{12} content of a meal; 500 mg can destroy an amazing 95 percent of the B_{12} content. Here again, it appears, the pill user who takes the 500 or 750 mg of C required daily to make her blood levels normal may be robbing Peter to pay Paul. In normalizing her C levels, she further jeopardizes her "iffy" folic acid and B_{12}.

In July 1975 an illuminating letter appeared in *Lancet*, from researchers at the Department of Food Sciences, Polytechnic of North London. These nutritionists, commenting on the work of Professor Wynn, pointed out that even 500 mg daily of vitamin C "may be too little for women whose vitamin C intake has been low for a long time, unless this dose is sustained for several months." Six pill users were given almost seven times that amount of C, a whopping 3,300 mg, to take each night at bedtime. Then they were carefully tracked. In the mornings, their plasma C levels improved greatly, but by evening they were down to the presupplementation levels. (Note that Pfeiffer and others stress the need to take C in divided doses, because it washes out so rapidly.) The London nutritionists concluded that in pill users "Large doses of ascorbic acid were quickly lost."

On the other hand, these investigators had some good news:

They had also examined nutrition students who, being knowledgeable about the pill, tried to compensate for the deficiency in their diet. "They deliberately increased their vitamin C intake for over a year with fresh fruit and vegetables," probably on the advice of their professors. These women revealed C levels that were not greatly disturbed.

Women who wish to protect or replace their vitamin C levels should be aware that the vitamin is much more biologically *available* in fresh orange juice than in either frozen or pasteurized. (This was recently demonstrated in research at Mount Sinai Hospital in New York City and is contrary to what was previously thought.)

DIETARY SOURCES OF VITAMIN C
High:
>   Broccoli, brussels sprouts, collards, horseradish, kale, parsley, peppers (sweet), turnip greens
>   Black currants, guava, rose hips

Medium:
> Cabbages, cauliflower, chives, kohlrabi, mustard, watercress, spinach
>
> Lemons, oranges, papayas, strawberries

Low:
> Asparagus, lima beans, chard, cowpeas, mint, okra, spring onions, peas, potatoes, radishes, rutabagas, turnips, dandelion greens, fennel, soybeans, summer squash
>
> Gooseberries, passion fruit, grapefruit, limes, loganberries, mangoes, cantaloupes, honeydews, red currants, white currants, tangerines, raspberries, tomatoes, kumquats

FOLIC ACID
> 400 mcg (.4 mg) to
> 800 mcg (.8 mg) daily for pill users and pill convalescents

Folic acid is a story in itself. Like B_{12}, folic acid is essential to the health of our blood and blood cells. At times, although rarely, the pill produces such acute deficiency that megaloblastic anemia ensues. One such case was reported recently by Dr. F. Bruce Lewis of St. Paul, Minnesota: His patient was a 29-year-old, single executive. She had been on Ovral for three years, and in this case had been eating a normal diet with adequate amounts of folate (folic acid). In time she developed a gall-bladder condition—now recognized to be another pill side effect—and had surgery for it. Following her operation, she was put on an oral iron supplement to compensate for lost blood.

Nonetheless, the woman continued to suffer from alternating diarrhea and constipation. No one took her off the pill. Six months later she was readmitted to the hospital with complaints of a pounding pulse in the ears, easy bruising, fatigue, and weakness. Her hemoglobin and white count were only half the lower limits of normal, which meant she had severe anemia. She also had many scattered black and blue marks, and two hemorrhages on the retina of her right eye.

"The contraceptive was stopped," he doctors reports, "and the patient was started on oral folic acid." At the end of a week her blood picture was much improved, and in time her eye healed also. Lewis's conclusion—and warning: "Periodic hemoglobin or hematocrit checks should be done on women who are using oral contraceptives. Even after administration of these agents for a substantial period of time without problem, there is still the risk of the insidious development of megaloblastic anemia. It would also seem wise to observe individuals on oral contraceptives particularly carefully after such stress as surgery, fad diets, or other events which lead to decreased dietary intake of folate."

Besides causing blood disorders, folic acid deficiency impairs metabolism of other B vitamins, and C, as well as nucleic acids. It causes intestinal disturbances, and also has the curious effect of lowering the pain threshold (the deficient person feels pain more sharply) as well as decreasing resistance to many infections.

Of special interest to pill users is the effect of folic acid deficiency on the reproductive organs. Without folic acid, the response of these organs to estrogen is blocked. Pregnancy is abnormal (some researchers think folic acid deficiency is the reason for the pill's association with birth defects) and the cells and glands of all the reproductive organs are altered.

Folic Acid, the Cervix, and the Pill

Changes in the cervix are easiest to observe and have been the most explored. Besides a chronic cervicitis (inflammation), small, irregularly formed glands are seen in many pill users. The Pap smear is often abnormal—1 in 5 pill users develops a suspicious Pap after three or four years—and there has been much controversy over *what* the abnormal cells portend. Some doctors construe this as a very early stage cancer, or precancer, and they advocate surgery. Others think it's benign—just a typical abnormality of the pill.

Progressively, as women stay on the pill, the lining of their uterus grows thinner, and the uterine glands look abnormal, too. Certain cells in the ovaries atrophy, and after a few years the ovaries themselves appear somewhat shrunken.

In time, a most provocative observation was made by research scientists: *The abnormal cells found in the Pap smears of many pill users much resemble those observed in patients with folate deficiency anemia.* In other words, these genital and reproductive aberrations might well be an expression of folic acid deficiency.

We do not know yet whether folic acid supplements could prevent *all* of the changes that occur. However, a team of researchers in New York City, hematologist John Lindenbaum and his associates, have demonstrated that abnormal Pap smears *can* be reversed with folate therapy.

The Lindenbaum group tried a daring experiment on pill users with abnormal Pap smears. Leaving the women on the pill, they treated them for three weeks with 10 mg daily of oral folic acid. This is a very high dose, as the recommended allowance is only 0.4 mg (400 mcg) or one twenty-fifth the amount these doctors prescribed. All of the Pap smears returned to normal, or near normal.

Three and a half years later, 4 women who had chosen to continue on the pill, but had taken no further folate supplements, were re-examined. In all 4 cases the abnormal Pap smear had returned.

Lindenbaum and his associates have been stingingly condemned in some quarters. One doctor ventured, in the *Journal of the American Medical Association,* that their work would lead to "an epidemic of neglect" of early cancer of the cervix.

But pill users who wish to avoid unnecessary surgery are entitled to know that three weeks of folic acid therapy *could* restore their Pap smears to normal—and spare them surgery on the cervix, or even hysterectomy. The truth of the matter is that many doctors don't fuss over these abnormal Pap smears anyway. They've become so used to finding them in pill users that they merely "watch" them, and don't operate.

Might extra folic acid also prevent—or reverse—the ovarian changes in women who take the pill? There is as yet no research evidence, but—in light of folic acid's effects on all the reproductive organs—it seems possible, or even likely.

We would place folic acid high on the list of supplements that women recovering from the pill should take. It could reverse much of the damage, speeding the return of fertility in women who fail to ovulate, and helping to ensure normal pregnancies in those who conceive while on the pill, or shortly after stopping.

We urge current and recent pill users to select a diet rich in folic acid. Folic acid is considered essentially nontoxic in humans. In fact, many nutritionists consider it one of the hardest of all vitamins on which to overdose. Seventy-five percent of ingested folic acid is excreted in the urine within twenty-four hours. In a controversial move, the FDA has limited the amount of folic acid that can be included in *one* nonprescription vitamin to 800 mcg or 0.8 mg. This is because certain symptoms of B_{12} deficiency anemia (rarer than folic acid anemia, it afflicts mainly vegetarians and people with the inability to absorb B_{12}) may be masked by high supplements of folic acid. However, the level at which folic acid may start to mask B_{12} deficiency anemia is over 1 mg daily, which is two-and-a-half times the recommended allowance, and also the same minimum level at which Lindenbaum believes cervical abnormalities can be reversed.

The recommended allowance of folic acid in pregnancy and lactation is 0.8 mg, and this also seems like a good level for pill users and pill convalescents to aim for. Such nonprescription pregnancy vitamins as Mead Johnson's Natalins contain 0.8 mg, and would be suitable for many pill users except for the inclusion of controversial A, and perhaps unneeded iron.

Doses of over 1 mg daily of folic acid should perhaps be avoided by epileptics, as it may increase seizures. Allergic rashes and such complaints are occasional side effects of folic acid also. Heavy drinkers require still more folic acid than others to correct deficiencies.

DIETARY SOURCES OF FOLIC ACID
High:
>   Liver (beef, lamb, pork, chicken); asparagus, spinach; wheat bran; dry beans (lentils, limas, navy); yeast

Medium:
>Kidney (beef)

Low:
>Lima beans, snap beans, broccoli, corn, beet greens, chicory, endive, kale, parsley, chard, turnip greens, watercress; almonds, filberts, peanuts, walnuts; barley, oats, rye, wheat; beef (muscle, heart), lamb, pork, chicken, turkey (muscle); all fruit tested; cheese, milk; brazil nuts, coconuts, pecans; wax beans, beets, brussels sprouts, cabbages, carrots, brown rice, cauliflower, celery, cucumbers, eggplant, escarole, mustard, kohlrabi, lettuce, mushrooms, okra, onions, parsnips, peas, peppers, potatoes, pumpkins, radishes, rutabagas, squash, sweet potatoes, tomatoes, turnips

Besides eating a folate-rich diet, pill users can purchase separate 0.4 or 0.8 mg supplements in health-food stores. Most B-complex or multi-vitamin preparations do not contain as much as they may need. A product called the Pill Pill, made by the Cosvetic Laboratories, does include 0.4 mg of folic acid.

ZINC (Taken with B complex, C, and E)
>15 to 30 mg daily
>For pill users—current and former—to help correct stretch marks, poor hair growth, fragile nails, acne, absent menstrual cycles, joint pain, bruising

In a June 1968 press release, the FDA defended the quality of U.S. soil with a quote from Dr. Frederick Stare, Chairman of the Department of Nutrition at Harvard and known to some as the "Cornflakes Professor" for his homages to prepared breakfast foods. Stare said: "Fertilizers, regardless of type, do not influence the nutrient composition of the plant in regard to its content of protein, fat, carbohydrates, or the various vitamins. These nutrients are influenced primarily by the genetic composition of the seed and the maturity of the plant at harvest."

What Stare (and the FDA) omitted is that fertilizers do influence the *mineral* composition of plants, the iodine content and trace elements such as zinc, cobalt, and selenium. Not until the mid-1970s did physicians and nutritionists wake up to the fact that much of the U.S. populace is borderline deficient in zinc. Though the recommended allowance is 15 mg daily, we consume only 8 to 11 mg in most diets. Soil exhaustion, food processing, careless cooking, and junk foods all leach from us our natural zinc allotment. Zinc is not "destroyed" in the same sense a vitamin is, but it can be removed or made inaccessible.

In calculating the vitamin and mineral content of most cooked foods, nutritionists usually start with the raw values and reduce them by 25 percent. This method may work for garden-fresh produce, but not for what happens to it in today's world. For example, in the freezing process, green vegetables are blanched with chemicals called "sequestrants" to ensure a beautiful bright color after they are cooked. Sequestrants reduce the zinc and manganese content to only 20 percent of normal. Zinc and manganese, as it happens, are also removed from white flour. We have amazingly few high-zinc sources left to us. A serving of Atlantic oysters contains 120 mg of zinc, enough for a week's supply if only we could store it that long. (We can't.) Unfortunately, even today's oysters may not suffice, for if they come from contaminated waters, they contain excess copper, which drives out zinc.

If you want to ensure getting what natural zinc you can (a matter of urgent importance to pill users), proper cooking will help preserve it and other nutrients:

• Use fresh vegetables—garden fresh (as opposed to market fresh) whenever possible.

• Use a minimum of cooking water and save it to add back to the meal. (One reason Europeans are less deficient in zinc than we are is that they consume much more homemade soup.)

• Cook slowly and use low temperatures.

• Keep food as cold as possible while storing.

• Eat raw foods as frequently as possible.

• Buy small quantities to avoid storage losses.

The best vegetable sources of zinc are peas (4 mg per 3-oz serving) and carrots (2 mg). Oysters, herring, and clams have an extremely high zinc content, but are often contaminated. Liver has a high content, but as it also has

DES and other drugs (see chap. 6), we would not recommend most U.S. liver nowadays.

Whole cereals, especially wheat bran, whole oatmeal, and wheat germ, are excellent sources. Ideally, a serving should supply a full day's requirement of zinc. Unfortunately, actual levels in food crops depend on adequate zinc in the soil, and many soils are deficient. Whole nuts and peanut butter are fair sources.

The widespread appearance of spontaneous zinc deficiencies has led to zinc enrichment of animal feeds. Cows' milk is presently one of our most reliable ways to get zinc. Although the content is variable, one glass daily, even from relatively low-zinc cows, may satisfy the average requirement.

Children who are zinc deficient, as many are, lose their appetites and sense of taste and smell, fail to grow, their wounds are slow to heal, and they lack zest for life. In extreme cases their sex glands are small (hypogonadism) and they themselves undersized. In a recent study of school children in Denver, an increase in daily zinc intake dramatically improved the health of many.

How much zinc should you use? For most conditions, 15 mg daily or certainly 30 will suffice, especially if B complex, C, and sometimes E are taken with the zinc, for they seem to help it along. You may have to purchase separate zinc tablets, for most vitamin and mineral preparations still contain far too much copper and far too little zinc. Willner Chemists, at 330 Lexington Avenue in New York City, makes a one-a-day product called Willvite Tablets which is quite economical (250 tablets for $5.95) and includes, besides the usual basic vitamins, 15 mg of zinc and no copper. It seems like an excellent supplement for women *recovering* from the pill, but is not suitable for those still on it. (Willvite Tablets contain 10,000 units of vitamin A, which pill users should perhaps shun, and only 200 mg of vitamin C, enough to speed recovery in a former pill user, but not to correct blood levels in a present one.)

Health-food stores now stock zinc tablets in various dosages. The 15-mg zinc tablet is the most popular since this represents the daily needed intake of zinc for an adult. Do not exceed this amount once deficiencies are corrected. Some scientists think that excess zinc diminishes selenium, which may have a protective effect against cancer.

The patient who takes too much zinc may slowly develop diarrhea, nausea, and vomiting. In that case, of course, she should cut way back. Be wary of megadoses, except under medical supervision. (In chap. 35 we explain the important distinction between mega- and therapeutic doses.)

VITAMIN AND MINERAL SUPPLEMENTS THE PILL USER DOES NOT NEED

Copper
Iron
Vitamin A (unless she is on a low-protein diet)
Niacin (B_4)

COPPER

In contrast to zinc we are saturated with copper, which, in excess, is now thought to be poisonous, like lead and mercury. We are getting so much copper that some of us can taste it in our mouths. The average adult need is 2 mg daily, and many of us ingest 3 to 5. Surplus copper can cause severe mental and physical illness.

There seem to be two principal factors in our dietary excess. One is the switchover from galvanized water pipes to copper plumbing. Some of us, depending on the condition of our water pipes and the source of water (acid well water tends to leach lots of copper from the plumbing), are getting more than our daily requirement with every glass we drink. A second factor is that copper sulfate is widely used today to promote growth in food animals. Extra copper—along with the other chemicals discussed in chapter 6—is often served up to us with our meat. Copper and zinc have a complex, somewhat antagonistic relation to one another. Zinc deficiency exaggerates copper excess, and vice-versa. And now—enter the pill.

Estrogens make the entire zinc-copper imbalance much worse. According to Dr. J. Cecil Smith, Jr., chief of the Trace Element Research Laboratory at the Washington (D.C.) VA Hospital, pill users ordinarily have a twofold rise in both serum copper and ceruloplasm, the blood protein to which most serum copper is tightly bound. (In late pregnancy, a woman has similar elevations, but they return to normal after she gives birth. Furthermore, it isn't pertinent to compare pill aberrations with those found in pregnancy, for the pregnant woman *is* in a sense "eating for two." Values considered normal for her, in her temporary state, are grossly abnormal in the nonpregnant.)

What, asked Smith, does the elevated copper mean? He examined a half-dozen women who showed other side effects from the pill, and found that all of them had even higher levels than the symptom-free pill user. Instead of being twice the norm, copper levels were tripled. Smith showed—for copper—what Wynn and others had shown for B_6, and still other researchers had shown for folic acid. *Most* pill users have some distortion in their normal copper levels. They tolerate these distortions for a while, although no one knows or will guess the aftermath or long-term effects. Excess copper has been linked to iron deficiency anemia, nausea, and vomiting, and also to heart attacks, where it is thought to be an additional risk factor.

Copper ions also may increase blood clotting. The "brain stimulant" effect of excess copper is also feared to cause constriction of the blood vessels contributing to the elevated blood pressure often found in women on the pill.

Migraine

Insomnia, depression, hypomanic states (like those produced by amphetamines), and migraine headache have also been linked to the excess-copper–low-zinc syndrome of women on the pill. Pfeiffer reports that he successfully treats migraine patients with heavy zinc supplements.

Most neurologists urge women on the pill who get migraine, or whose previous headaches worsen, to give it up at once. Women who have this reaction appear to be in danger of stroke. Altogether, any neurological or eye symptoms should be viewed most seriously. However, as Pfeiffer points out gloomily, there are some women who insist on taking the chance.

Pfeiffer recommends the following for migraine:

• Two Bufferin and one Benadryl at night. The aspirin in the Bufferin will keep the blood more liquid and possibly help to prevent clots. (Benadryl is a prescription antihistamine made by Parke, Davis in Detroit.)

• 100 mg of niacin morning and night.

• 500 mg of calcium gluconate in the morning, and occasional potassium supplements as needed.

• A high zinc-magnesium tablet morning and night. Two such preparations are Vicon C and Ziman C. If the patient has abnormally low blood pressure, Vicon Plus (which includes 4 mg of manganese chloride) or Ziman Fortified should be used instead.

• For menstrual migraine, Pfeiffer adds a water pill to be taken each morning at the time of the period.

OTHER TRACE ELEMENTS

Serum iron increases in pill users. This used to be thought due to decreased menstrual bleeding, but the changes are too marked for that. Hemoglobin levels remain as before, which means the increased plasma iron is probably due to "mobilization from iron stores." Nonetheless, the rise in circulating iron does not seem to deplete bone marrow, as some researchers feared. Most agree now that the need for dietary iron in pill users is slightly *decreased*.

Magnesium is involved in many metabolic functions, including blood clotting. Magnesium deficiency may cause thrombosis and, since the pill lowers serum magnesium, Smith fears this may be another factor in the clotting disorders that come with the pill. Magnesium is also an essential part of many enzyme systems, and is important for nerve and muscle activity. Severe deficiency causes tremors, convulsions, and sometimes behavioral changes.

The recommended magnesium allowance for women is 300 mg. Many of us are slightly deficient to start with, again because of convenience foods. Processed wheat has almost no magnesium. Softening agents remove magnesium and calcium from our water. Four tablets a day of dolomite (calcium and magnesium) will provide your magnesium requirements.

Milk, nuts, seeds, whole grains, seafoods, and some green vegetables remain good sources of magnesium. Beware of spinach, which has oxalic acid that "ties up" this important mineral.

VITAMIN A

For unexplained reasons, serum vitamin A levels are raised in pill users by 30 to 80 percent. It is thought that this may reflect a shift of the vitamin from the tissues to the blood. In theory, this could have untoward effects on women who are already deficient. Symptoms include night blindness and other visual disturbances, as well as lowered resistance to infection.

On the other hand, scientists fear that the excess might cause birth defects, as it does in other mammals, especially in rats. Since A levels take two to three months to return to normal when the pill is discontinued, it is strongly advisable for a former pill user to avoid conceiving right away.

The daily requirement of A is 5,000 units. Doses of around 100,000 units can be fatal. It is generally thought best for a woman on—or recently off—the pill to avoid taking A supplements, although *if the vitamin has indeed shifted from her tissues to her blood*, she may, in some senses, be deficient in it. No one is actually sure whether the pill user should be considered to have a simple excess— as her serum levels indicate—or a deficiency, if, as is postulated, her blood is drawing on *other reserves*.

All that can be said for certain is that estrogens are known to be "antagonistic" to vitamin A. Too much estrogen keeps A from performing normally in the body, and, at the same time, A is needed for proper steroid synthesis. Perhaps every woman starting on the pill should be tested for her vitamin A levels first. Some scientists believe that if she is *deficient in A to start with*, the subsequent transfer from tissues to blood might *so harm her tissues* that she needs supplemental A to protect them, even though serum levels will get too high. Others deem such supplements dangerous in this murky situation.

For the time being, and until the situation is better clarified, the following seems like a sensible compromise:

The pill user whose regular diet is low in A and also protein—this could apply equally to poor women and to college students eating dormitory food—might as well take a product like Feminins, which includes the daily allowance of A. But women who are getting lots of dietary A

and protein should avoid further supplements, especially
if they have symptoms of A excess. These include irritability, nerve lesions, fatigue, insomnia, painful bones and
joints, hair loss, jaundice, itchy skin, loss of appetite, blood
clotting changes, and possible birth defects.

If disturbances in A utilization were *the only side
effect of the pill*, we would be afraid to take it, as a long-
term drug, on this basis alone.

DIETARY SOURCES OF VITAMIN A
High:

   Liver (beef, pig, sheep, calf, chicken); liver oil (cod),
      halibut, shark, sperm whale; carrots, mint, kohl-
      rabi, parsley, spinach, turnip greens, dandelion
      greens, palm oil

Medium:

   Butter, cheese (except cottage), egg yolks, margarine,
      dried milk, cream; white fish, eel; kidneys (beef,
      pig, sheep); liver (pork); mangoes, apricots,
      yellow melons, peaches, cherries (sour), nectar-
      ines; beet greens, broccoli, endive, kale, mustard,
      pumpkin, sweet potatoes, watercress, tomatoes,
      leek greens, chicory, chives, collards, fennel,
      butterhead and romaine lettuce, squash (acorn,
      butternut, hubbard), chard

Low:

   Milk; herring, oyster, carp, clams, sardines; grapes,
      bananas, berries (black-, goose-, rasp-, boysen-,
      logan-, blue-), sweet cherries, olives, oranges,
      avocados, prunes, kumquats, pineapples, plums,
      rhubarb, tangerines, red currants; summer and
      zucchini squash, asparagus, beans (except
      kidney), brussels sprouts, cabbages, leeks, arti-
      chokes, peas, corn, cucumbers, lentils (dry),
      peppers, lettuce, celery, cowpeas, rutabagas,
      okra; hazelnuts, peanuts, black walnuts, cashews,
      pecans, pistachios

THREE B's

   B_1 (thiamine) requirement for pill users:
      5 to 15 mg daily
   B_2 (riboflavin) requirement for pill users:
      10 to 15 mg daily

B_{12} (cobalamin) requirement for pill users:
  6 mcg to 250 mcg daily

Three further B's (besides B_6 and folic acid) may be required in greater quantity. These are B_1 (thiamine), B_2 (riboflavin), and B_{12} (cobalamin).

B_1 (thiamine): Though the recommended allowance of this vitamin for those not on the pill is 1.5 mg daily, pill users and those just off the pill should take 5 to 15 mg. Small as these doses may sound, thiamine is essential. Thiamine has a diuretic effect, but may also be constipative. Sodium nitrite and nitrate, so widely used in processed meats, cause a substantial decrease in the thiamine content (as well as riboflavin and vitamin C) when foods are stored for two weeks or longer. Deficiency symptoms include fatigue and weight loss, circulatory and cardiac involvement, muscular atrophy, and, perhaps most notably, mental disturbances such as depression and irritability. Another clue to thiamine deficiency is oversensitivity to noise.

Thiamine deficiency is a common and serious complication of alcoholism. Treatment with large doses of thiamine corrects hallucinations and DTs. The pill user who is a heavy drinker and also relies heavily on "delicatessen" meats such as franks and salami may be in serious trouble with her thiamine supply.

Wheat germ, rice bran, soybean flour, and yeast are the best dietary sources of thiamine. Ham (without nitrites and nitrates) is also very good.

B_2 (riboflavin): Working synergistically with the other B vitamins, riboflavin helps maintain normal estrogen functions. While pill users are somewhat deficient, they are not so strikingly lacking in riboflavin as they are in other nutriments. However, the recommended supplement for pill users is 10 to 15 mg daily. Deficiency symptoms include sore mouth, lips and tongue, dandruff and scaly skin, and eye problems, especially sensitivity to light. Dietary sources include organ meats and yeast, as well as many vegetables—for example, asparagus, beet greens, broccoli, spinach; and kidney, wax, snap, and lima beans.

B_{12} (cobalamin): Half of pill users have B_{12} levels below the normal range, while 15 percent are strikingly deficient. This reduction occurs quickly, within a few

months after starting the pill. In some subjects, the levels reported are so low they are indistinguishable from patients with B_{12} deficiency anemia. Curiously, however, no clinical cases of B_{12} anemia have been observed—unlike the situation with folic acid. These extremely low B_{12} levels, without anemia, are considered most puzzling.

B_{12} has a central influence on the blood, the brain, and nervous system, and, perhaps, energy. It is said to influence the electrical activity of the heart, as well as carbohydrate and fat metabolism.

Some people have trouble absorbing B_{12}. The molecule is too large to pass through openings in the digestive tract and must link up with a carrier. In such cases, increasing the oral dose does not seem to help, and this is why injections remain popular despite widespread skepticism about them.

It can be difficult to get sufficient B_{12} on a vegetarian diet, as plants are very low in it. B_{12} occurs in organ meats, clams, sardines, salmon, crabs, oysters, herring, cheese, eggs and milk. The recommended allowance is 6 mcg daily, but under special circumstances extremely high doses are prescribed. Alcoholics as well as pregnant women, old people, and new pill users may need extra B_{12}.

Two Case Histories

Ideally, when a woman gives up the pill, she should consult a doctor who'll run blood tests and prescribe a diet and supplements for what *she* lacks. Regrettably, few doctors have the interest or equipment to do so.

Grace D., a Canadian economist, took the pill from 1965 to 1972. Toward the end, her hair was getting thin on top and she noticed brown spots on her skin. The whole time, she now acknowledges, she was "a driven person." But when she stopped she felt wretched. She developed breast and chest pains, plus "extreme anxiety and depression."

After several false starts, she found a doctor, Louise Gilka in Ottawa, who prescribed a regimen including the following: 3 g of C; 800 units of E; B complex, including 250 mg of pyridoxine; and 250 mg of bone meal three times daily.

The vitamins worked almost immediately. "I couldn't believe how different I felt. I didn't tell anybody. Instead, I went off for three days, and the symptoms came back. Two weeks later I tested it again." On her own, Ms. D. has added minerals, and over time has tapered down to one-third of her original supplements. But she says, four years later, "I expect I'll always have to take some vitamins. I went on holiday for a week without them recently. I was suffering."

While most of Ms. D.'s post-pill syndrome disappeared quickly, her hair, she says, took a year to recover.

Louise Lacey, author of *Lunaception* (see chap. 16), was 32 when she gave up the pill. "Until I stopped, I had no idea what it was doing to me," she states. "It was only when I had a standard for comparison that I could see how profoundly my system had been affected. The first and most obvious change occurred in my menstrual cycle, which became very irregular. Figuring it would be a while before it settled down, I didn't give it much thought at first. But then other strange symptoms of imbalance began to force themselves on my awareness.

"About six months after I stopped taking the pill, dozens of new wrinkles suddenly appeared on my face, my buttocks 'fell,' my waist thickened without any increase in weight, and my whole torso changed shape. These are all aging changes that normally are gradual and culminate in menopause. I can only conclude that the hormonal balance of my body had been hyped up for so long, relying on the artificial crutch of the pill to supply its essential ingredients (which otherwise would have been manufactured at home, so to speak), that when I stopped taking it, my system collapsed, literally. . . .

"A nutritionist friend suggested that I might get my own glandular system working again by priming it with extra doses of vitamins B and E. She recommended that I take vitamin pills, until I could work out diet supplements. . . .

"I didn't want to be a pill-popper, I protested. She reassured me that first, all the B vitamins could be found in one pill, and the E vitamins [600 units] in as few as two; and second, I could do it for a couple of months and judge the result for myself. If the regimen turned out to be of value, I could learn something about nutrition myself and eat my vitamins in my food instead of taking pills. Otherwise I could just quit doing it. In any case, I had only the price of the pills to lose, as these vitamins, particularly in such moderate doses, could have no harmful effect.

"So I did as she suggested. Inside a month, the new wrinkles had disappeared and my shape reverted to normal. Even my fanny, to my astonishment, climbed back up. The mood flashes disappeared and my normal personality pattern . . . reasserted itself.

"My delight at my success in getting my hormonal processes working again was marred only by the fact that when I stopped taking the vitamins, thinking everything was fine again, some of the symptoms returned. So I did have to work out diet supplements for myself, and I am resigned now to the necessity of boosting my glands indefinitely. I can't help but think that my metabolism certainly was permanently altered by the pill, no matter what the medical profession declares."

After the Pill—Summary

Women with pronounced post-pill symptoms are grateful for—and sometimes astonished at—the benefits of vitamin therapy.

Grace D. was taking real mega-doses, but was under a doctor's supervision; Louise Lacey was following the advice of a nutritionist familiar with her case.

For most women, moderate supplements will do. Further information about vitamins, when and how to take them, their interaction with hormones, and relationship to symptoms is included in chapter 35.

Our Suggestions

When recovering from the pill, or even taking it, many women are able to reduce or cure their discomforts by means of dietary supplements. Deficiencies vary. One woman may be highly deficient in folic acid, another much more so in other B's or C or zinc. Thus, the user will have to adjust her own daily intake according to the response she gets.

The basic regimen below is for pill users and those recovering from the pill.

1. High potency therapeutic "stress formula" B complex with C including folic acid and a minimum of 5 mg of B_6.
   One tablet twice daily
   • If depressed or showing symptoms of diabetes or hypoglycemia, add separately one 50-mg tablet of B_6 daily or even two.
   • If showing symptoms of bleeding gums, easy bruising, or spider veins, add one tablet of vitamin "C complex" containing the citrus bioflavonoids, hesperedin, and rutin, or else take a daily bioflavonoids pill (available from Nature's Plus), along with the normal stress supplement.

2. *One* Selene-E (25 mcg selenium and 200 units of E) tablet *three times a week*, or 100 to 200 units of E daily. If vitamin E cannot be taken after a meal with fats, a couple of lecithin tablets should be swallowed with it.

3. Four hundred mcg of folic acid *once a day* if stress supplement contains less than this amount.

4. 30 to 50 mg of zinc *three times a week* if deficiency is suspected.

For women who cannot abide more than one daily vitamin, there are several individual products that may fill their needs.

A new Pill Pill can be ordered for $7.95 for 30 from Cosvetic Laboratories, P.O. Box 14009, Atlanta, Georgia 30324. It is also available at some drug and department stores. The Pill Pill is overpriced, in our opinion, but soundly designed. The formula follows:

B-1	5 mg
B-2	10 mg
B-6	50 mg
B-12	20 mcg
Folic acid	400 mcg

Vitamin C	300 mg
Bioflavonoids	50 mg
Inositol	100 mg
Magnesium	150 mg
Zinc	15 mg
Vitamin E	500 units

Cefol, a prescription vitamin by Abbott, also contains ample folic acid and 30 units of E, as well as the needed C and other B supplements. (An Abbott spokesman told us that the company may soon be making this vitamin available without prescription. Check with your pharmacist.) Similar products, containing E, the B's and C, but with less folic acid than Cefol are available with no Rx.

An advantage of the Pill Pill over Cefol is that it includes the minerals zinc and magnesium, as well as the bioflavonoids or "C-complex" (capillary) factors. These may be especially helpful to the pill user with skin or gum disorders. On the other hand, the 50 mg of B_6 in the Pill Pill, a hefty dose, could cause sleep disturbances in women who don't require that much. It's desirable, however, for those with depression or impaired carbohydrate metabolism. The E may be excessive for women with high blood pressure, diabetes, or heart disease.

Feminins, by Mead Johnson, discussed earlier in the chapter, probably contains too much A for women whose diets are abundant in this vitamin. The product may be helpful for some women on low-A diets, but watch for symptoms of A excess.

Convenience notwithstanding, the soundest approach to compensating for pill-caused deficiencies is to take a good stress supplement, twice daily after breakfast and dinner. The Plus Products Company's Formula 72 is a safe and sane example, the Cadillac among such products. It is available at most health-food stores. C and the B's in *divided doses* help maintain consistent blood levels.

Then, as needed, and depending on her own deficiency symptoms, the pill user or convalescent may well wish to add additional E, B-6, folic acid, bioflavonoids and/or minerals.

Vitamins seem to work better in the long run if the user "vacations" from them for brief intervals. Some women stop on weekends, or for one weekend day. Others stop for a few days or a week out of each month.

Some Special Considerations About Supplements

• E has extremely complex interactions with the pituitary hormones. Moderate E supplements, of up to the recommended allowance of 30 daily units, often suffice for *women who are presently on the pill*. When they stop, however—during the recovery period—women may benefit dramatically from adding more E.

• If a woman stops the pill in order to have a baby, it is crucial to avoid A and add folic acid. Excess of the former and deficiency of the latter are suspected to be associated with birth defects. If she has any history of seizures or epilepsy, however, she should eat a *diet* rich in folic acid instead of taking supplements. It's slower, but safer.

• Women who are close to menopause age or have menopause-type complaints—like Louise Lacey—may want to increase their E supplements from 100 to 600 mg, or even (preferably under medical supervision) slightly more. Also, a woman whose diet is high in polyunsaturated fats needs more E.

• Women who suffer from muscle and leg cramps or breast tenderness and premenstrual congestion might be helped by extra E along with dolomite.

• Health-food products such as organic desiccated liver (which contains no DES), yeast, wheat germ, and lecithin contain associated factors which may boost the effectiveness of the B tablets and E. See chapter 36 for further information and discussion.

• The pill disturbs sugar metabolism—mildly in most users, severely in up to 15 percent. The consequences may include weakness, dizziness, and even fainting, as well as irritability and some depression. The longer a woman stays on the pill, the more marked her sugar metabolism disturbance is apt to be. While pyridoxine (B_6) helps modify such effects, it may also be necessary to adopt a special diet. Consult your doctor or a nutritionist.

• Pyridoxine is not the only B vitamin deficiency

associated with both pill use and mental symptoms. Thiamine (B_1) and B_{12} deficiency—to name two others—both have well-established psychiatric effects, and both are depleted by the pill.

• Women who are plagued with hair loss should avoid copper, add zinc and ample B complex to their diets, and eat foods containing sulfur, such as egg yolk. Hair loss after stopping the pill has been compared to the loss some women experience after childbirth. There are similar nutritional factors, especially copper excess.

A different pattern of hair loss occurs in some women who are still taking the pill. Here actual bald spots, instead of a general thinning, are more apt to occur; this hair loss is similar to male baldness. For this condition we advocate stopping the pill. The progestins used in most brands of pill are testosterone derivatives which, according to Dr. Wynn, can create a more "male" biochemical pattern. But one progestin, norgestrel (used in Wyeth's Ovral Lo/ovral and Ovrette) may be less masculinizing.

After-care for Skin

A college freshman was pleased with himself, for he'd gotten a job as a night clerk in a drugstore. He was learning medical and sexual "secrets."

"Here's how you can tell if a girl's on the pill," he confided to his friends. "Watch for girls whose boobies get bigger and whose acne clears up."

There's some truth to it—and there's also another side. Lots of women's skin has been ruined by the pill, ruined in ways that cannot easily be corrected. The young man might also have cautioned his friends:

"Watch out for girls who get brownish patches on their skin, like butterfly marks across the cheeks and forehead, or a pseudo mustache. These patches appear gradually after a year or two on the pill. They don't usually fade when she stops. You'll see them most often in brunettes and women who get a lot of sun. After weight gain, fluid retention, breakthrough bleeding, and depression, patchy skin discoloration is the most common side effect of the pill."

If brown patches—also called melasma, chloasma, or

the "mask of pregnancy"—develop, it's imperative to stay out of the sun. The vitamin PABA may help; topical bleaching agents may also. Pills with low estrogen and progestin are less associated with this effect. Sometimes the patches fade, but often not.

If oily skin and acne occur after stopping the pill, diet and nutritional measures (B complex, C, E, and extra zinc), combined with proper skin care, can usually reverse them quickly. (See instructions for steaming in chap. 35.) Vitamin A is essential for skin health, and, as we have explained, the pill disturbs it in a most curious way.

Former pill users *who are not planning to have a child in the near future but who are troubled with skin disturbances*—excessive dryness as well as oiliness—might try adding 10,000 units of A daily to their vitamin regimen. This can be obtained in an A and D tablet, or a multivitamin supplement.

If adding A makes the skin more oily, itchy, or discolored, drop it. The effects are somewhat unpredictable. An unusual feature of A is that it *decreases* basal metabolism.

Other skin conditions our night clerk might mention are hair loss, severe herpes infections, or a dreadful condition called porphyria cutanea tarda that affects the liver as well as the skin. Hairy ears and wild, bushy eyebrows are early symptoms. The skin bumps and pits that come later leave permanent scars.

Some pill users grow so sun-sensitive that they get a rash just from light streaming in through a window glass. Spider veins, and bleeding under the skin are other dermatological effects, as well as monilial infections of the vagina, which doctors consider "dermatological." Skin cancer, including malignant melanoma, has been tentatively linked to the pill.

Yeast or monilial infections in the vagina are hard to get rid of on the pill. Try eating a lot of yogurt, the type with lactobacillus acidophilous culture, and also apply the same kind of plain yogurt vaginally. Lactobacillus acidophilous tablets are also available—take six or more daily. Stop wearing pantyhose and slacks until the condition clears up. White cotton underpants (or none) are recommended.

* * *

Does the brand of pill influence side effects? Possibly. Pills with a higher balance of certain progestins (Ortho-Novum, Norlestrin, Norinyl, Norquen, Loestrin, Zorane) may produce more androgenic, or "mannish," effects such as acne, hairiness, scanty periods, and permanent weight gain. More estrogen-dominant pills (Enovid, Demulen, Ovulen) can improve acne, but be more apt to cause fluid retention, heavy periods, and the breast swelling so valued by our pharmacy clerk.

At present some doctors believe that pills containing less than 50 mcg of estrogen cause fewer blood clots than those with greater amounts. They may be less reliable, however, and they cause more spotting between periods. These "low-dose" pills include such brands as Loestrin, Zorane, Modicon, and Brevicon.

When a woman has side effects on one type of pill, her doctor may switch her to another. True, more estrogens may cure breakthrough bleeding, or acne, and less may reduce edema and breast swelling. But, as we have mentioned, the most serious side effects such as blood clots or complete loss of periods seem to occur more often following a brand switch. When trouble arises, the safest policy is to stop.

AID (Agency for International Development) buys pills from the lowest bidder for shipment overseas. Women receiving birth control under these programs are frequently subject to brand switches. They have served as guinea pigs for us.

CHAPTER 11

Help for Post-Pill Menstrual Problems

Thomas Jefferson had periodic migraines; Abraham Lincoln had periodic depression. . . . Richard Nixon's "raging hormonal imbalances" may have caused the Watergate morass. Even John F. Kennedy . . . had a serious hormonal disorder, Addison's disease [adrenal insufficiency].

Janice Delaney, Mary Jane Lupton, and Emily Toth, in *The Curse: A Cultural History of Menstruation*

As many pill users have learned—to their regret—infertility and/or increased menstrual problems may occur after stopping. One of the ugliest chapters in the pill's history is Dr. John Rock's long denial that such consequences exist. In the early and mid-1960s, as honest and concerned doctors sounded the alarm about infertility, Rock got after them with all the power and prestige his name and Harvard position could command. He continued to maintain that women would be superfertile after quitting the pill. One of Rock's major targets was a California fertility specialist, M. James Whitelaw, who, in 1966, published a major alarm in the *Journal of the American Medical Association* on the "oversuppression syndrome" that follows after the pill. Later, at the Nelson pill hearings, in 1970, Whitelaw testified:

> Although it is five years since I originally submitted my report to the *Journal of the American Medical Association* on my observations of amenorrhea and infertility following administration of the oral contraceptives, and four years since it was published, there was over a two-year-lag period before these observations were confirmed. During

this interim it was vehemently denied by all pharmaceutical concerns and by those connected with the investigation of these synthetic hormones that this syndrome ever existed; and, even if it did, they maintained it made little difference and was the same as that seen after a normal pregnancy. . . . Since my original publication of my observations there have been ten other reports confirming my findings in the world literature. . . .

When you demonstrate something and it is clearly scientific and you bring it out and it does not sit well on somebody else's shoulders, and they scream the loudest like Hitler, why then, they win. . . .

Then the following dialogue ensued:

Senator McIntyre: "Doctor, in your research . . . what is the longest period of time you have known a previously fertile woman to be infertile following use of the pill?"

Dr. Whitelaw: "Forever. Forever from the time I first saw her up until today. By that I mean five years, and there are lots of them."

By the 1970s the "oversuppression syndrome" was widely acknowledged, and so was the comforting news that the "spontaneous cure rate" was very high. A textbook, published in 1969, urged that post-pill fertility treatments be delayed for at least a year, as ovulation is likely to resume.

But sometimes normal fertility takes still longer. A not unusual case was reported in the *American Journal of Obstetrics and Gynecology* by Dr. R. Pinkney Rankin. His patient was on the pill for one year, and did not menstruate for a month after she stopped using it. Then she menstruated infrequently for a number of months, and then not at all. After seventeen months she began to menstruate spontaneously, conceived two months later, and now has a healthy baby.

The conservative approach to post-pill sterility is just "watchful waiting," but of course this requires emotional stamina. On the other hand, fertility agents are nothing to take lightly. The most popular is Clomid, a drug originally studied as a possible contraceptive. Next are gonadotropins —ovary-stimulating hormones, extracted from either the pituitaries of cadavers or the urine of menopausal women. The leading U.S. product (from urine) is called Pergonal.

Sometimes when drugs fail a surgical procedure called ovarian wedge resection is performed.

Dr. Raphael Jewelewicz of Columbia University recently summarized the management of infertility. "In properly selected patients," he said, "the success rate is quite high, but treatment has undesirable side effects that occasionally may be severe."

The side effects of Clomid include ovarian enlargement, sometimes with cyst formation (14 percent), hot flashes and menopause symptoms (10 percent), abdominal discomfort and bloating (7 percent), and occasionally nausea, vomiting, fatigue, dizziness, mental distress, rashes, hair loss, and visual symptoms including blurring spots and flashes of light.

Clomid appears to *induce ovulation* in about 70 percent of patients, but the subsequent pregnancy rate is much lower, ranging from 27 to 40 percent. This discrepancy has never been explained, according to Jewelewicz.

Gonadotropin therapy is more dangerous than Clomid, and is also very costly. In Jewelewicz's series of 142 patients, there were 89 pregnancies (63 percent), 62 live births (44 percent), 21 miscarriages (23 percent of pregnancies), 15 multiple pregnancies (17 percent of pregnancies), and 7 women were still undelivered when he compiled his report.

Three-fifths of the multiple pregnancies involved only twins, the remainder triplets to quintuplets. Mrs. M. K., a mother of quintuplets (three daughters and two sons), all of whom survived, commenced complete bed rest at home in her twenty-second week of pregnancy, and was admitted to the hospital in her twenty-sixth.

A major complication of gonadotropins is a condition called the "hyperstimulation syndrome." About 30 percent of fertility patients have it in mild or moderate form, with ovarian enlargement and lower abdominal cramps. In severe form (2 percent) the patient grows seriously ill with fluid in the abdominal and chest cavity, scanty urine, thickened blood, low blood pressure, and other blood disturbances including electrolyte imbalance and significant weight gain. Several deaths have occured from arterial thrombosis following gonadotropin therapy.

Nutritional Aids for Amenorrhea

Instead of drugs or hormones, a woman who is infertile after stopping the pill can try a high-protein diet with appropriate supplements. For post-pill amenorrhea (absence of menstruation), follow the recommended basic regimen from the previous chapter, and include the additional B_6, zinc, folic acid, C complex, and E with selenium supplements suggested.

On this regimen, ovulation and menstruation usually return within three or four months unless the amenorrheic woman is underweight as well. If she is, however she values her thinness, she must recognize that this is a *frequent* factor in absent menstruation. It is usually corrected by a *higher calorie diet, including wheat germ oil* (see chap. 35) and other forms of vitamin E, or even E alone.

Fat cells make a central contribution to the normal production and distribution of sex hormones. Young girls do not start menstruating until they reach a critical body weight, and women of fertile age who are anorexic usually lose their periods as well as their appetites. Older women who are too thin produce so little estrogen (for their age requirements) that it may affect their vaginal condition and, secondarily, normal maintenance of their skin and bones. Older women who are too fat get more cancer, diabetes, heart and gall-bladder disease, and other illnesses associated with estrogen excess, which Premarin users get too.

E—especially in the form of wheat germ oil—was demonstrated—long before the era of the pill—to induce menstruation in women who are malnourished or extremely stressed.

Charlotte C. started taking the pill in her sophomore year at Radcliffe, the point at which her active (i.e., potentially pregnancy-inducing) sex life began. Charlotte, an excellent student, had been a grind until age 19. She was considered a "serious" young woman and had been valedictorian of her high school class.

When she fell in love, and started taking the pill, she also started caring more about her looks and style. She knew better (she says now) than to go on a crash diet, but the college food was so starchy that she had little choice.

Charlotte adopted an extreme Stillman-type diet of rabbit foods, occasional lean meat or fish, and cottage cheese. She kept the rabbit food (mostly carrots and cucumbers) on the window sill outside her room, and got the meat whenever she was invited out to dinner. She lost thirty-five pounds in two months, a quick transition from twenty pounds overweight to fifteen pounds under.

Charlotte stayed underweight, although many people told her she looked *too* thin. When she met her boyfriend's family his grandmother observed, "She's lovely but so skinny. She might not have children." (Note: The folk wisdom has always been correct on this point.)

When Charlotte gave up the pill her periods did not return for a year and a half. The doctor at the student health service gave her a progesterone prescription, which he said he would follow with Clomid if the progesterone failed. Charlotte was a little suspicious. "Don't those drugs give you twins and quadruplets?" she asked. "I don't even want one baby at present. I just want my period back."

"Take it or leave it," the doctor shrugged.

Charlotte was pondering what to do when her roommate, who was attending a Know Your Body course at a Cambridge women's center, invited her to come along and meet the local nutritionist. Charlotte's roommate, like her boyfriend's grandmother, had long been concerned that she was unhealthily thin.

Charlotte agreed to give the nutritionist's regimen a six-week trial. It consisted of a 2,500-calorie diet plus a 200-unit E capsule, swallowed twice daily with a teaspoon of wheat germ oil, a stress formula vitamin capsule (B complex with C, also taken twice daily), and separate zinc and selenium capsules to be swallowed several times a week.

Charlotte got her period fourteen days later and has been menstruating normally ever since. She has not yet tried to have a baby, but there is no reason now to anticipate any special difficulty. She gained eleven pounds (leaving her four pounds underweight by the life insurance tables) and is still a thin and fashionable-looking woman, but her bones do not stick out as much. In Charlotte's case it is impossible to say whether the pill itself or her poor diet had been the critical issue in her loss of menstruation.

Many women, like Charlotte, go on the pill and also diet when their mating instincts are aroused, but we have no research that distinguishes the relative influence of the two factors in producing amenorrhea.

In time, Charlotte discovered that she still "felt too fat" premenstrually, when her face, her ankles, and her abdomen swelled up. She controlled the swelling with a low-salt, diuretic premenstrual diet, and also learned that by doing ten sit-ups daily throughout the month she sufficiently strengthened the muscles in her abdomen and lower back so that her "tummy" did not pop out at menstruation. Charlotte found that during exam week, and other crises, the sit-ups regimen could be reduced to every other day. When she fell below *that*, some of her skirts and pants stopped fitting right. Ten daily sit-ups can be accomplished in about forty-five seconds. Performed on only alternate days, for maintenance, the time requirement is three minutes or so a week.

Women who suspect that their failure to menstruate may be connected with underweight should check the life insurance tables, which remain a good businesslike guide. The normal latitude, which is not too likely to produce serious symptoms, is about ten to fifteen pounds above or below what up-to-date insurance tables indicate. For older women it's probably more dangerous to get *above* this normal latitude, but for younger women it may be more dangerous to fall below it. Infertility is but one of the associated conditions.

Post-pill amenorrhea has been said to occur most frequently in women who were irregular before taking the pill. A recent study of 311 women in Providence, Rhode Island, suggests that a late menarche (beginning of the menstrual cycle) coupled with early use of the pill are predisposing factors. This is another reason why the pill is so dangerous for teen-agers—it can destroy their fertility forever.

Overall, the risks of *permanent or long-term infertility are highest for women who have not borne a child prior to taking the pill.* Long suspected, this sad fact was statistically established by 1976 in an ongoing study of 17,000 diaphragm, pill, and IUD users, performed by Dr. Martin Vessey and his associates at Oxford University. (In the course of this research it was also clarified that the diaphragm remains a highly reliable method. Vessey and his group are counted among the most scientifically responsible birth control researchers in the world.)

What emerged from the Oxford study was this: Initially, when contraception was stopped and pregnancy desired, pill users, as a group, had notably more trouble conceiving in the first two years than women who had been relying on other methods. After that, the fertility of those *pill users who'd borne previous children* was usually restored. Comparing them to the diaphragm and IUD groups, some differences remained, but these were "negligible."

Among pill users who had not borne previous children, the tendency to impaired fertility persisted.

The Vessey report also confirms Melamed's earlier finding that diaphragm users enjoy a virtual immunity to cancerous conditions of the cervix. By contrast, about 1 in 1,600 young pill and IUD users develop such conditions annually. Whether cervical problems might have any bearing on infertility remains unclear.

On the whole, the picture is reassuring. Most cases of post-pill infertility or amenorrhea correct themselves spontaneously within a few months to two years. With the proper nutritional stimulus, many such cases can right themselves much more quickly than that. When time and nutrition fail, fertility drugs are often effective in the last resort. Here are 2 cases from the files of Dr. Robert Kistner:

"Mrs. R.T., a 22-year-old, was first seen in 1971 because of secondary amenorrhea of twelve months' duration. Her menses had begun at age 11 but had always been irregular, the cycles varying between fifty and ninety days. She had used an oral contraceptive for twelve months and did not menstruate after discontinuation. Progesterone did not produce withdrawal bleeding." After nine cycles on various fertility drugs, in combination, Mrs. R.T. conceived, delivering a normal five-pound, nine-ounce boy.

A second patient, Mrs. M.P., was 27. She had started menstruating at age 13, and always had regular periods until her second go-around on the pill. She had used the pill for seventeen months, discontinued in July 1969, after which her menses resumed promptly, and then took the pill again until January 1970. This time her periods did not come back, and it took her two years to conceive. During most of the second year, she, like Mrs. R.T., received monthly Clomid, Pergonal, and sometimes additional drugs. In time she delivered a healthy seven-pound, three-ounce daughter.

After the birth of her daughter, Mrs. M.P. failed to menstruate again. When ready for another child, she resumed fertility treatments and conceived, this time after only three cycles of effort.

A few former pill users are hopelessly sterile. Whitelaw and others have recorded cases where total sterility has occurred even in women who had easily borne children prior to the contraceptive. Others, like Mrs. M.P., can only ovulate and menstruate under the influence of the drugs. However, the majority of amenorrheic women do return to normal by the end of two years whether they have any treatment or not. After that, it is most often the non-mothers who are left with enduring infertility.

Some fertility treatments, aside from the nutritional regimens we've mentioned, are so dangerous in themselves that no woman should agree to them just to get her periods back. Unless she wants a child very badly, it's a safer policy to wait. If she cannot bear the anxiety, her doctor may suggest Provera after three months, and low doses of Clomid after six.

Post-Pill Menstrual Cramps

Elena M., now 27, had used a diaphragm confidently since the age of 16. However, Elena, who began menstruating at 11, always had severe periods, and in her late teens they got worse instead of better. The reason—in the opinion of her current doctor—may be that her uterus is exceptionally small.

By her last year of college, Elena was grounded for most of her period—up to three days—instead of just one, as before. She suffered acute nausea and vomiting, as well as pain.

Elena went on the pill, more for her menstrual cramps than for contraception. She never felt better in her life. But, after a time, she developed a severe vaginal herpes infection that would not respond to any treatment. Neither she nor her doctor connected it with the pill, which Elena continued taking as menstrual medication. However, the nature of her infection was such that she had to remain sexually abstinent for many months.

After two years, Elena's cautious doctor suggested she stop the pill for a few cycles. This was his custom with all patients. Elena fought it, for she feared the return of her menstrual cramps. When she stopped, however, the cramps did not return too severely, and, amazingly, her herpes infection cleared up promptly.

Elena was curious and did some research. She learned that severe herpes infections in pill users are thought to be linked to pyridoxine (B_6) deficiency, and sometimes respond to pyridoxine treatment or treatment with other B vitamins. She also learned that people who once have a herpes condition (even cold sores) are feared to harbor the virus thereafter, and face danger of recurrence. She never went back on the pill.

After several years, Elena's severe menstrual periods crept back upon her. Dysmenorrhea (difficult menstruation) rarely begins with the onset of menstruation but rather a number of months or up to two years later. A young girl's first periods are rarely severe. Similarly, childbearing often cures dysmenorrhea, but after some years it may recur, though less severely.

By now Elena had moved. She consulted a new doctor, who wrote out a prescription for the pill. Elena protested. "It's the only solution," he said.

The doctor was wrong. Not only is the pill *not* "the only solution" for dysmenorrhea (admittedly, it works in the short run for many women, although for others it makes their periods *worse*), but to prescribe the pill for this purpose is not considered good medical practice.

"As part of the treatment of primary dysmenorrhea, endocrine (hormone) therapy or surgery may properly be employed, but the physician who depends upon these entirely and who takes no notice of other possible factors is sure to meet with failure in a large proportion of cases," says *Novak's Textbook of Gynecology*.

When endocrine therapy must be used, cautious physicians still steer away from the pill, for as *Novak's Textbook* further explains:

"Some progestational drugs, without estrogen added, can be used to control dysmenorrhea. . . . Side effects are minimal. . . . By avoiding the estrogen which is incorporated into most of the oral contraceptive regimens, many of the complications and clinical symptoms associated with these drugs can be obviated." Careful doctors prefer products specifically designed for menstrual disorders, such as Norlutin and Gynorest.

In most cases, however, hormones can be avoided altogether, for there are many safer measures that help substantially.

As *Novak's* concludes: "Certainly a part of the treatment of every case of dysmenorrhea should be to outline a regimen calculated to raise the patient's general health level in every possible way, and these measures alone will in some cases cause disappearance or marked amelioration of the dysmenorrhea."

Home Remedies for Dysmenorrhea (Difficult Menstruation)

For the premenstrual week, it's advisable to go on a high-protein or even a "hypoglycemia" diet, with a reduced intake of sugar and starches, and to avoid spicy foods and salt. Foods that are naturally diuretic, such as cranberry juice and eggplant, should be added to the diet. Other such foods include artichoke, asparagus, cucumber, corn silk, grappa, parsley, parsnip, strawberry, watercress, and watermelon. A woman who likes to take a drink might try sloe gin fizzes, comprised of sloe gin, club soda, and lemon juice—the sloe gin berry, like the cranberry, is naturally diuretic.

It's also helpful to keep the bowels loose, as constipation can worsen menstrual cramps. For that, one can eat some prunes or figs or drink senna leaf tea. Ripe bananas and fresh orange juice add beneficial potassium.

When her period begins, a woman may prefer a light or high-liquid diet, with lots of fresh vegetable juices and herbal tea. Some women find it helpful to avoid coffee. But apricots, eggs, milk, whole grains, and molasses help to replace the iron that is depleted at this time. (Iron supplements also should be followed with vitamin E.) It's best to get iron from natural sources such as organ meats, clams, oysters, kelp, kidney beans, and soybeans. Prune juice and kelp are two double-barreled menstrual supplements, for the prunes are laxative and also contain iron (the same applies to dried apricots), and the kelp may be diuretic. For people who do not care for the taste of kelp, it is available in pressed tablets at health-food stores. For women who find iron-rich natural foods unappealing, Lederle makes a product called Stresstabs 600 with Iron that is soundly formulated to meet premenstrual and menstrual needs. It includes the daily allowance of E and folic acid, 600 mg of C, and 25 of B_6, as well as iron and threapeutic amounts of the other B's. Stresstabs are available at pharmacies without prescription.

Many people believe, mistakenly, that a high protein diet must include lots of meat. We suspect that there may be elements in meat which aggravate menstrual cramps as well as menopause complaints. In any case, both conditions are rarer in vegetarian societies, and American women who cut back on meat often report improvement. Directions for high protein meatless eating are included in two excellent books: *Diet for a Small Planet* by Frances Moore Lappé, and *Recipes for a Small Planet* by Ellen Buchman Ewald, both available in paperback from Ballantine.

Calcium and Other Supplements

Of all supplements advisable to take for menstrual distress, calcium may be most important. Calcium blood levels drop about ten days before menstruation and remain low until it is nearly over. Calcium deficiency is associated with a host of premenstrual and menstrual symptoms, including muscle cramps, water retention, headache, and nervous symptoms. Many menstrual sufferers report dramatic improvement from taking calcium pills (dolomite, plain calcium or a calcium-magnesium combination such as the Plus Company's Formula 184) throughout the premenstrual week and during menstruation. In her useful book *Healing Yourself*, Joyce Prensky recommends a calcium pill every hour when cramps are severe. However, this, she cautions, may sometimes cause diarrhea.

If calcium intake is more than twice as high as magnesium, a magnesium deficiency will occur and calcium will be lost. Dolomite, a naturally occurring mixture of calcium and magnesium, has the right proportions of each. Americans may be borderline deficient in magnesium to start with. There is tentative new evidence that it is not advisable to take large quantities of dolomite over long periods of time. Calcium alone, or calcium with magnesium may be more digestible.

Each person will have to determine her own best supplement, but around three to six tablets a day, premenstrually and during menstruation, seem to help most people. Some need to go up to ten or twelve tablets, which somewhat exceeds the recommended allowance of 1 g of calcium.

A woman who eats much chocolate, or takes more than 250 mg daily of vitamin C, may need to use more calcium than that. Cooked greens that release oxalic acid—spinach, beet greens, dock, and sorrel—may also interfere with calcium and iron absorption. Alcohol, refined foods, and hydrogenated fats cause loss of magnesium. Calcium cannot be used properly without vitamin D, so on days when calcium is taken, 400 to 1,200 units of D should be added also.

Among the B vitamins, pyridoxine, or B_6, is reported to be especially valuable in reducing *premenstrual and menstrual edema.* If you have this problem, *be sure* that your B complex supplement contains *at least* 5 to 10 mg of pyridoxine. If the edema is severe, or if 10 mg of pyridoxine do not provide sufficient relief, consider buying separate B_6 tablets and take 25 to 200 mg daily during the premenstrual week and menstruation. Some women with edema so severe that it cannot even be controlled by potent diuretics respond dramatically to B_6 therapy. Pyridoxine can also provide speedy relief for breast engorgement, and sometimes nausea and vomiting. (Fibrocystic breasts, on the other hand, are improved in five cases out of six by vitamin E, 600 daily units, according to a recent report by Dr. Robert London, director of obstetrical and gynecological research at the Mount Sinai Hospital in Baltimore. Symptoms such as lumps, sores and tenderness are substantially relieved in half the patients who try this regimen, while another one-third show some improvement. It's interesting—and probably *not* coincidental since E is involved in estrogen secretion—that Dr. London's ratio of success is identical to that reported by investigators of E treatment for hot flashes of menopause.)

Women who develop premenstrual acne flare may also benefit from these higher levels of B_6 supplementation. The vitamin does not control the acne altogether, but about 3 women in 4 report a significant reduction.

The technical term for *excessive menstrual flow* is menorrhagia. Women who suffer from this symptom are advised to be sure and find a C supplement that includes the bioflavonoids. These factors, sometimes called the P vitamins, or "C complex," are usually found with C in nature. They occur in the peel and white pulpy portion of citrus fruits. Green peppers are a vegetable source. In addition to the citrus bioflavonoids, the P, or C complex, vitamin group includes at least two other factors, called rutin and hesperidin. The P factors strengthen blood vessels in persons resistant to C therapy alone and have a specific strengthening effect on capillaries. Medical dictionaries list them as the "capillary vitamins."

As with most nutritional and exercise remedies for menstruation, a three-month trial is required before the full effects can be ascertained. Vitamins and exercise work more slowly than drugs, *and* more safely.

Some women who get acne in association with their periods find that it may be worsened by C, *and especially C with the associated factors we have mentioned* (a clue to this is whether natural foods cause skin eruptions), and so there is a delicate balance to maintain here, which the user can only establish for herself. The woman who has heavy bleeding but not acne should certainly try C complex. The woman who has acne but not heavy bleeding should probably pass it up. The woman who has both will develop her own best regimen, through trial and error.

Iron deficiency can be a factor in *menstrual fatigue,* but has been somewhat exaggerated or singled out by vitamin advertisers. The woman who, in addition to having a heavy flow, feels and looks anemic throughout the month may indeed lack iron. But IUD users—as opposed to pill takers—are apt to develop iron deficiency because they lose up to five times the amount of iron as other women during menstruation.

The woman who suspects anemia should take supplements of about 25 mg daily throughout the month and also increase her intake of B_{12}, folic acid, and E. Too much iron irritates the gastric mucosa, and may even produce bloody vomiting.

Vegetarians should be especially alert to possible B_{12} deficiency as there are very few plant sources of this crucial blood vitamin. Pill users should be alert to folic acid deficiency, as the pill severely depletes this one.

Liver should be an excellent source, but don't forget that the liver is the body's filter. Today's commercially grown liver is apt to contain residues of DES, antibiotics, and other undesirable chemicals.

We personally do not eat liver very often, nor would we recommend it. The woman with possible anemia may especially profit from organic desiccated liver products. These products are defatted and dried, so they have a further advantage for cholesterol watchers. Three or four tablets a day provide the equivalent of the weekly liver serving nutritionists used to advocate.

To summarize, a good diet for the premenstrual week should include high-protein foods, somewhat diuretic and bowel-loosening, with supplements as needed, especially dolomite or calcium. By eating carefully, it is usually possible to get what is needed naturally, but for those who are uncertain about their diets, here is what we suggest:

Dolomite or other calcium product—6 tablets daily

B complex (with folic acid and PABA if you don't have cystic mastitis; without these if you do)—1 or 2 tablets daily

Add 50 (or sometimes up to 300) mg of separate B_6 for severe premenstrual acne flare or water retention

E—30 to 200 units daily. Stay on the low side if you have high blood pressure

C with or without bioflavonoids—250 to 750 mg daily in divided doses

Extra boosters—organic desiccated liver tablets 3 or

4 daily; kelp tablets—3 to 12 daily; soy products such as lecithin tablets—4 to 12 daily; zinc, up to 15 mg; potassium gluconate, about 500 to 600 mg.

Patent Medicines, Herbal Teas, and Ginseng

Aspirin-based products such as Midol are most effective if taken *before* cramps start or at the first twinge.

Several traditional herbal teas for menstruation are available at health-food stores. One of the most popular is pennyroyal or squaw mint tea. Some women say they can prevent cramps by drinking one cup daily, starting several days before their periods. Taken during the period, it reduces pain in about one-half hour. Directions are on the packet.

Motherwort and/or raspberry leaf tea are other favorites, as are camomile, cramp bark, rosemary, valerian, or comfrey root with a bit of peppermint added toward the end of brewing time.

Kiehl Pharmacy, established in 1851 at 109 Third Avenue, New York, N.Y. 10003, manufactures a Cornseal Compound (Herb Tea no. 42) with the following ingredients: pleurisy root, gentian root, helonias, aletria, dandelion root, camomile, cramp bark, squaw vine, black cohosh, peppermint, and golden seal root; available by mail order.

Women respond differently to these various compounds, and their own stand-bys are usually arrived at through trial and error. Taste is important, as is odor (valerian smells awful, we think). When you're not feeling well you will hardly be drawn to an unappealing brew. The Kiehl compound tastes highly medicinal to us, although many women swear by it and order it from all over the world. Squaw mint is described as pleasant or palatable by most people.

Ginseng—1 to 1½ g daily in two or three divided doses—is excellent for the menstrual "blahs." (See chap. 31 on ginseng, for you must exercise care in purchasing it.)

Remember that effective herbs have pharmacological properties, and should always be used in moderation. (See p. 556, note 28, for important cautions.)

Exercise and Body Care

Saunas and steam baths, as well as orgasms, increase menstrual flow, relieve congestion, and often bring dramatic relief. On the other hand, a few women feel *worse*, not better, from the increased flow that heat (including hot baths and heat pads) precipitates. Strenuous exercise is usually excellent for cramps, if a woman can bring herself to do it. Swimming is the best compromise activity as it is not *too strenuous*. Many women have cured fairly severe first-day cramps just by joining a Y or health club where they swim and take saunas. Swimmers have a dramatically lower incidence of menstrual problems than women who are not athletic.

Some women feel menstrual pain more in the back than the abdomen. A moderate regimen of regular exercise that strengthens the back and abdominal muscles can dramatically reduce menstrual backache within a few months. (See Charlotte C.'s experience with sit-ups earlier in this chapter.)

The back exercises described either in *Miss Craig's 21-Day Shape Up Program* (Random House) or Dr. Hans Kraus's *Backache, Stress and Tension* (Simon & Schuster/ Pocket Books) are easy to follow and highly effective. Miss Craig and Dr. Kraus both urge their readers to follow a daily program, and while this is best, it's useful to know that ten-minute sessions three times a week still do the job.

A third good guidebook for stretch exercises is *Orthotherapy*, by Dr. Arthur Michele (Evans).

After sit-ups, the next best simple exercise for prevention against menstrual backache may be the knee-chest stretch. You lie on your back with your legs bent and a pillow beneath your head, your feet about twelve inches apart. You grab one knee and pull it as close to your chest as you can, then bounce it toward your chest about twenty times or more. Repeat with the other knee. Finally, pull both knees toward your chest and hold for a count of ten.

Americans are perhaps the most sedentary people on earth, and this is one reason we have so much dysmenorrhea. When Kraus and his associates tested the muscle condition of 5,000 healthy American youngsters, aged 6 to 16, about 60 percent failed one or more of the six basic tests. In contrast, when comparable children in Austria, Italy, and Switzerland were tested, less than 9 percent failed.

Kraus states: "The basic sports, those that will put you in condition and give you good physical and emotional workouts, are swimming, calisthenics, gymnastics, hiking, running and bicycling. . . . By far and away the best thing you can do is a lot of running. There is nothing that can match running—hard running—as a conditioner."

Before and after running, it is essential to walk and jog, working up a light sweat. All exercise programs should be started gradually and slowly, and increased in steps.

Incidentally, if one's undergarments—or outerwear—bind the body uncomfortably, it's silly to try any menstrual remedy without a prior vacation from such clothes. Young women today don't wear corsets or panty girdles, but tight-fitting jeans—that you have to "lie down to zip up properly"—can interfere with circulation and thus contribute to menstrual distress.

It's long been said that women have to "suffer to be beautiful." Why? In truth they suffer profoundly from remedies prescribed fro beauty's sake. A "natural look" achieved artificially, from excessive dieting and corsetlike jeans, is as bad for menstrual symptoms as tight corsets themselves.

We have noted that it's easier to stop menstrual pain before its inception than after it is established. Medication is usually started at the first sign of menstruation and repeated every three to four hours. Some patients get good results by starting aspirin *before* the menstrual flow. Here are the treatments doctors prescribe preceding or during a difficult period:

• Analgesics such as aspirin and sodium amytal to induce sleep. Morphine and Demerol are highly effective, but are considered too addictive for a regular purpose of this sort, except in extreme cases. Some doctors are willing to prescribe aspirin with a dash of codeine, but this can be constipating. Other remedies combine pain killers with stimulants or tranquilizers. Some patients are relieved by what are called anticholinergic drugs (atropine-like products that affect the central nervous system) such as Trasen-

tine, and others, by smooth muscle relaxants such as Vaso-
dilan. Some respond to Indocin, a strong anti-inflammatory
analgesic. Antispasmodic drugs are often helpful.

• The nauseated patient can retain rectal suppositories, if not oral medications. The point is that there are
many treatments available. Flexible, careful doctors work
with their patients to arrive at the best program, and avoid
surgery and progesterone therapy (mentioned earlier) except in extreme cases. There is no need to push birth control pills on women, like Elena, who are reluctant to take
them. For some uterine conditions that may underlie dysmenorrhea—fibroids are an example—the pill may make
things worse. Women who did not have severe menstrual
cramps prior to the pill but who developed them only
after stopping should be extra cautious about accepting
further hormone treatment.

We wish to emphasize that no woman will need to
use *all* of our proposed home remedies. Only through trial
and error can the individual determine what works for her.
Elena's solution was a diuretic, semi-liquid diet on her last
premenstrual day and first two days of bleeding, vigorous
bike riding, lots of calcium lactate (which worked better
for her, personally, than dolomite), some D, and three daily
ginseng capsules.

It took Elena almost a year to arrive at her regimen,
but now she feels fine. In desperation she had started "with
everything" (many supplements, an extensive program of
exercise) and gradually eliminated all but the essentials.
She was not, as she discovered, deficient in the B's, C, or
E, but was deficient in calcium. Other women take the
opposite path from Elena. They begin with a few obvious
health boosters (based on their particular symptoms) and
then add more if needed.

Physician Remedies for Premenstrual
Tension and Edema

Some 30 percent of women show a gain of three or more
pounds premenstrually; occasional patients have gains of
as much as fifteen pounds from fluid retention. There is
often marked puffiness of the face and eyes, as well as

swelling of the feet and ankles. Many women grow nervous, depressed, restless, and cry easily. By school age, perceptive children sometimes guess, correctly, that "Mommy is getting her period."

Some feminists deny the existence of premenstrual tension, which is understandable since it's used against women to keep them out of high-level jobs. However, men have cycles too—which in a way may be more dangerous because they are *not* linked to a concrete event like menstruation. Monthly cycles in normal males have been reported for body temperature, weight, pain threshold, emotion, and even beard growth.

While premenstrual tension is not universal, it nevertheless occurs, in varying degrees, in 33 to 40 percent of women. It may be more pronounced in cycles where the woman has eaten injudiciously or failed to get normal exercise. Other circumstances, such as sunburn, travel, or emotional crisis, can also aggravate fluid retention and "PMT."

For milder edema, a chemical called ammonium chloride is prescribed in the last two weeks of the cycle, along with a low-salt high-protein diet. For more severe cases drugs such as Diuril are given. In cases of severe emotional disturbance, lithium or other psychiatric drugs, along with psychotherapy, are sometimes effective.

Be on guard against doctors who propose surgery for premenstrual tension. It is drastic and usually ineffective. Symptoms such as edema remain after all that, according to *Novak's Textbook of Gynecology.*

Menstrual Problems Summarized

The pill can cure them—because it eliminates the monthly cycle and substitutes withdrawal bleeding—but it's like using a cannon to kill a sparrow, and the potential price is high. It includes, for example, the possibility of dropping dead from side effects like pulmonary embolism, stroke, or heart attack, as well as the risk of *severely* abnormal menstruation and sterility when the pill is stopped.

Women who are considering the pill to treat menstrual cramps should try the following measures first: exercise as described, diet and vitamin therapy as described, more comfortable clothing, mild pain-killers and diuretics, or even progesterone alone.

Such patients should, of course, have a checkup with a careful, conservative doctor who takes a thorough history, does an unhurried physical exam and blood tests, and considers anatomical and nutritional factors *before* he or she prescribes the pill. The pill is the lazy or ignorant doctor's catchall panacea for menstrual problems. There are many who, like Elena's physician, won't even be bothered to seek and find other solutions.

In rare cases, such as some instances of endometriosis, the pill is the best prescription for menstrual distress, but most of the time this end can be achieved more safely by other means.

Birth Control: Alternatives
to the Pill

If new patient labeling prepared for the pill is put into effect, many women who read the negative disclosures on the label will opt against the pill.

This certainly will prove stressful to drug manufacturers, and possibly to doctors as well, since it will encourage prolonged discussions with patients as to alternatives—causing more interruptions in their busy days.

The question of stress for all concerned should be borne in mind in reading this section. For some women the dangers associated with the pill or IUD are highly disturbing. For others, abortion is more so (although in our abortion chapter we suggest how the stress of abortion can be reduced). Still other women find that local methods diminish their sexual spontaneity, and this is highly stressful to *them*.

A final note: Proponents of various methods may disagree with our presentation of them. In all cases we have balanced medical pronouncements against input from satisfied and dissatisfied users. The Billingses themselves (see chap. 16) do not favor combining their mucous technique with the use of the condom at mid-cycle. However, this is precisely what many American couples (who have no religious objections to birth control) are happily doing.

There is not and will probably never be any one best method for everybody. We can only find the most acceptable methods for us, as couples or individuals, when we know ourselves and know the facts.

CHAPTER 12

Pain and Perforation: The Inside Story of the IUD

We like to send the patient out of the operating room with the device taped to the back of her hand. When she wakes up, she can be assured that her abdomen is nice and clean.

Dr. Charles Debrovner

The forerunner of the modern intrauterine device was a 19th-century invention called a "uterine stem pessary." These were buttons or caps that covered the opening of the cervix, constructed of ivory, wood, glass, silver, gold, ebony, pewter, and even—for the very few—diamond-studded platinum. Attached to stems that extended into the cervical canal, some also had flexible arms or wings that opened into the uterus.

Since birth control was frowned on, the ostensible purpose of these pessaries was to "regulate" menstruation, or hold the uterus in place. One product, called the Sterilette, was sold with instructions for self-insertion. It was designed, obviously, to bring about abortion, and often caused serious complications. In 1909 a German physician named Richter devised, from silkworm gut, the first intrauterine device that was enclosed within the uterus. Other models followed and were prescribed by selected physicians, especially in Germany and Japan. IUDs did not become widely available until the 1960s, when the Population Council and other family planning groups began to promote them.

How It Works

A curiosity of the IUD is that its mode of action varies from species to species. In sheep it reverses the direction of uterine contractions, preventing sperm from ascending the Fallopian tubes. In the cow and the pig, it produces abortion, destroying the embryo *after* fertilization and implantation have occurred. Research has still not clarified how it works in humans. Somehow it interferes with implantation of fertilized ova, perhaps by creating a chronic inflammation. The uterus changes markedly in women with IUDs and contains, in the words of one researcher, "colossal numbers of macrophages." These are "garbage-eating cells" that emerge in response to infections or inflammation.

Reliability

The pregnancy rate for women who retain IUDs is 1 to 6 pregnancies per 100 users a year. *The average, with most devices, is 2 or 3.* But this is only part of the story, for many women cannot tolerate IUDs at all. Under the best circumstances, no more than 2 women in 3 keep IUDs for a year or longer. The number still using them after four years drops to 1 in 3. What has happened to all the others? Some IUDs—7 to 20 out of 100 (this varies with the device in question, the skill of the inserter, and the age and number of pregnancies of the patient)—are spontaneously expelled. Most women notice when they've lost their IUD, but 1 in 5 does not, and assumes incorrectly that she is still protected.

Three to 35 IUDs in 100—a wide variance, depending on model, clinic, and population group—are removed at the patients' request because of pain and bleeding. The typical user has a two-day to four-day increase in her period, while the amount of blood she loses doubles or even triples! For this reason, anemia is five times more common among women who choose this contraceptive method. *All* women with excessive or lengthy bleeding should be counseled to take iron supplements—five times the recommended daily amount, and C complex with bioflavonoids to shorten their periods. How women view prolonged menstruation varies with their culture and sexual customs. In Israel it was found that orthodox women are much more likely than nonorthodox to give up the method because of long periods (orthodox Jewish men must not associate with menstruating women). Copper-based IUDs and the new Progestasert may control the excess menstruation to some extent.

In addition to removals for pain and bleeding, another 4 to 15 users annually, out of each 100, must give up their IUDs for "other medical reasons," including infection.

Generally, older women and those who have had children tolerate IUDs with least discomfort. The new copper and hormone devices perform best in young or childless women but pose special problems and dangers of their own.

The fact is that for a motivated women, *whose doctor has fitted her diaphragm carefully*, the diaphragm with jelly *is more reliable!* Studies at clinics with doctors who believe in it and who take pride in their good diaphragm fitting show that with motivated patients the diaphragm is a 99.4 percent reliable method. Even the condom and foam alone do as well, *in motivated self-reliant populations*, as the IUD. In combination, condom and foam rate better. There are personal and cultural differences that make such local methods hard to use for some people or distasteful to them, but many others use dangerous methods (like the IUD) only because they've been falsely led to think the local ones are unreliable. With a barrier method like the diaphragm, a woman doesn't risk anemia, perforations, longer and more painful periods, associated infections that cause sterility and death, or pregnancies that are medically problematic.

Safety

Some IUDs are worse than others, but no one model is ideal.

To quote from "IUDs Reassessed—A Decade of Experience," a recent Population Report from the George Washington University Medical Center:

> Research on the IUD has focused on eliminating, or at least reducing the major adverse side effects—accidental

pregnancy, expulsion, voluntary removals for bleeding, pain, and other medical reasons, and perforations [perforation is the protruding of the IUD into the uterine wall or even passing entirely through into the abdominal cavity]. The development of a "bloodless, comfortable IUD" is a first priority of research as funded by USAID. Bioactive ingredients such as trace metals and hormones are being added to the IUD to increase contraceptive efficacy and to reduce side effects. Also, modifications in IUD configuration, rigidity, area of contact with the endometrial walls, and location in the uterus are under study. *Unfortunately, however, a modification which helps one side effect may aggravate another. For instance, rigid devices decrease the likelihood of expulsion but increase* both the risk of perforation and bleeding [italics ours].

A good example of the latter was the Majzlin Spring, an expulsion-resistant stainless-steel device, which was removed from the market because it tore up so many uteri.

The IUD is less deadly than the pill, according to FDA figures. In nine years of use, from 1965 to 1974, FDA received reports of "only" 39 IUD deaths in the United States out of an estimated 3 to 4 million users a year. But while the IUD is not as likely to place women in the morgue, it is just as apt to place them in the hospital as the pill is. Here is FDA's official calculation:

". . . The mortality rate from the intrauterine device is between 1 and 10 deaths per million women years, while with oral contraceptives it is 22 to 45 per million women years. [This estimate has of course risen sharply,—up to a minimum of 20 annual deaths per 100,000 pill users, or at least 200 per million,—with the official recognition, in 1975, that in addition to blood clots the pill is implicated in cardiovascular and liver disease, as well as cancer of the endometrium.] The hospitalization rates with intrauterine devices are in the same order of magnitude as with oral contraceptives: .3 to 1.0 per 100 women years of use."

In short, both IUD and pill users face a risk of associated hospitalization ranging from 1 in 300 to 1 in 100 per year. The IUD hospitalization figures would be higher yet if more doctors were conscientious about removing these devices whenever perforations occur.

The usual perforation rate among IUDs inserted by skilled doctors averages about 1 per 1,000 insertions. In amateur hands it is very much higher. Complicating the issue, some perforations are asymptomatic. Neither the woman nor her doctor can be sure whether a missing IUD simply fell out or migrated through her uterus. Most perforations occur or begin at the time of insertion, but this misfortune can happen at any time, even after five or six years. No IUD wearer should ever ignore a pain in her abdomen. Some doctors and clinics have much worse perforation records than others, perhaps because they do their insertions too hastily.

When should a woman suspect perforation? She may have pain, but sometimes she does not. If she cannot find the device and was not aware of expelling it, she should go to her doctor for x-rays. It is essential to remove closed devices (rings and bows) promptly, for they may strangle the bowel (intestine). Copper IUDs in the peritoneal cavity may cause dangerous inflammation.

How does a doctor remove a perforating IUD? This is one of those medical "gray areas." Some IUD specialists say that if the device is still in the process of perforating (making its way through the uterus but has not yet completely worked itself into the abdominal cavity), it's all right to pull it out via the string. Others believe this is a very dangerous procedure and maintain that laparoscopy or laparotomy should always be performed. (See chap. 17 for a description of these surgical techniques.) Still other IUD doctors are willing to let nature take its course. If it isn't a closed or copper device, and the woman has no pain or fever, they say not to worry.

The problem is that IUDs are foreign bodies, alien to the uterus, and more alien yet to the abdomen.

In 1966 a 23-year-old Spanish woman in Brooklyn, New York, was brought to a hospital emergency room by her husband. She claimed that her IUD had moved into her abdomen and was giving her severe cramps.

The gynecologist on duty said that this was not possible. He referred her to the psychiatrist, who hospitalized her in the psychiatric ward, where the psychiatrists and social workers were fascinated by her "fantasy." She died, leaving an unemployed husband and three preschool children. Her "fantasy" was right: The IUD was found in her abdomen at autopsy.

Pregnant with an IUD

A recent medical survey flatly claimed that "IUDs are more effective in preventing pregnancy than any other nonsurgical method except oral contraceptives." This is one of those half-truths circulated about by people who are convinced that women are too stupid to use diaphragms or other local methods.

What they really mean to say is that, next to surgical sterilization, the IUD is the most effective method for the half-witted female. Once it's installed, the patient need do nothing herself except check the string of her device, if it has one. If it stays in place, her IUD is a 94 to 99 percent reliable method.

The string is an interesting "control" issue in itself. The typical IUD has a string that extends into the vagina. The patient is advised to check it after each menstrual period, if not oftener. The missing string reveals the loss of the device or its perforation. In addition, the string makes it easier for the doctor himself to remove the IUD when called for. In its absence, he must use a fairly treacherous hooked device and "fish" it out.

Yet some doctors are opposed to the string, and some IUDs are inserted without them for fear that patients who can check themselves regularly may be less inclined to schedule medical visits. Another argument is that insertion of fingers into the vagina may lead to infection.

When IUDs first grew popular rumors abounded about the failures. Frightened patients—and doctors—said that when pregnancies did occur, the outcome was messy. There were miscarriages and infections of a sort that jeopardized the mother's health and very life.

Echoes of the pill—these early critics were absolutely right, but at first they were laughed at and called alarmists, sexual puritans, or ignoramuses who disregarded the population problem.

In 1974, after a decade of widespread IUD promotion, two important studies clarified the facts. Ordinarily, about 15 percent of pregnancies end in miscarriage. When pregnancy occurs with an IUD in place, *the miscarriage rate rises to 50 percent or over*. In addition, IUD miscarriages tend to occur later, making them more dangerous, and to involve more risk of serious infection. *Getting pregnant with an IUD in place is often a medical emergency!*

Population controllers argue that any unplanned pregnancy is a medical emergency, but the facts of life are sometimes different. For a married couple spacing their children, but hoping to have more in time, a contraceptive failure, while inconvenient, may not be a tragedy at all. If the pregnancy occurred using a benign method (the diaphragm, condom, foam, or rhythm) which does not damage mother or baby, the woman's options are still open. She can abort, if she wishes, or she can go on to have a normal pregnancy and healthy child. A serious drawback to the extreme methods (the IUD, pill, and female sterilization) is that *when they fail they leave mother and embryo in a precarious position.* The medical pressures toward abortion are high. Not only has the pregnant woman lost her options, but her health or future fertility may also be endangered. (The complications connected with the pill and sterilization are explained in chaps. 9 and 17.)

During the years of rumors, U.S. population controllers seemed indifferent or unwilling to perform the pertinent studies, but finally British investigator Martin Vessey and his associates published the results of their important research in *Lancet* in 1974. His findings compared 320 women who had unplanned pregnancies while using different contraceptives: Among IUD wearers, 54 percent had miscarriages (spontaneous abortions), while the figure was only 17 percent for those using other methods. Thus, *an IUD increases the risks of miscarriage threefold.* Curiously, Dr. Vessey and his group were the same researchers who established in 1968 (also after years of argument) that the pill *does* cause fatal blood clots. Both their pill and IUD studies were classically simple—and sound. It cannot be that we lack equivalent talent in this country: It appears that we *do not wish to know.* We wait around for a decade or longer until English researchers—who have a much smaller budget for this type of investigation—clarify the most obvious side effects of contraceptives that *we* devised or popularized.

Finally, in a U.S. study involving 46 women who became pregnant with their IUDs in place, it was established again that about half—49 percent—had miscarriages.

Obstetricians admit they have no sure guidelines for handling IUD pregnancies. At first it was advised that the device be left in place and the pregnancy treated as normal. Then in August 1974, after the British study, ACOG (The American College of Obstetricians and Gynecologists) issued a technical bulletin suggesting that "the IUD should be removed if the string is visible, or interruption of pregnancy should be considered or offered as an option."

Ectopic pregnancy and septic abortion are especially serious matters for IUD users. A fertilized egg may implant in the Fallopian tube instead of the uterus, where it belongs. Should this happen, it constitutes a grave medical emergency, for the conceptus may grow to a point where it ruptures the tube. To make matters worse, ectopic and other rare "extrauterine" (outside of the uterus) pregnancies are difficult to diagnose before emergency occurs.

Unfortunately, new research compiled by Dr. Howard Tatum, Dr. Martin Vessey, and other investigators indicates that, perhaps because of "ascending infection," IUDs directly encourage ectopic pregnancies. The rate of ectopic pregnancy is 1.2% in the first year of IUD use, but rises to 3% by the second year. It remains higher than normal even after removal of the IUD. Normally, only 0.2 to 0.5 percent of pregnancies are ectopic.

A septic abortion is a critical infection in a pregnant woman that can and occasionally does cause her *death*. IUD users also may get septic uterine *infections* causing death even if they are not pregnant, especially in the early months following insertion.

The Lippes Loop and the Dalkon Shield

The dangers of one IUD, the Dalkon Shield, were highlighted when the FDA acknowledged in 1974 that 14 U.S. deaths had been reported in association with pregnancies among wearers. A panic ensued: The Dalkon Shield was banned, then unbanned, and the device ended up with a bad reputation. Persons who read the FDA report carefully—and we ourselves—were not at all sure that it *did* indict the Dalkon Shield beyond other IUDs. In reviewing septic deaths attributable to IUDs *called to the FDA's attention* (it should be repeated here that the FDA gets reports of only a fraction of possible drug- or device-associated deaths), here is what FDA reviewers discovered:

• There were 15 septic deaths associated with the Lippes Loop, 6 of which involved pregnancy.

• There were 14 septic deaths associated with the Dalkon Shield, 13 of which involved pregnancy.

• There were 6 septic deaths with other devices, 1 of which involved pregnancy.

To complicate the problem, the FDA has no precise figures on *how many of each type of IUD are in actual use.* This is a serious scientific problem. You cannot define the magnitude of a risk, obviously, unless you know how many patients are exposed to it.

In 1974 the FDA concluded that septic deaths involving IUDs were far higher for the Lippes Loop and Dalkon Shield than for other models. But these two types were by far the most widely used models in the United States. Other devices seemed to cause an equivalent number of septic deaths, in proportion to their popularity. The Loop was more likely to cause septic death at the time of insertion; the Shield later on, if pregnancy should occur. With other devices, the chances of septic infection were more concentrated at insertion than during pregnancy. The Saf-T-Coil was an exception, being implicated in 14 serious pregnancy infections, a rather high figure considering its limited popularity.

The modern IUDs were brought to the United States by a few European physicians fleeing Hitler, who had introduced their use almost in secret. Drs. Ernst Graefenberg, Hans Lehfeldt, Herbert Hall, and Lazar Margulies were among these early pioneers. By the 1960s these men interested the late Dr. Alan Guttmacher of Planned Parenthood, and also the Population Council, in testing the devices more widely.

In time, two U.S. gynecologists, Jack Lippes of Buffalo Planned Parenthood, and Hugh Davis of the Contraceptive Clinic at Johns Hopkins in Baltimore, designed or co-designed their own IUDs, the Lippes Loop and Dalkon

Shield. The Loop became the standard for older women whose uterus has increased in size, and the Dalkon for younger ones. Although the Loop is made in several sizes, the larger are traumatic for the young uterus, and the smaller are insufficiently effective.

Dr. Davis was one of the first U.S. obstetricians to violate the "diplomatic immunity" that was granted the pill in its early years. At the 1969 convention of the American College of Obstetricians and Gynecologists, Davis took the negative in a "Great Debate." Among his comments:

"It is perfectly true that we all have to die of something, but there is no need to be in a hurry about it. When the apologists for the pill told me that the risk of death from taking the pill is really insignificant because it is no greater than the risk of dying in an auto crash, far from finding this reassuring, I rushed out, bought an extra set of safety belts, doubled my disability insurance, bought a St. Christopher's medal to be on the safe side, and took my wife off the pill."

Then, in January 1970, Davis was the kickoff witness at Senator Nelson's pill hearings. He emphasized the need for informed consent and indicted birth control clinics—and doctors—for failing to apprise patients of the risks.

Dalkon Shields have now fallen into disrepute, and as young patients still do not adapt well to the Loop, most are given copper devices, which have their own dangers. Some of the copper is excreted in urine and menses. The possible long-range effects of any extra copper retained by the body is a source of concern to some physiologists. One observed wryly: "[The copper device promoters] will think up some reason why it's beneficial. They'll say it protects against arthritis of the uterus." The effects of intrauterine copper on a developing fetus are totally unknown.

Davis says he has always cautioned family planners against leaving the Dalkon in place in a pregnant woman, and that any doctor who did so was a "damn fool." ACOG now recommends removing *all* devices if pregnancy occurs.

The controversy surrounding the Dalkon has made it a Lieutenant Calley among IUDs, and lulled users of other models with false reassurances. While the Dalkon may be associated with higher infection rates, other models have other flaws.

American women are now most frequently fitted with the Cu-7, about which there has been some discussion. For years Dr. Howard Tatum and others at the Population Council worked on developing and testing a device called the Copper-T. Then through a series of maneuvers the Searle Company rushed to market with its Cu-7 first, and also obtained exclusive distribution rights (for copper devices) in many areas. The Copper-T was shouldered aside by Searle, just as Syntex's hard-won progestin had been some twenty years earlier. The 7 is, incidentally, as the name suggests, a T (more or less) with one of the arms knocked off. (Searle's progestin was but a few molecules changed from the earlier Syntex entry.)

Were the products always equivalent, such "competitive practices" might be of little concern to the *patient*. But studies at the Sanger Institute and other reliable research centers where both devices were tested indicate that the T may be a better model, with fewer expulsions and perforations.

According to a Searle press release dated March 29, 1977, the Cu-7 has "accounted for more than 80 percent of all intrauterine contraceptives inserted in the United States during 1976."

The IUD and Infection

Infection rates second, after pain and bleeding, as the leading cause of IUD removal. Serious IUD infections are most apt to occur in association with insertion or with venereal disease.

During the first fifteen days after insertion, 1 user in 12 develops an infection just from the process of *getting* an IUD. After that the rate declines. In the fourth through sixth years of use, serious IUD-associated infections afflict at least 1 out of every 100 women per year.

IUD users are cautioned to be alert for such symptoms as fever, abdominal or cervical tenderness, or a foul discharge.

Some infections are caused by the IUD itself. Bacteria are introduced upon insertion, and may also be introduced later by, perhaps, the tail. These facts *were not established by family planners or birth control clinics,* but by emergency-room physicians in the mid-1970s. Acute PID (Pelvic Inflammatory Disease), requiring at the least emergency outpatient treatment and, very often, long hospitalization or sometimes extensive surgery, is *5 to 9 times as likely to occur in IUD users as in other women.* In populations with a high incidence of VD (and VD complications), the increase in PID risk is manyfold.

Antibiotics usually get PID under control, but alarming numbers of young women—in their twenties and even in their teens—fail to respond to antibiotics and need surgery, most often of the Fallopian tubes, which renders them sterile. Few of these women die, so many family planners still view it as a minor complication, rarely explaining to clients who visit their clinics the risks of illness and possible permanent infertility.

As the lame leg, from a blood clot, has become an emblem of pill victims, excised tubes and ovaries are battle scars of women who gambled—and lost—on the IUD.

When infections develop in IUD users, it may be tricky to diagnose them precisely. In the early 1960s, many doctors treated these infections without removing the IUD, but present wisdom usually advises taking it out.

One infection frequent in IUD users is *endometritis,* an *inflammation* of the uterine lining, which may remain painless and unsuspected until the time of a pelvic examination. The cervix may produce a thick, unpleasant discharge. Treatment includes antibiotics, rest, and sexual abstinence.

Endometriosis, on the other hand, is a condition in which endometrial tissue *grows* in a place it doesn't belong, such as in other genital areas or in urinary or intestinal organs. Severe menstrual pain is the most common symptom. When allowed to progress, endometriosis may produce infertility, for the ovaries or tubes may become blocked. Neither the cause nor the cure of endometriosis is well understood. The studies of pathologist Nikolas Janovski of the National Naval Medical Center in Bethesda, Maryland, indicate that sometimes an IUD may help stimulate this condition. Certainly no woman suspected of having it should use this method of birth control.

Pelvic Inflammatory Disease (PID)

PID is a catchall term for a variety of pelvic infections that may invade the uterus, the tubes, and sometimes the ovaries. Before the widespread use of the IUD, 60 percent of cases were associated with gonorrhea. Among the poor and malnourished, tuberculosis is sometimes a cause. A third group of PID conditions are due to streptococcus, staphylococcus, *Escherichia coli*, or other organisms. Such infections may occur after childbirth, abortion, or surgery, as well as in connection with an IUD.

Laura R. had a Dalkon Shield for several years. Over that time, intercourse and orgasms became somewhat painful, but, says Laura, "I was foolish—I didn't connect the pain to the IUD."

At Laura's checkup, her doctor suggested removing the Dalkon Shield and substituting a Cu-7. Laura agreed. (Note: More conservative doctors often urge patients to skip at least a month in between IUDs.)

When her doctor tried to insert the Cu-7, Laura screamed in pain. The doctor investigated. "Oh," he said, "you have scar tissue all over your cervix." He sent Laura home.

The pain continued, along with a low-grade fever. Laura called her doctor and asked if some leftover Bactrim tablets she found in her refrigerator might help. He said to try them. (Bactrim is a sulfonamide type of product used to treat urinary tract infections. It was inappropriate, ineffective, and may have complicated the course of Laura's PID.)

Two weeks later, having failed to try a more suitable antibiotic, Laura's doctor suggested hospitalization for a laparoscopy so he "could see what's going on inside." Laura fled to another doctor, who tested and cultured her, ascertaining that she had a strep infection associated with IUD, which he treated successfully with Ampicillin. During her lengthy recuperation, Laura had to rest and abstain from sex.

It is suspected, but still unproved, that gonorrhea is more likely to progress to PID if a woman uses an IUD. With other infections, it is easy to understand how bacterial contamination might occur at the time of insertion, but it is not clear why PID should develop after years of IUD use. Perhaps the chronic inflammatory reaction in the uteri of all IUD wearers just makes them more susceptible. Perhaps the strings *are* a wick for bacteria, as some doctors think.

IUD–PID is often unilateral, occurring on only one side. Thus it may be difficult to distinguish from ectopic pregnancy, for the symptoms are similar. Increasing pain with intercourse and orgasm and/or menstruation, chills, fever, and irregular bleeding may mark either condition. For that reason, a cautious doctor may wish to perform a pregnancy test, as well as take cultures, blood studies, and antibiotic sensitivity tests. The PID patient is fortunate if the infection occurs unilaterally, for her fertility is likely to be spared. Although one tube and ovary may be destroyed, the other pair continues to function.

Many PID patients respond well to oral antibiotics if the right ones are used promptly. The most common choices include penicillin, penicillin with streptomycin, or broad spectrum antibiotics.

Rest, adequate fluids, a highly nutritious diet (perhaps with yogurt or acidophilus tablets to mitigate antibiotic side effects), and painkillers are usually prescribed. We also advise taking therapeutic B complex, as these vitamins are depleted by antibiotics. *Novak's Textbook of Gynecology* further states: "It is our feeling that heat in any form increases comfort and promotes resolution of the inflammatory process, and douches or sitz baths are utilized except in the extremely ill patient."

Once controlled, PID may never recur, or may flare up repeatedly. Adhesions or internal scar tissue may leave the patient in chronic pain, for which surgery is sometimes advised. Mercifully, the newer antibiotics may effect a complete cure, without any residual of closed tubes, infertility, reinfections, or exacerbations. The course and outcome in a given case are not easily predictable.

Patients are less likely to respond well to antibiotics if the ovaries as well as the tubes are involved. Also, any abscessed areas are likely to be "walled off" from the antibiotic, and cannot easily be reached by it. After a ten-day trial of home care, the patient who is not responding may be hospitalized and given intravenous antibiotics.

Abdominal surgery is not usually advised in the presence of active infection ("I don't like to cut a 'hot' belly," one doctor confided. "It could spread the mess.") but laparoscopy and other exploratory procedures may be used. Sometimes, suction curettage is performed (see chap. 18) to evacuate the uterus. Abscesses may be drained. When the infection quiets, one or both tubes and sometimes the ovary(ies) may have to be removed. Occasionally—and this is a most critical situation—selective surgery must be performed in the acute stages, particularly if an abscess ruptures.

Infection sometimes spreads to adjacent tissues, such as the intestine or bladder. Associated blood clots may form in the pelvic veins and then move on to the lung.

With vigorous treatment (and luck), PID is just an unpleasant episode, or perhaps a series of them. But a few women die from its complications, and some are left severely handicapped, especially if the digestive system gets involved or clotting ensues. Many women are left sterile. Many suffer mild discomforts that drain their vitality for years. Should PID settle into its "chronic" form, the symptoms include aching in the lower abdomen and pelvis, backache and rectal discomfort (perhaps from adhesions), bladder irritability, severe menstrual cramps, and shortened menstrual intervals. As one woman told us, "I've just had to learn certain *not to's:* not to do much bending, not to have sex before my period (the pains get worse at that time), not to get stuck too far from a bathroom. I often feel 60, but I'm only 31."

PID that is gonorrheal may respond to drugs faster than strep, and strep responds better than staph. But staph infections may be curable too, with certain antibiotic combinations. With the nongonorrheal infections the fever, as one textbook puts it, "is apt to persist, dragging along for weeks." On the other hand, sterility is a more frequent outcome of gonorrheal PID.

Sometimes nutrition succeeds in curing PID where antibiotics fail. One case was Crescent D., a 24-year-old writer, who had her first IUD, a Lippes Loop, inserted when she was 17. She hemorrhaged badly and had several serious infections.

A friend told Crescent that the Dalkon Shield was

supposed to be better than the Lippes. "It hurt much more than the loop when they put it in, but after that it seemed ok. I had an occasional discharge and some cramps, but no more serious infections."

One day Crescent tried LSD. She felt her body "telling her" to eject the Dalkon, and she started to bleed. Then she did eject the Dalkon spontaneously.

The next day Crescent was fitted for a diaphragm, but the damage had been done. Soon she developed high fever and excruciating pain. Her doctor, fearing that she might have an ectopic pregnancy, operated at once. "He removed my left ovary and tube and pieces of my right tube, leaving me sterile," Crescent reports solemnly. "I know that everything they say about adoption is true. You do love the child as if it were your own. Nevertheless, childbirth is an experience I would have chosen to have."

Crescent's pain and complications continued. She was treated, unsuccessfully, with massive doses of antibiotics, hormones, and enzymes. She even tried acupuncture, but was told that the PID scar tissue had blocked her "energy channels."

When her newest doctor recommended more surgery, Crescent, who had written several books on food and nutrition, turned away from orthodox Western medicine and decided to meditate and fast. Through her study of natural healing she arrived at the following five-day regimen, which she went through twice with a break in between:

• Fresh-squeezed vegetable and fruit juices (no other food).

• Herbal teas of the standard remedies for "women's troubles," including blue cohosh, black cohosh, pennyroyal, licorice root, and ladies' mantle. Most of these have been described as uterine sedatives or cleansers in old herb books.

• A daily enema with herbal water.

A few weeks later her doctor, who had expected to schedule a laparoscopy, said, "This improvement is medically impossible. It cannot be the same pelvis."

Among other effects of her diet, the natural vitamins in the juices and teas replaced those lost through antibiotics. Crescent has not required antibiotics for a year now. If the pains start to recur, she returns to a short juice fast.

Another young woman, Sandra K., had recurrent PID for more than two years after her IUD was inserted. She too had been hospitalized and laparoscoped, but her reproductive organs were spared. Traveling in India, after a six-month course of antibiotics, she was referred to a doctor whose cure consisted of fresh raw milk direct from his own cows, hot oils, tonics, and herbal pills soaked in more raw milk. In six weeks, the last traces of her infection were gone.

Our friends Crescent and Sandra may seem unconventional, but nonetheless we would advise any woman who has been dragging along with chronic PID to consult a nutrition specialist. The importance of rebuilding the body's natural defenses cannot be denied.

Women who deem the diaphragm "too much trouble" should make friends with a PID victim. They're easy to find in this IUD age.

The IUD and Perforations

As a dancer, 28-year-old Jeanne C. is highly aware of her own body and well informed on health. She has also read up on contraception. When her IUD string disappeared, she quickly made an appointment to see her doctor.

"Glad you came in," he said cheerfully. "You could have gotten pregnant. Let's just put in another, and I won't even charge." "Wait a minute," said Jeanne. "Aren't you supposed to x-ray me, or something? I would have noticed if the IUD fell out." "Probably didn't," the doctor replied. "But with two you'll have double protection. There's nothing to worry about."

Jeanne didn't believe him. She declined his free offer, and made an appointment for a second opinion the following week. Meantime her dance troupe had an engagement on the West Coast.

Jeanne was not yet in pain when she boarded the airplane. Over the Grand Canyon, abdominal cramps overwhelmed her and she fainted. An ambulance met her at the airport. Luckily her roommate, who knew of the IUD problem, was on the plane and accompanied her to the hospital.

Emergency surgery was successful—all of Jeanne's organs were spared. The last we heard she started a suit against her original doctor.

IUD technology, like DES, has brought its own tragic or bizarre subspecialties of surgery. In New York City, gynecologist Charles Debrovner has recovered dozens of lost IUDs. "We like to send the patient out of the operating room with the device taped to the back of her hand," Debrovner told us. "When she wakes up, she can be assured that her abdomen is nice and clean."

Most IUDs can be located and removed by laparoscopy, or culdoscopy (see chap. 17), he explained further, but the copper models require real abdominal surgery. The Lippes is the device most likely to perforate, in his experience. He had to open the abdomen of one Majzlin Spring victim and disentangle the wires from the uterine muscle in which they'd become embedded.

Debrovner feels that under some circumstances, with some models (those made of inert materials—or in an open design—as opposed to the circular closed model that may strangulate the bowel), it may be harmless to leave an IUD in the abdomen after establishing that it is there. However, he generally advises getting them out, for the patient's peace of mind, as well as the doctor's protection.

Who Should Not Get an IUD

IUD complications could be reduced if doctors were more selective and more cautious. Arthur Davids, a diaphragm advocate, at the Mt. Sinai School of Medicine in New York, gives IUDs to no more than one-half of the patients who ask for them. To others, he explains that the risks are too high for them personally.

Our Bodies, Ourselves offers the following good summary:

"IUDs should not be used by anyone with the following conditions: pregnancy, endometriosis, venereal disease, any vaginal or uterine infection, pelvic inflammatory disease, prohibitively small uterus, excessively heavy menstrual flow and/or cramping, bleeding between periods, large fibroids, uterine deformities, use of anticoagulants, cardiac disease, anemia and sickle cell disease."

To this list, we would add the following: *Any history of VD* even if it is no longer active (this because of the possibility that IUDs make it flare up again), and recent childbirth or abortion.

How small is a prohibitively small uterus? Many doctors believe that if the uterus measures less than 6.5 centimeters (discovered by sounding—a process for taking internal measurements) the patient is likely to experience intolerable pain and may also expel the IUD.

When to Get an IUD

At many hospitals and abortion clinics, women are encouraged to accept IUDs at the time of their confinement. This is a cynical practice, for as Dr. Marvin Zuckerman explains:

"The incidence of perforation on insertion increases markedly during the immediate post-partum and post-abortal periods. Consequently, insertion of an IUD should be postponed until six to eight weeks after a birth or abortion, to allow enough time for complete involution [of the uterus] to take place."

Since perforations are a serious emergency, any circumstance that "markedly increases" them should surely be avoided.

Despite the perforation problem, some family planners still argue that "the ideal time for IUD insertion seems to be immediately after abortion. . . . Women are strongly motivated to prevent another pregnancy and as a result are more willing to tolerate minor discomfort or bleeding irregularity." And some doctors maintain that insertion is *easier for them* postabortion since the cervix is already dilated.

When IUDs are inserted just after childbirth, the expulsion rate is very high, more than 1 in 4.

The safest time to insert an IUD is during normal menstruation. The possibility of undetermined pregnancy (which greatly increases the complication rate) is minimal then, and the softening of the cervix makes insertion easier.

Before agreeing to insert any kind of IUD, a doctor should perform a thorough physical to rule out any contraindications, and determine the exact depth, shape, and position of the uterus.

A Pap smear must be performed, and a gonorrhea culture and—ideally—a blood test for anemia. A precise medical history, including all pregnancies and infections, must be taken.

It's advisable to use a painkiller—Tylenol or Darvon, codeine—about twenty minutes before IUD insertion. In theory, aspirin might increase bleeding. A thoughtful doctor may anesthetize you further with paracervical block (a local injection) and/or the application of Cetacaine spray, applied with a cotton-tipped applicator, to the cervical os and canal.

After the uterus has been sounded, the cervix must be cleaned with antiseptic solution and then grasped with a tenaculum. Traction on the tenaculum holds the uterus straight, which decreases the risk of perforation. If the cervical opening is narrow, the doctor may wish to enlarge it with a dilator instrument.

Most IUD models are applied with an inserter, a plastic tube shaped like a straw. If the doctor loads the inserter more than two minutes ahead of time, the IUD may lose its "memory" and fail to resume its original shape when nestled in the uterus. This, too, invites expulsion, as well as pregnancy.

After insertion, at least one and one half inches of the string or tail should be left dangling below the opening of the cervix.

In most cases, the bleeding from IUD insertion lasts from a few hours to several days. Of course, if a woman has her period, the bleeding is masked. About half of all new IUD users continue to have intermittent bleeding for one or two more menstrual cycles. Zuckerman prescribes vitamin C, 1,000 mg daily, to help control the spotting and staining. If the bleeding is heavy, he adds vitamin K, 2.5 mg daily. (We would personally counsel that the vitamin C be in a form that contains C complex or bioflavonoids—the capillary factors—and that a B complex supplement and dolomite [6 tablets daily]—as well as an iron supplement be added in the weeks just before IUD insertion. These vitamins may sound expensive, but the total cost would be under $10, which is very much below the average exorbitant fee for IUD insertion. The vitamins can help protect against excessive bleeding and pain and perhaps infection, as well as other symptoms such as associated fatigue which leads to IUD removals—often at an additional cost.)

Many patients require codeine preparations to keep them comfortable the first few days after insertion. Since so many IUDs are expelled in the earliest weeks, some manufacturers now recommend that a second method of contraception such as foam or condoms continue to be used. Spontaneous expulsion is most likely to occur at the time of the first or second menstrual period.

It's best to get an IUD from a seasoned expert, one who has inserted a great many. And beware of the doctor who is testing new models, the superspecialist, for he may select a device that is not necessarily the best for the individual woman. We would place the most trust in a doctor who informs a woman that he or she *can't be sure the patient is a good IUD candidate* until her uterus has been examined. The careful doctor hesitates to do an IUD insertion on the spot: It *should* require two appointments. He or she usually keeps several models on hand, selecting one, after thorough examination, that seems best suited for the individual. Even so, subsequent emergencies or failures cannot be totally avoided.

New Models

The long-range effects of the IUD are still unknown. Most cancers take ten to twenty years to develop, so no definitive studies have yet been completed. Still, cervical cancers appear at a notably higher rate among current users of both the pill and the IUD than among diaphragm users.

Copper devices, such as the T and 7, may have extra reliability that comes from the copper itself. But these devices must be changed often, pose special dangers when they perforate or if pregnancy occurs, and raise unanswered questions about where the copper goes.

Devices containing hormones, such as the Progestasert, are finding current favor. The Progestasert, which is

T-shaped, contains a core reserve of progesterone, dispersed in silicone oil, in the vertical section of the T. Again, the hormone may increase contraceptive efficiency, but any long-range complications remain to be clarified. Early reports suggest that the uteri of the wearers show adverse effects from the hormone as well as from the IUD itself. For these reasons, many doctors still prefer the older models.

The Lippes Loop ranges in length from 22.5 mm for size. A to 30 mm for size D. Generally, the smaller the device, the easier the insertion, and the less the rate of pain and bleeding. Larger devices, on the other hand, have lower expulsion and pregnancy rates. The usual rule has been to select the largest device that each individual uterus can accommodate.

The size and type of the inserter are pertinent factors, too. When the Alza Corporation, manufacturers of the Progestasert, reduced the diameter of its inserter, expulsion of the device by childless women declined. The Cu-7 inserter has a width of only 0.3 cm (the diameter of a wooden matchstick), while the Saf-T-Coil inserter is only slightly larger. These are said to be among the easiest to apply.

Moreover, bleeding and pain may be significantly reduced when narrower inserters are employed. This factor is most crucial for childless women whose cervical canals are narrow and inelastic.

How Long Can an IUD Be Kept?

Pathologists do not treat living patients directly. They work in laboratories where they perform autopsies or study tissues that a surgeon has removed. Pathologists have a loftier view of medicine than other doctors, both more objective and less personal. Unlike gynecologists, they do not have to deal with everyday disasters like unwanted pregnancy.

Pathologists who have studied the changes in the uterus caused by the IUD generally loathe it and have consistently warned against it. Many family planners are unaware of these studies or are indifferent to them. If the method works, they consider it a luxury to worry about possible hysterectomies, or cancer, twenty years hence.

The patient's position is somewhere in between. If the method works for her, she is happy with it, but she probably would like to know *what pathologists fear*. She wants to make her own choice, based on knowledge of the long-term as well as the immediate risks. Our own belief, derived from prudent findings of pathologists, is that five years should be the outer limit of IUD use. After that, the uterus deserves a rest, a chance to heal and return to normal.

An early alarm was sounded in 1968 by Commander Nikolas Janovski of the National Naval Medical Center in Bethesda, Maryland. Janovski collected 18 hysterectomy specimens and 21 endometrial curettings from IUD patients, a total of 39 cases.

Janovski's report, delivered at a congress of the International Academy of Pathology in Milan, was highly technical. "It is beyond any doubt that the duration of IUD insertion is proportional to the anticipated morphological alteration of the endometrium and myometrium. . . . *Prolonged and persistent use of the intrauterine device is not recommended*," he said.

The endometrium is the mucous membrane comprising the inner layer of the uterine wall. The myometrium is the muscular wall of the uterus. Part of the endometrium sheds with the monthly menses, but the lower layers do not. Thus changes in the lower layers, or in the myometrium, may leave permanent effects.

One of Janovski's most dramatic findings was the presence of visible indentations or ridges, 3 to 4 mm in depth, caused by pressure of the devices. The microscopic changes, which he described as "striking," were observable in all layers of the endometrium. Such changes included overgrowth (reactive hyperplasia), erosion, metaplasia (cells that have started altering in character, which may mark the beginnings of cancer), "structures indistinguishable from polyps," necrotic (dead or dying) cells and—in fully 95 percent of the cases examined—chronic endometritis (inflammation of the endometrium).

In 10 percent of the cases there was an absence of

glands in the deep basal layer of the endometrium, occurring beneath the deepest ridges or indentations observed on the surface. There were signs of beginning endometriosis and two unusual tumors. "We do not believe that these lesions, once established, can regress," Janovski cautioned dimly. "But," he added, like a good scientist, "this is only a point of speculation to which, nevertheless, the clinician must be alerted."

Janovski proposed that all IUD users have regular and "strict" cytological checkups (endometrial biopsies, etc.), a practice rarely observed. He feels that women over 30 should not use IUDs at all. He also believes that the barium salt coating (now included on most IUDs to make lost ones visible on x-ray) may be adding to the damage, and to risks of cancer.

Six years after Janovski's warning, in 1974, pathologist William Ober of New York's Beth Israel and Mount Sinai hospitals reported a larger study that confirmed and clarified many of Janovski's findings. Dr. Ober collected biopsies from 209 IUD patients. His vivid collection of medical slides, used to illustrate his lecture, amply demonstrated the mischief these devices make in the uterus.

Ober began his lecture straightforwardly: "When the original papers came out describing IUDs, they said there was no alteration in the endometrium. It was perfectly clean, looked beautiful, etc. Nonsense, I said, this can't be, and when I looked closer I discovered that these biopsies had been performed after six to nine months of exposure to inert polyethylene [plastic]. So I said, 'Let's wait,' and, in collaboration with Dr. Aquiles Sobrero, I waited for a good period of time."

Ober and Sobrero's patients were divided into various subgroups: those who had symptoms beyond pain and bleeding, and those who did not; those who'd had IUDs for three years or longer, and those who'd had them for only one and a half to three years. (All told, 112 of the 209 patients, more than half, were considered symptomatic —that is, they had discomforts beyond heavier menstruation.)

Of the women who tolerated their IUDs well, who remained free of symptoms, only a small percentage had "significant lesions." Of those who *did* report symptoms but whose IUDs had been in place for three years or less, 20 percent had significant lesions. Finally, of the symptomatic group, whose devices had been in place for three years or longer, 40 percent had significant lesions.

"If you leave a foreign body in the endometrial cavity, after a period of time significant lesions will develop," Ober concluded. "They might not be enormously significant, like cancer, but they will be significant."

Ober's slides—a chamber of intrauterine horrors—included placentas with IUDs entangled in them, and one uterus, after hysterectomy, that contained both a fetus and an IUD.

Take a tip from the pathologists.

The FDA Hedges Again

In addition to patient labeling on the pill and estrogens (see p. 103), the FDA now requires a warning to IUD users. At first there was talk that the warning would be dispensed in two stages, the first to occur when the patient requested an IUD and came in for her gonorrhea culture, Pap smear, and anemia test. Then she was to read the warning and think it over. *If* she still wanted the device, and *if* her test results were negative, insertion could take place after the patient signed a consent form.

The procedure was condensed, and the consent proposal eliminated. Doctors are merely required to give out the leaflet, and many don't. If you do not get the IUD warning from your doctor or clinic, write to the FDA Commissioner and the National Women's Health Network, at the addresses mentioned on p. 104.

Two Women's Experiences

Concerning the side effects of the IUD, painful, heavy periods are not considered by doctors to be "unusual trouble." But in an article called "Me and My Diaphragm: Love at Third Sight," writer Adele Clark observed:

"Within two months of the removal of the IUD, I had returned to a 'normal' cycle. It is now five months since I began using my diaphragm. I no longer bleed half of every month—I have a five-day period with one day heavy and crampy. In contrast, what I used to call the 'discomfort' from my IUD I can now see as real pain—pain that I could not acknowledge because I would have had to take responsibility for myself by using a diaphragm."

Women whose troubles are worse than Ms. Clark's, who think they might fall into Dr. Ober's "symptomatic" group, are apt to be experiencing pathological changes in their uterus. These get worse with time. The outcome of these changes in long-term users—cancer, endometriosis, benign tumors, or infertility—will not be clarified for many years.

Women in the lucky minority, who have little trouble with their IUDs, nevertheless may not want to keep them for more than five years. More subtle adverse changes occur in symptom-free women, too. These may suddenly "explode." Take caution from the story of Caroline S., a 39-year-old Long Island woman who had "few symptoms" for her first six years of IUD use. Indeed, she felt so well that she neglected her checkups. Then, quite suddenly, she lost her uterus, ovaries, and part of her intestine, too. We interviewed her a few weeks later:

"I got nauseated one morning, I had extreme pain in the abdominal cavity, and I realized that there was something wrong. I went home, went to bed, and called my gynecologist, but he was on vacation. When the pain got so bad that I couldn't stand it, I asked to see the doctor who was covering for him. He had me go into the hospital emergency room, where he examined me and said that I had an infection due to the fact that the IUD had been in too long. He gave me antibiotics and a pain medication, which I took for about a week. When my own doctor came back, about five days later, he removed the IUD and told me to stay on the medication and to keep track of what was going on. The pain just didn't diminish, and in a couple of days I was admitted to the hospital, where they started to observe what was happening.

"After some five or six days, they decided to do an exploratory. I think my husband knew that there was a possibility that I might need a hysterectomy, but the operation was logged in as an exploratory with permission. *When they opened me up, they found I did need to have my uterus, my ovaries, and my tubes all removed. In addi-*

tion, *because of the infection, the small intestine had somehow joined with the uterus, so they had to cut a piece off to make that right.* I was in the hospital twenty-seven days, all told. They never told me exactly what had happened— I don't think the IUD had migrated, because my doctor hadn't had any trouble removing it. I think the problem was the length of time that I had had it, and the fact that I hadn't gone for my checkup in, I guess, two years. Even though the IUD was the cause, I have to take equal responsibility. I don't know the prescribed length of time for keeping an IUD. My doctor no longer recommends the IUD at all. He said the reason is that something like this can happen.

"I haven't been back for my follow-up, but so far he hasn't prescribed any medication whatsoever, and I'm hoping that it's going to stay that way. Now, whether my body will accept the fact that I am missing all these parts, I don't know. This is something that I'm going to have to cope with."

CHAPTER 13

The Diaphragm: Queen of Contraception

The sexual revolution of the sixties was no liberating experience for us: we got the pill, blood clots, an increased chance of cancer and a prevailing attitude that now we were obligated to have sex on men's terms. The birth control pill and the IUD obliterated "our problem" and made us highly marketable objects for men's exploitation, with the lust shred of male responsibility removed from the relationship. . . . It is our belief that the diaphragm is the best of the existing options, and offers for women the safest, most effective, and least exploitive method available.

Holly Burkhalter of the Ames
(Iowa) Women's Community
Health Project

Cosmopolitan magazine announced it with exclamation points: "The Diaphragm Is Back in Town!" *Country Woman* called its article "Me and My Diaphragm: Love at Third Sight." The *Woman's Day* article was entitled "Update on Birth Control." Soon the news spread beyond the women's magazines—*Newsweek* had an article on the diaphragm's return, and it was candidly discussed on many talk shows. Manufacturers lagged months behind on filling orders. It was 1976, and "the old rubber parachute," as a friend from Indiana calls it, was The Method of the Year.

The Sanger Research Bureau Study

There were two reasons. One was disenchantment with the pill and the IUD. The other was a study—the largest ever made of contemporary U.S. diaphragm users—that proved

214

it to be a highly reliable method, even for unmarried women and teen-agers.

Contrary to popular myth, the diaphragm, *if fitted and used properly, is more reliable* than most IUDs or the mini-pill, and almost on a par with conventional, medically dangerous oral contraceptives. At the Margaret Sanger Research Bureau (which operated in New York City for fifty years—from 1923 to 1973) 2,168 diaphragm users were studied for two years. Only 2 percent suffered accidental pregnancies, but of these 37 women, 22 admitted that "they had used the diaphragm inconsistently or not at all." Thus, for disciplined women, *the diaphragm is a better than 99 percent reliable method.*

Of course there's another catch. Even with all the patient's good intentions, if her doctor or paramedic has failed to fit her properly, or instruct her with precision, the diaphragm will fail. For years, during the 1960s, diaphragm fitting—which takes less than a day to master—was dropped from the medical school curriculum, and at present there is a shortage of personnel who are truly skilled in the method.

As Judith Wortman, R.N., has explained in George Washington University's *Population Reports:* "Since the advent of the pill and the IUD, medical schools in many parts of the world have devoted little or no time to teaching students about the diaphragm. As a result, recently graduated physicians may not only lack proficiency in fitting the device, but also they may lack knowledge about proper use. On the other hand, nonphysicians throughout the world are being trained to provide the method."

As Ms. Wortman says, often the most experienced diaphragm fitters are not physicians at all, but paramedics, midwives, or nurses. In Philadelphia, one nurse-practitioner who is a staunch diaphragm advocate told us that on reviewing her clinical records *there were fewer accidental pregnancies among her diaphragm users than her pill patients.*

"I don't let my diaphragm patients out of the office," she explained, "until they, and I, are absolutely confident they're getting it right. If they don't like the springy models, I let them take the old-fashioned flat ones. We schedule a second visit the next week to make absolutely sure no insecurities or hassles have developed. Sometimes it takes hours, but all my patients make friends with their diaphragms. On the other hand, you can't guarantee anyone she's going to make friends with those pills. No sir, not with some of the side effects I've seen around here. A lot of my patients are black, you know, like me. My people have enough trouble with high blood pressure to start with. For that reason alone, I especially hate to see a black woman take those pills. Kill-pills, I call them, and I guess my patients can tell how I feel. They're mighty happy with their diaphragms—most of 'em, anyway—and they sure don't get pregnant when I'm their coach. I have a lot of fancy degrees, an R.N. and a master's, but basically I think of myself as a Diaphragm Coach. I feel very good about my work, helping women to help themselves."

Getting a Diaphragm

A woman who decides to get a diaphragm should make sure that her source is of good reputation and experience. *This is essential.* Above all, *she should not accept a diaphragm from a doctor or paramedic who has tried to talk her out of it.* She should seek out the specialist who says with pride that his or her diaphragm patients scarcely ever get pregnant. (One such example is Dr. Harold Davidson of New York City, who states that in 50 years of practice *no patient* for whom he prescribed a diaphragm has ever to his knowledge conceived while using it!)

The woman should also be sure to use the strongest spermicide that she finds agreeable.

The downgrading of the diaphragm's reliability, in the mid-20th century, was a scandal. Studies that showed high failure rates were popularized, while those showing the opposite were scarcely heeded. Even the decisive two-year Sanger study was published not, as one might expect, in a mainstream medical periodical, such as *The Journal of the American Medical Association,* but in a relatively obscure publication called *Family Planning Perspectives.* Luckily, the popular press picked it up, so doctors read about it, like patients, in their newspapers. In 1974, the even larger study of 4,052 British diaphragm users by

Dr. Martin Vessey and his associates showed results similar to the Sanger findings, but the news was not publicized here. Thus, until 1976, most U.S. women believed that the diaphragm wasn't reliable. Many scarcely knew that it existed!

In her book *First Do No Harm,* Natalee Greenfield tells the story of her young daughter, Kathryn, who died from breast cancer apparently caused or exacerbated by the pill.

Kathryn, who was a Ph.D. candidate at Harvard, surely had the wit to master the diaphragm. After her death, her family won a legal settlement instigated by Kathryn, who had explained, "If I must die, and die so terribly . . . I want to feel I've done everything I can to expose this secrecy of silence that exists about the pill. . . . I want to warn others so they won't be misinformed or have to suffer the pain and agony I've had. . . ."

At the conclusion of *First Do No Harm,* her mother states:

"Kathryn was denied information she sought, and that denial in a democratic society made a mockery of the right of self-determination, the right to informed consent, the right to individual freedom of choice, and the right to knowledge. That denial was immoral and unethical on the part of all those who played a role in it. . . . Every dollar received from the settlement in Kathryn's case was donated to libraries."

Kathryn and her parents believed that if women have *honest information,* they will make sensible choices for themselves. It was never honest to downgrade the diaphragm. Thousands of women like Kathryn, who could have used it happily, have died from other methods of birth control instead.

What's especially poignant now, in retrospect, is that so many pill and IUD casualties failed to trust their own mothers. As *Our Bodies, Ourselves* point out:

"Until the 1960s . . . the diaphragm was the safest precaution women had; at one time, one-third of American couples practicing birth control used the diaphragm." (That time, incidentally, was the 1930s, when we had the lowest birth rate ever achieved before the legalization of abortion.) "Many of our mothers used the diaphragm for thirty years without a slip."

Types of Diaphragms

There are four basic styles of diaphragms to choose from, and each behaves quite differently. All do their job well *if* the right size has been selected by the technician.

The four commonly used diaphragms are called:

- The coil-spring
- The flat-spring, or Mensinga
- The arching, or Findlay
- The "bowbent"

Ideally, every diaphragm candidate should have the chance to sample all four. At least, she should be offered a choice between the coil- or flat-spring models and the arching. Some women find the arching easier to insert, while others deem it more difficult.

A few women have special conditions of the vagina that will incline their doctors or technicians to recommend one model over the others. The arching spring, for example, may be better retained by women who have difficulty with vaginal muscle tone, or a tilted uterus. On the other hand, some women find this model decidedly uncomfortable compared to others because it may exert pressure against the urethra, causing pain or difficulty in voiding. The ideal diaphragm is easy to insert (for the particular woman!) and so unobtrusive that neither she nor her lover is troubled by its presence, or inhibited by it in any way. The ideal diaphragm *can be found for almost every woman*—the recent Sanger and British studies both proved it—but the patient must participate in the selection.

A writer, Adele Clark, describes her own experience: "At the clinic, my friendly woman paramedic, Nancy, and I talked for a while and agreed that the diaphragm should be fitted before she 'pulled' the IUD. We tried one kind and it wouldn't fit; tried another and we both could get it in and out, and it fit properly. Success. The use of the word *we* is crucial. I was a participant, not a patient or a *victim*, in this process of fitting my diaphragm, just as I am when I use it to prevent conception.

"This was the third diaphragm in my life, but my first as a feminist and my first with supportive information about its use from a woman. It is the first diaphragm I have loved."

And now we come to the real reason the diaphragm was dumped—from medical school curricula and most family planning clinics—when the pill and the IUD came on the scene.

The diaphragm is costly to the doctor, *in terms of his or her time*. Fitting and teaching its proper use are more of a coaching than medical procedure, comparable to training a child to use her first toothbrush.

But the time of paramedics is less valued, and growing numbers of clinics—as well as some private practitioners—engage non-M.D. personnel to help with birth control services. Why haven't paramedics been fitting more diaphragms, since mastery of this utterly safe method does not require long medical training?

The dismaying truth is that even today, even with the diaphragm's new bloom and recognition, few population programs subsidize the distribution of diaphragms, while the pill, IUD, condom, and foam are *all widely subsidized* with government and foundation monies. We, in fact, help —through our tax dollars—to buy pills and IUDs for poor women, but no such money is allotted to buy them diaphragms or pay paramedics to train them in proper use. From the viewpoint of clinical personnel, the diaphragm is "less available and more costly" than other methods, according to *Population Reports*. When clinics can get financial support for pills and IUDs, they are scarcely apt to talk up the diaphragm.

The average price of a diaphragm is about $4.50. Fitting fees start at around $15 in private offices, but may be less at clinics. Diaphragms should be changed every year or two and whenever there is:

• childbirth, abortion, or pelvic surgery

• any evidence that the diaphragm was improperly fitted

• Some experts say the diaphragm should be refitted whenever there's a weight gain or loss of more than fifteen pounds. But one doctor told us: "In hundreds of cases, I've never found diaphragm size to change because of a change in body weight. The vagina is not involved in body fat!"

A diaphragm that is too small will slip around, and one that is too large will buckle, producing discomfort.

Sometimes a too-small size may be prescribed if (a) the woman was exceptionally tense during the original fitting, causing her vaginal muscles to tighten, or (b) she is a virgin. Sexual experience expands the tissues in the vagina. Sometimes, after a long period of celibacy, the vagina may also shrink. Thus a woman who has been sexually inactive may have fitting problems similar to those of a virgin. In either case, the second visit is *essential*, and perhaps a third as well. The condom and foam are probably better methods to use during one's first few weeks or months of sexual activity. The cervical cap is also a suitable method, if it can be obtained. Cervical measurements are less likely to alter.

Spermicidal creams and jellies, used with the diaphragm, sell for $2 to $3 for a 2½-ounce tube, good for about a dozen applications.

Use of the Diaphragm

While barrier contraceptives, and cervical caps in particular, were an ancient idea, the modern diaphragm is of unique design in that it divides the vagina, more or less vertically, into two compartments, protecting the cervix, or pathway to reproduction, from the arena where sperm is deposited.

The diaphragm was devised in Flensburg, Germany, in 1882 (forty-four years *after* the modern cervical cap or pessary described in the next chapter), by a physician named Hesse, who adopted the pseudonym Wilhelm P.J. Mensinga to protect his reputation.

Mensinga diaphragms, made of rubber, soon grew popular in Germany, Holland, and England. In the latter country they came to be called "Dutch caps," and were ordinarily fitted in the back rooms of apothecaries. Due to our prohibitive Comstock laws, they were not accepted for import into the United States. Early in the 20th century, Margaret Sanger visited a Johannes Rutgers in Holland. He instructed her in the use of fourteen different sizes and styles of diaphragm. In the 1920s, after a long and colorful struggle by Sanger and her associates, several U.S. companies began to manufacture diaphragms, and the device became widely available here. It remained prominent for about forty years.

Then in 1962, just as the pill was gaining widespread acceptance, research by Masters and Johnson shook medical confidence in the diaphragm. To summarize what they discovered: When a women is sexually excited, the inner two-thirds of the vaginal canal expand. The diaphragm then fits more loosely. If under such conditions the penis escapes from the vagina and is reinserted, it may either displace the diaphragm or enter the wrong portion of the vagina (contraceptively speaking), the "danger zone" between the diaphragm rim and the anterior or vaginal wall. Such misadventures are apparently more apt to happen in sexual positions where the woman is on top.

Thus, it appeared that under the following circumstances the diaphragm, however well fitted, might still fail:

• if the woman is highly excited

• if the man has a tendency to slip out during intercourse, or a preference for withdrawing and re-entering

• if the couple like what is called "the female superior" position.

However, Mary Lane, former clinical director of the Sanger Institute, later demonstrated that even allowing for "occasional loss of correct diaphragm positioning during the excitement and plateau stages of sexual response," the failure rate of a diaphragm used without omissions or errors is extremely low. Presumably, then, the spermicidal jelly usually succeeds in its fail-safe mission.

Before inserting the diaphragm, at least one teaspoonful of spermicide should be liberally applied to the side of the diaphragm that goes toward the cervix, and more spread around the rim. As Dr. Marcia Storch has cautioned: "Using a spermicide sparingly is a classic case of false economy." Storch also points out that while some brands are made especially for use with diaphragms, it is likely that better protection results from using a spermicidal jelly or cream *that was designed to be used alone.*

Gynecologist Hans Lehfeldt believes a *small* amount of jelly or cream spread on *both sides* of the diaphragm is just as effective and may appeal more to women who dislike the texture of spermicide.

Health Advantages and Drawbacks

The safest method of contraception, from the standpoint of a woman's health, is a barrier method backed up by the availability of a legal abortion in the case of failure. Few women are aware of this fact. They fear abortion more than they should (from a health standpoint) and the pill and the IUD *less.*

We would not urge abortion on anyone who finds it immoral. For such a patient the issues are different, and the very slightly greater protection afforded by the pill may be worth the greater health risks.

Then there is the matter of convenience. If a woman is willing to trade off the very real risks of the pill and IUD in return for the bonus of spontaneity that they offer, that too is her own decision.

Serious health drawbacks to the diaphragm simply do not exist. Very rarely, a woman finds she is allergic to the rubber, but she can be switched to a plastic model. Some women—and some men—are allergic to ingredients in the spermicides, but again, a simple brand change usually solves the problem. Occasionally infections occur in women who leave the diaphragm in place for more than twenty-four hours, because microorganisms trapped by the diaphragm multiply. These infections are not of a serious order and can be avoided by remembering to take the diaphragm out. A diaphragm that is too large may cause painful intercourse, but a properly fitted softer-rimmed model disposes of this problem.

On the positive side of the ledger, spermicidal jellies and creams, as well as foam, seem to decrease the likelihood of infections when used properly and left in place the recommended length of time. Studies indicate that there is a lower incidence of vaginitis and cervicitis (inflammation of the cervix) among diaphragm-and-jelly users, and that in general they enjoy better vaginal health.

Diaphragm users get less cervical cancer than women who select the pill or IUD, but no one is yet certain why. It may be that the newer methods directly promote such cancer. Evidence further suggests that women who select the diaphragm over the pill take better general care of their health (they smoke less, for example). A third possibility, however, is that *if* cervical cancer is caused by a virus, as some researchers think, the diaphragm provides an actual physical barrier against it.

The Sanger Clinic Success Story

At the Sanger clinic, all new clients selected their contraceptive method following a half-hour group discussion with a nurse. The actual diaphragm fitting was accomplished by a number of attending physicians, medical fellows in training, or a nurse practitioner. The model selected depended on the anatomical characteristics of the woman's vagina and cervix, as well as her own preferences concerning manageability. Also, it was important that the woman have no sensation of its being in place. Five to ten minutes was the average time required to select and fit the diaphragm. After that, a nurse-counselor instructed the patient further, helping her to recognize her "anatomical landmarks" with the aid of a three-dimensional model and "through her own exploration of her vagina." The patient was required to demonstrate that she was able to place the diaphragm properly and remove it. A second appointment was scheduled for the following week. In the interim the patient was advised to use an additional contraceptive with her diaphragm.

This bears repeating. Sanger patients had such excellent success rates with their diaphragms *because they were instructed not to rely on them until they'd had a week's practice—under normal "use" conditions—and then returned for a second coaching session and checkup on technique.*

Donna K., a TV newscaster, is 28 and unmarried. She says she is pretty certain that she doesn't want children. She took the pill for five years, and stopped when a breast lump developed. She tried an IUD and "nearly died from the pain." Then she asked us about different kinds of sterilization. "I've made up my mind to do it," she exclaimed.

We tried to talk Donna into giving the diaphragm a chance, but she was appalled. "The diaphragm is fine for married women. It's not for me."

We didn't see Donna for another six months, then ran into her at a party.

"You look wonderful," we said. "What kind of sterilization did you have?"

"I didn't," she grinned, and, digging into the good-sized pocketbook that she, as a traveling reporter, always seems to have in tow, she gave us a peek at her diaphragm compact.

"I got cold feet," she said, "and went to Sanger. The diaphragm fits in fine with my life-style—in fact, it improves it. See—it takes up less room in my purse than my hairbrush or make-up, not to mention my reporter's notebook. So, I have my diaphragm if I need it, but it also gives me time to say 'no'—a few minutes to think things over. I'm more selective now, and I like it that way. I like it a *lot*. I don't think it's good for a woman to be an Eveready Battery concerning sex."

Donna is not at all unusual. Many women who come home to the diaphragm make similar observations.

The Sanger clinic instructed patients "to insert the diaphragm and spermicide as long as six hours in advance of anticipated need" and to leave it undisturbed for a minimum of six hours afterward.

There has been confusion and debate on whether spermicides remain active long enough to permit inserting the diaphragm many hours before intercourse. For many women, using a diaphragm at the start of a romantic evening is far preferable to interrupting the culmination. But some diaphragm advocates caution that no more than an hour should elapse between insertion and intercourse.

The Sanger research is highly reassuring on this matter. Apparently 99 percent results can be obtained even by women who adopt the up-to-six-hours insertion schedule.

A majority of the Sanger patients—7 out of 10—were single, and most were young. Even girls of high school age used the Sanger diaphragm effectively. Indeed, the clients under 18 had an especially *low* failure rate. It is for single women, particularly, that the convenience of being able to insert the diaphragm up to six hours in advance may be a decisive issue.

Multiple Intercourse and the Diaphragm

The diaphragm raises complex questions for users who, like potato chip snackers in the TV ads, can't stop at one.

We put the question of diaphragms and multiple intercourse to Dr. Aquiles Sobrero, a co-author of the Sanger diaphragm study and an expert on spermicides in his own right.

Sobrero is always candid about the limits of modern contraceptive knowledge.

"We stick to the rule," he explained, "that you do not remove your diaphragm until six hours, even if a second exposure will take place. Which I think is longer than necessary. It's difficult to believe that in the presence of spermicidal jelly, the sperm would stay alive in the vagina for more than three or four hours. But—we stick to this rule.

"Privately I would say that if the woman is going to have a second intercourse after four hours, she will feel better—if she has the facilities—to remove the diaphragm, wash it and wash herself, and place it back. It will be less messy, it will be more protective, and probably she will feel more at ease.

"Less than three hours, no—you do not take out the diaphragm, for the sperm might still be living from before. I would say that she can add an extra amount of jelly that she can put a couple of inches into her vagina with her index and middle fingers. If she squeezes and presses down, the symphysis pubis will, so to speak, brush the spermicide out from the fingers. That should be enough."

What Sobrero believes, then—and his opinion is most informed—is that when repeat intercourse *occurs within four hours the diaphragm should not be removed.* Instead, a condom can be employed or an extra dollop of spermicide added to the vagina.

Adding spermicide with the fingers may seem too

messy for some women, especially if they cannot or do not wish to wash. The Ortho Company manufactures paperboard disposable applicators which are ". . . designed to provide a simple, clean, accurate method for inserting tubed vaginal jellies and creams into the vagina." "The applicator," says Ortho, "may be readily filled directly from the tube, used and then discarded." Additionally, good spermicidal products, such as Conceptrol cream, come in prefilled disposable applicators which may be even handier. (However, as we explain in chap. 15, creams and jellies should not be used alone, even when they are manufactured for that purpose. Only foam disperses well enough for solo employment.)

Foam should not be used with the diaphragm on initial insertion; it does not adhere. Whether or not it's suitable as an encore spermicide is still unsettled. Sobrero finds it to be effective, but there have been reports that it may gradually corrode the rubber in the diaphragm.

Choice of a basic spermicide, to be applied at the same time as the diaphragm, or as a backup for encores, is highly personal. Preference will vary with body chemistry, sexual practices and tastes, and a woman's or her lover's possible allergies. (See chap. 15 for a description of the textural differences among jelly, cream, and foam.) Some women are happiest with whichever product they find least "runny," while others are more concerned with smell and flavor.

The FDA and Consumers Union are both in the process of reevaluating spermicides. Watch for their conclusions.

Diaphragms Used Without Spermicides

There are some models of diaphragm—including the Koroflex hinge—that some women believe they can use confidently without spermicides. For example, Muriel S. explains:

"In about 1960 I got my first diaphragm and was revolted by the jelly, so I was very glad to get a doctor who recommended using a well-fitted diaphragm alone, no jelly. . . . It was a whole lot nicer, so you were a lot more likely to use it. I had my diaphragm *checked for fit every six months* . . . had two pregnancies, planned and easily achieved.

"I have always had bad feelings about telling anybody about this, because people get upset and say that doesn't work. But for me it did, and apparently it did for many patients of my doctor."

Until the 1930s, diaphragms were generally used without spermicides, although a few pioneers, such as Dr. Hannah Stone of the Sanger Bureau, did combine them with "medicated jellies." In its earliest incarnations, the diaphragm worked fairly well without spermicides, but in most social circles women were not *expected* to experience much sexual excitement, so perhaps the "vaginal ballooning" observed by Masters and Johnson was more rare.

Even today, in point of truth, women rarely reach orgasm at the same time as their lovers. Many women reach climax before or after their partners, and often in connection with direct stimulation of the clitoris. It may be that couples who enjoy the much-vaunted mutual orgasm are those who need worry the *most* that the jelly or cream is there as backup. In other words, if he is thrusting hardest and deposits semen at the moment that her diaphragm is bouncy and dislodgeable, spermicides could make all the difference. If, on the other hand, his orgasm follows hers, the bouncy diaphragm will have settled back in place. If his highest excitement precedes hers, the sperm he has already deposited might sneak through, but there is still less danger than if the force of his ejaculation occurs *while* her diaphragm is bouncing.

Incidentally, some diaphragms—about half—apparently do stay firmly in place during sexual excitement and orgasm. There appears to be no research that clarifies whether this is due to the woman's personal anatomy, the style or brand of diaphragm, or the technician's fitting skills. About half of diaphragm users really need that spermicide—especially when they orgasm simultaneously with their lovers—while the other half do not. Nobody knows which is which, although the matter should be easy enough to settle, with appropriate and inexpensive research.

But why would anyone who has the funds and technology to do this research be interested? All it would mean for the drug industry is the sale of less cream and jelly to go with their diaphragms. The larger profit is in the cream and jelly, which must be frequently renewed.

All it would mean for clinicians is that they would have to become even more exacting in determining the right diaphragm—and instructions—for each individual patient. Extra time is what they don't wish to spend.

Women who can contracept by the diaphragm *without* jelly seem to have had to discover it for themselves. Here and there an exceptional doctor or technician tries to provide astute coaching.

In the meantime, for those who dislike jelly, the cervical cap or pessary seems like a safer alternative. Held in place by suction, the cap is less likely to go askew during sexual excitation. The cervix, unlike the vaginal walls, is not so affected.

Diaphragm Insertion

This can be accomplished in any one of several positions: sitting on the edge of a chair, lying flat on the back with knees bent, squatting or propping up one leg on the seat of a chair or toilet.

The diaphragm, containing spermicide, is pinched together and inserted into the vagina as far as it will go. (Unlike the IUD, it cannot "get lost" or perforate.) The forward rim of the diaphragm is pressed behind the ridge created by the pubic bone. Then the user checks with her forefinger to ensure that her cervix is covered. A specially designed plastic "introducer" or "inserter" is preferred by some women to their own fingers.

Arching-spring models, such as Ortho's All-Flex, are extremely popular, but difficult to use with an introducer. Some patients deem arching-spring models the clumsiest to insert, but once in the vagina, they slip into correct position most reliably.

Coil diaphragms can be used with an introducer, but have a tendency to slip around while being inserted. The flat-spring, or Mensinga, models lend themselves best to use with an introducer, and are still deemed easiest to manage by some women who've tried the more modern styles.

The "bowbent" diaphragm has an irregular shape, and is more difficult to fit than other models. Many doctors and clinics have not bothered to stock these diaphragms at all. Sobrero predicts that they may make a comeback, as they are good for certain women who have cystoceles (a weakening of the bladder walls after childbirth) or poor vaginal tone. "As many women give up the pill or the IUD because they have become afraid," he comments, "I think we will see a new interest in the diaphragm, and probably some of these forms that many people have discarded will be needed again. There will be a demand."

The diaphragm is removed by hooking an index finger behind the forward rim and pulling gently downward. The blunt hook at the end of an introducer can also be used for this purpose.

Diaphragm Care

A gently preserved diaphragm may last two years or longer, but it's safer to change it annually, or whenever defects are suspected. A still-in-use diaphragm should be flexible and soft, free of cracks or holes, and healthy-looking.

Before each insertion it should be inspected, especially near the rim, either by holding it up to a light or placing water in it, to check whether any tiny perforations have developed. If drops collect on the *underside*, or if the diaphragm puckers, it should be thrown out.

Upon removal, the diaphragm should be washed with mild unscented soap and clean warm (not hot) water, dried, dusted with cornstarch, and returned to its plastic case. Avoid exposing it to heat, bright lights, oils such as Vaseline or cocoa butter, metals such as copper, silver or zinc, or newsprint. It should be kept in its container.

Women who can't adjust to the diaphragm usually discover it within the first three months. Most often they give it up for "personal reasons." They find it too messy or inconvenient. On the other hand, women who discontinue the IUD or pill usually do so for "medical reasons," some of them crippling or indeed fatal.

It makes no sense, as Sheldon Segal has noted, for women to try the dangerous methods *first*. They should be reserved as backup for those who truly cannot adjust to barrier birth control.

The Vessey and Wiggins Report, from England, was of married women, aged 25 or older, who were already using the diaphragm when they entered the study. Vessey and Wiggins concluded that "women attending family planning clinics who are already established users of the diaphragm need not be encouraged to change to a more modern method of birth control with its attendant risks."

And now the Sanger report has placed the matter in a still more optimistic perspective. "We believe," Mary Lane of Sanger stated, "that since our largely young and unmarried population, all new users of the diaphragm, experienced rates of pregnancy consistent with contraceptive efficacy of around 99 percent, this method can be offered to these women as well, with high expectation of success."

And so, women are returning to the diaphragm, and with good coaching, most of them can adapt. But a feminist has stated the real crux of the problem: "There has been no birth control method developed that is at the same time safe, effective, and esthetically satisfactory. The patriarchy has put a man on the moon, but has yet to take seriously our problem of responsible birth control."

CHAPTER 14

Gone but Not Forgotten:
The Cervical Cap

Putting it in is, well, no harder than slipping a thimble on your finger with your eyes closed.
                    Lady R.B., cervical cap user

The perfect contraceptive is one that is highly reliable, convenient, and free of harmful side effects. It hasn't been invented yet, or so the experts claim. However, satisfied users of cervical caps beg to differ, for this excellent device is highly reliable, can be left in place between menstrual periods, and is far superior to the diaphragm in both convenience and lack of mess.

The cervical cap, or pessary as it is sometimes called, is a thimble-like object made of lucite, rubber, or polyethylene, which fits tightly over the cervix and is held in place by suction. (The cervix is the neck of the womb extending into the vagina.) Until recently, some caps were constructed of ivory, gold, platinum, or other metal, and some of these lasted a lifetime. The cap can be used with or without a spermicide. Unfortunately, it is almost unavailable in the United States.

We interviewed Lady R.B., a British mother of four ("all planned"), who has used the cervical cap for thirty years, conceiving only when she wished to, and always in her first unprotected cycle.

"Ordinarily," she explained, "I remove it once or twice a week at my convenience, when I am taking a tub bath rather than a shower. It just seems more hygienic. It only takes a few seconds to put in or take out.

"Taking it out is a little trickier than putting it in, actually; you have to tilt the rim away from the cervix to break the suction. Putting it in is, well, no harder than slipping a thimble on your finger with your eyes closed. Once while we were visiting the States I misplaced it. I had to get a diaphragm temporarily. Too springy for me— it was always bouncing away and rolling across the bathroom floor. I didn't like having to muss with the jelly all the time, or taking it in and out whenever we made love.

"Speaking of jelly, I did use it until I was about 45, but only at mid-cycle. What you do if you want that extra protection—or rather, what I did—was take out my cap every night at bath time, just for those few days around ovulation, and fill it about one-third up with jelly. It's important not to use too much or it interferes with the suction. Just a dollop for extra insurance, you know."

Had the Englishwoman had any side effects in thirty years? "No—well, yes." She was mildly embarrassed, "At first, I left it in all the time until my period was due, but sometimes I got a discharge that smelled unpleasant. That's when I got the habit of removing it now and then. My cousin avoids the problem by adding a dash of chlorophyll when she puts in her spermicide."

We asked Lady R.B. a question that concerns many women when they learn of the cervical cap: "What if you get your period early, and you've forgotten to take it out?"

"You leak a bit," she explained, "and then you remember to pull out your cap and rinse it. Nothing terrible occurs."

Then she warmed to her subject. "Actually, it's quite handy when you have your period—you can make love without any mess. And if you're caught without, er, supplies, you just wash out your cap and put it back on your cervix. I believe they're making a menstrual cup now that's based on the same principle. I always thought that they should. It's more economical, and it saves a lot of space if you're traveling."

The Cap Then and Now

The cervical cap is thousands of years old. In ancient Sumatra, women molded opium into a cuplike device and fitted it over their cervixes. In the Orient, a kind of oiled silky paper called *musgami* was used in the same manner.

European women, especially in Hungary, melted beeswax into cervical discs, and in the 18th century Casanova himself proposed the most "organic" variant of all—a squeezed-out half a lemon. As an extra bonus, the citric acid served as a spermicide.

The modern cervical cap was perfected in 1838 by a German gynecologist named Adolphe Wilde. It was an excellent device, highly personalized, for Wilde took a wax impression of each patient's cervix, and then custom made each "pessarium" out of rubber. Thus, they fitted *better* than a glove. At about the same time, a New York physician, E. B. Foote, devised his own version of the modern pessary, or cap. It never caught on here as well as it did in Europe.

Properly fitted, a cap will not make direct contact with the cervical os, or opening. Caps are "self-adjusting" to slight changes that occur in the cervix over the course of the monthly cycle. As the cervix swells, the cap descends slightly; as the cervix decreases in diameter or length, the cap ascends.

In New Delhi, India, a gynecologist named Muang Sein has developed a new flexible polyethylene cap, and reports that there have been *no pregnancies* among 300 British and Indian women he fitted with the device.

In the United States, the Ortho Pharmaceutical Corp. used to make what gynecologist Hans Lehfeldt of New York considers an excellent lucite cap. It was discontinued, but revival of interest in barrier contraception may convince Ortho to bring it back. Then again it may not, for Ortho makes a full line of contraceptives, including the pill, diaphragm, and spermicides. The profits on a single diaphragm aren't much, but the profits on the spermicides for use with it mount up. Ideally, a diaphragm should be renewed every year. A cap may well last for two years, or much longer, and women use less spermicide with it, if any at all. Thus in bringing back the cap, Ortho might reduce sales of its own spermicides. Delfen Foam, an Ortho product, has grown increasingly popular with women who want a barrier method but dislike the diaphragm. Were the cap available, it might cut into the foam sales, too.

A recent George Washington University roundup on

barrier methods of birth control concedes that there are few clues as to why the cervical cap has been rejected by doctors in the United States. However, it's clear enough that, from the manufacturer's viewpoint, the cap is not a high-profit item. During the 1960s and early '70s, the demand for barrier birth control was low. Of all barrier methods, the cap is the biggest bargain, averaged out over time, so it's understandable that it was dropped.

By contrast, women have *not* rejected the cap, if given this option. At the pioneering Marie Stopes Clinic in London, one of the first great birth control centers in the world, the cap was stocked in favor of the diaphragm, based on patient preference.

Only one detailed U.S. study of cervical caps was performed in the last quarter century, in 1953, by Christopher Tietze and Hans Lehfeldt, who rank among the most distinguished names in modern family planning.

Tietze and Lehfeldt ascertained that the cap remains effective as long as it stays in place, no matter how much time has gone by since the spermicide was inserted. Some years later, Lehfeldt, working with Aquiles Sobrero, investigated the staying power of spermicides within the cap. In general, the creams lasted longer than the jellies. In almost one quarter of the subjects, the creams were still active after a full week.

In Germany, original home of both the cap and the diaphragm, the cap achieved much greater popularity. In 1926, a U.S. physician, Robert Latou Dickenson, visited surgical supply houses in German-speaking countries and learned that caps outsold diaphragms four to one. The device has remained fairly popular in England.

In the past, when women were more squeamish and less informed about their own internal anatomy, it was the custom of many to visit their gynecologists monthly or semimonthly for insertion of the caps, removal, or both. Today, Lehfeldt still has some patients who observe this custom. There are women who have trouble mastering self-insertion, but most catch on to it in one or two training sessions.

In 1972, the Medical Committee of Planned Parenthood Federation of America concluded that the cervical cap is "about as effective as the diaphragm." Yet, Planned

Parenthood did not take steps to order cervical caps for its clinics. A scattering of U.S. doctors continue to stock and prescribe cervical caps that they obtain from abroad. But most American women who have had them got their prescriptions from foreign physicians or midwives.

The Cap Versus the Diaphragm

In the opinion of many who are familiar with it, the cap is quite possibly the best of the harmless barrier methods of birth control. There are very few women who can't use it —on the contrary, it is suitable for more patients than the diaphragm for the following reasons: A substantial number of women—as many as 3 out of 10 in developing countries —have a uterine prolapse or severe relaxation of the pelvic muscles, as a result of poor obstetrical care. Women with such damaged vaginas cannot well accommodate the diaphragm, but *can* be successfully fitted with a cap. Another advantage: There is less variation in cervical size and condition than in vagina size or tone. Thus, suppliers need stock only about six sizes of caps (or could even get by with three), while a dozen or more diaphragm models are normally required.

Like Lady R.B., many women find it quicker and simpler to insert than the diaphragm. Others do not. Every woman deserves the choice, and a chance to take her own anatomical and sexual measure.

Occasionally lovers complain that they can feel the cap during penile thrusting, especially when it is made of a hard material like lucite instead of flexible rubber or polyethylene. But sometimes women rejoice that the cap— almost like a tickler—enhances their own sexual response.

An American professor, now in her late thirties, reminisced as follows:

"In high school and college I had a cap. It was called a 'silver pessary' by the woman doctor—a German-Jewish refugee named Erna—who prescribed it for me.

"I never got pregnant and I had a super sex life. . . . Did I use it with spermicides? No. This was in the 1950s. Erna never said anything about that. It was just me and my cap.

"About the time I graduated from Holyoke—and

incidentally, I was Phi Beta Kappa in my junior year—my 'silver pessary' got dented. I tried to call Erna for a new one, but she wasn't at the old number. I couldn't locate her, so that was that. I went to my mother's gynecologist, a very sweet man who had delivered my kid brother, and he said that he didn't prescribe caps, and the diaphragm was better anyway.

"The diaphragm has been all right. I have one daughter—planned—and had one abortion, following quadruple intercourse when I did not stop to renew my spermicide. The diaphragm, with fresh spermicide, works perfectly for me.

"One drawback—when I had my 'silver pessary' I never needed clitoral stimulation. I can't explain it, but, for me, it enhanced intercourse. I'm sure you know that in Vienna, when Freud first described the 'vaginal orgasm,' most of his women patients were using some sort of pessary or cap.

"I've never found another American woman who had what Erna called the 'silver pessary.' What I think now is that it was an Austrian product she snuck out when she fled from Hitler. I bet I'm one of the last living American women who ever had one. If I could find my old one again I'd use it—dents and all—since abortion is legal now, and not a big deal. Erna told me that if my pessary got dented, it could break the suction, so I gave it up."

Today, few women are even aware of the existence of the cervical cap. Many confuse it with the diaphragm because of an unfortunate semantic coincidence—in England and other countries, the diaphragm itself, as mentioned, is often called "the Dutch cap," since, although it was invented in Germany, it was improved and popularized in Holland.

Some physicians formerly objected to the cap, sincerely, on the grounds that it might cause cervical erosion. These fears seem to have been groundless, although women with pre-existing erosion—or infections—might be better suited to the diaphragm.

Women for whom the cap is unsuitable include those with deep cervical lacerations or cysts. A cap should not be fitted if a temporary infection is present. Once these are treated and cleared up, the device can be prescribed.

The wonder of the cap is its versatility. The woman who does not wish to walk around with something artificial in her body at all times can use it like a diaphragm, inserting it as needed. The impulsive or spontaneous woman can wear it all month, or only remove it at her convenience, like Lady R.B. The woman who finds spermicides messy or irritating can eschew them. The woman who desires backup protection can combine the cap with spermicides.

The cap is inserted while the woman is in a squatting or half-reclining position. It must remain in place six to eight hours following intercourse, when a few live sperm remain in the vagina. Douching should be avoided with the cap in place.

On removal, the cap requires less care and grooming than the diaphragm. It is rinsed with soap and water but, being fashioned of sturdier material, it need not be stored so tenderly, nor monitored so carefully for holes.

If the diaphragm is regarded as the Queen of birth control, the cap might be called the Anastasia, or lost Princess. We hope that clinics and women's health centers will start ordering caps from England, and that American firms will soon resume manufacture.

The cervical cap is manufactured today in England by Lamberts (Dalston) Limited, 200 & 202 Queensbridge Road, Dalston, London E8, England. Lamberts makes two brands at present called Prencap (for women who have a normal-sized or short cervix) and the Prentif Cavity Rim Model (for women with longer cervixes). Like the diaphragm, the cervical cap must be individually fitted to the woman by a doctor or trained technician.

The cervix is so much less variable than the vagina that most women can be properly fitted with one of the three cap sizes—large (35 mm), medium (30 mm), or small (24 mm). A properly fitted cap is less likely than the diaphragm to be displaced during the excitement phase of intercourse. In hot climates, plastic caps are superior to those made of rubber, for they do not deteriorate.

Failure of the cap may occur if the user has an unusually long or short cervix, which interferes with the necessary suction. For women of exceptional vaginal or cervical anatomy, Lamberts makes two additional devices, called the Vault Cap and the Vimule Cap. These, like the diaphragm, cover an area beyond the cervix, but like the cap, they are held in place by suction. They are suitable for women who have very poor vaginal tone, cystocele(as mentioned, a weakening of the bladder walls after childbirth), or unusual conditions of the cervix.

At Chicago Lying-In Hospital gynecologist Uwe Freese, and his colleague Robert Goepp, an oral surgeon, have conceived the idea of a custom-made cap with a one-way valve, allowing for uterine discharges. It would fit as closely as a denture, and also allow for the timed release of spermicides. It would stay in place for many months, or perhaps a year.

Freese and Goepp have designed a little device, or "tray," for taking an impression of the cervix. Within a few days the cap is fabricated from heat-vulcanized silicone rubber.

The total cost of manufacturing this customized cap is $1.35, for impression material, rubber, and disposable "trays." However, state the designers hopefully, "supplies purchased in large amounts should appreciably lower this small cost."

CHAPTER 15

Vaginal Spermicides: The Contraceptive That Improves Vaginal Health

People in ancient times, who obviously could not have known about actual sperm, nevertheless knew a thing or two about contraception. Formulas for vaginal spermicides appear in early writings as far back as the 19th century B.C., and modern chemists think they must have been fairly effective. Probably through trial and error, the ancients discovered that environments that were either strongly acidic or strongly alkaline were hostile to sperm. In the 4th century B.C., Aristotle suggested oil of cedar, and frankincense in olive oil, to block the cervix. Cleopatra, and other prosperous Egyptians, used a vaginal paste mixed from honey, sodium carbonate, and dried crocodile dung. And in Europe, a sponge moistened with diluted lemon juice was a popular contraceptive.

Salt in an 8 percent solution is deadly to sperm. Eighth-century Indian writers describe the use of rock salt, dipped in oil or honey. By the 12th century, the Moslems had suppositories or tampons based on these ingredients.

The English feminist Annie Besant, a late-19th-century Margaret Sanger, advocated the use of sponges soaked in quinine solution and inserted in the vagina before intercourse. An English pharmacist called Rendell devised a commercial preparation of cocoa butter with quinine sulfate, but Besant's homemade method must have been more effective than Rendell's, for cocoa butter inhibits the sperm-killing properties of quinine. Besant, whose notorious 1877 trial in London established the right of Englishwomen to get birth control information, was also scientifically sound in her advocacy of *sponges*. A century later, in

1977, *Medical World News* reported a "new" birth-control method devised by Dr. Milos Chvapil, head of surgical biology at the University of Arizona. Chvapil's intravaginal sponge, made of collagen, is able to absorb ten times the average ejaculate, trapping sperm in its cellular structure. It is normally left in place for a few days, removed, washed, and reinserted. Developers claim that it causes no infections or irritation, and "has proved completely effective in blocking sperm." Actually, say the developers, their sponge can remain in the vagina for as long as twenty-eight days without creating any problems. Thus, if the market price is low enough, some women may prefer to throw out their collagen sponges, upon removal, and put in new ones.

Gradually a selection of adequate contraceptives became available, including condoms, which were first devised in 1564 by an Italian anatomist.

But then, before the turn of the century, the flow of information and products faltered and stopped in the United States. At the YMCA's urging, New York State enacted the first antiobscenity law, and contraceptives were among the "obscene" articles that were banned. The Y hired Anthony Comstock to press for national legislation, which was enacted in 1873. Contraceptives became scarce because it was illegal to sell or display them, or send them through the mail.

Mary Ware Dennett and Margaret Sanger

Half a century later, also in New York, two women started a battle for the public return of contraception. One was Mary Ware Dennett, who founded the National Birth Control League, and the other was Margaret Sanger.

Dennett has been forgotten, while Sanger remains a folk heroine, an ever enlarging mythic figure, the subject of a recent television special, several new biographies, and even a TV advertising campaign by Planned Parenthood.

Dennett made a serious mistake. She failed to reckon with the economic interests of physicians. In the 1920s, obstetricians had pretty well won a long state-by-state battle to ban midwives, a victory that had terrible consequences for poor immigrant and country women, for there were not enough doctors to serve them. (Consequently, their maternal and infant mortality figures were rising.) Having staked out control over parturition, doctors were not about to support anything that might cut back on business, unless there was something in it for them. Sanger saw this immediately, and issued a call for birth control *by prescription only*, in order to attract the support of some influential doctors. Dennett, on the other hand, called for total repeal of the laws banning contraceptives, including those contraceptives that people can manage on their own. She favored not only the diaphragm, which had to be fitted by a specialist (not necessarily one with long medical training—as we have said, a technician can easily do it) but also the condom, spermicides, and anything else.

In those days, before the practice of *combining* the diaphragm and spermicides, the condom alone or spermicides alone were better methods than the solo diaphragm. The high effectiveness of the diaphragm as it is used today may be principally due to the fact that it holds the spermicides in place. Diaphragms were first marketed in the United States in the early 1920s, but jellied spermicides to be used with them were not widely distributed until some years later. Other spermicidal agents, mainly suppositories and foaming tablets, were available for solo use, and some women probably used them in tandem with their diaphragms. The active ingredients in these products included mercury, quinine, chinosol, lactic acid, boric acid, and burnt alum. They were available by mail and at drugstores, but in the 1920s and '30s most physicians *still refused to endorse birth control.*

Sanger's advocacy of the diaphragm was political, not scientific. Since doctors could control the diaphragm, some rallied to her support. But they saw Mary Ware Dennett as dangerous—not to the health of women, *but to the fees of doctors.* The argument employed by the prescription advocates—then and now—was that only a "skilled professional" could provide instructions, protect the patient from getting ineffective or poor quality products, and answer questions.

Contraception for Teen-agers

The increasing medical control of contraception has had adverse consequences for numerous women, especially the very young. In our culture, it is most unusual for a virgin to seek birth control before her sexual debut. When such a young woman does show up at a family planning clinic, counselors hardly know what to offer her. The pill may induce premature bone closure in young adolescents, and, as we have said, most IUDs are not well tolerated by this age group. Since sexually active teen-agers may switch partners frequently, they are at substantial risk of VD exposure, and, as a new report from National Center for Disease Control in Atlanta confirms, IUD users are more likely to get pelvic inflammatory disease (PID), an advanced complication of gonorrhea, which often causes sterility and sometimes death. A diaphragm cannot be fitted in a virgin with an intact hymen, nor can the proper size be established until the young woman has some sexual experience.

The teen-age pregnancy rate and the incidence of venereal disease have been rising sharply. This is commonly attributed to changes in sexual mores, but the family planning movement must take some of the blame for its pernicious downgrading of "drugstore methods" in order to retain doctor control. Condoms, once a status symbol to the adolescent male (remember the hilarious condom-buying scene in the movie The Summer of '42?), are now held in contempt. A recent study of high school boys in Pennsylvania showed that even those who use condoms did not want their friends to know. A majority of these boys agreed, however, that "using a condom shows respect for your girlfriend."

The drugstore contraceptives such as condoms and foam (in our opinion they should be available in vending machines everywhere) are often the most suitable for young teen-agers. The condom—and foam also, as we shall see—protect against venereal disease as well as pregnancy, and (were they both widely sold in vending machines) could be obtained in complete privacy. In a recent study of teen-age boys who do use condoms (some girls, as well as boys, have the sense now to carry them), it was pathetic to learn that many had either stolen them or persuaded an older friend or sibling to make the purchase. In a number of communities it is illegal to sell contraceptives to minors, and a good many pharmacists still require proof of age. Most family planners have done nothing to ease this situation, nor to campaign for improved availability of contraceptive-dispensing machines. Adolescents say they would use these doctor-free methods much more regularly if they could buy them anonymously. It seems Machiavellian to force a not-yet-developed early adolescent to choose between the IUD and pill when condoms and foam could serve her so much more safely.

Contraceptive Advertising

Until 1970, foam and condom manufacturers both had great difficulty placing print ads, even in magazines such as *Playboy*. Most magazines and newspapers are still unwilling to run such ads (the *San Francisco Chronicle* was a pioneering exception), nor are they approved by the TV code for advertising on that medium.

On November 1, 1972, the National Association of Broadcasters (NAB)—while maintaining its blanket prohibition against contraceptive advertising—began to allow *all other personal-care products, including vaginal douches and hemorrhoid preparations*, on the airwaves. Stations that wish to remain members of NAB *still* may not accept contraceptive ads. At the May 1972 meeting of the Code Board, the Emko Company and, on behalf of Ortho, McCann-Erickson, presented personal appeals that were denied. In 1976, when the question was reopened at an NAB meeting, Dr. Louis Hellman, a gynecologist and our chief population officer at HEW, testified against such advertising nonetheless, although tasteful campaigns in Canada, and on a few nonmember stations, especially in Hawaii, have brought favorable results, and few if any complaints from viewers.

The laws against *display* of contraceptives in drugstores are slowly being changed. Thus the conspiracy of silence, as if to keep young women from knowing that these products exist and can be purchased, is being lifted in fits and starts, though with little help, and sometimes with the actual opposition, of our family planning physicians. But, by 1976 the Department of Health of the City of New York wrote an open letter to pharmacists requesting that they prominently display condoms as a public service in the fight against VD.

Foam Compared to Other Contraceptives

Some of today's spermicides, especially aerosol foam, work a lot better than most people probably realize.

In the 1950s, chemists added a new and extremely useful group of products to the long list of spermicides. These were "surface-active agents," which are commonly used in household detergents. Earlier products, which tended to be strongly acid, might produce vaginal or penile irritations, but the new spermicides, especially Nonoxynol-9, were more benign. By the early sixties, both the Emko Company in St. Louis and Ortho in New Jersey were manufacturing spermicidal foams in pressurized containers.

The first studies of effectiveness were highly contradictory. Some showed pregnancy rates of *less than 1* per 100 woman years—that is, the rate of 100 women on contraceptives for one year—while others recorded 5 to 35 pregnancies! In one study at the Sanger Institute, postcoital sperm counts were taken of 32 females who had used the new foam; 29 revealed no motile sperm in a standard sample of their endocervical mucus, while the remaining 3 had a total of only five sluggish and sickly spermatazoa, hardly the stuff of which babies are made. For contraception to occur, such a sample would have to reveal hundreds of active sperm, for the average healthy ejaculate contains 80 million or more.

Another study, which was to prove presaging, was performed at the Washington University School of Medicine by Dr. J. Barlowe Martin. Interested in safety and side effects, rather than efficacy, Martin tested 50 Emko users for an average duration of twenty-three weeks, during which there were no complications, not even minor irritations, and no pregnancies. Most interesting, 8 women who had minor vaginal infections at the start of the study were in good vaginal health by the end of it. This was the first hint that Emko and other such products might be *anti-infective* as well as spermicidal. No death and no disturbance more serious than an itch have ever been attributed to aerosol foam products. Even the itch is more benign than that associated with vaginal deodorant sprays and douches, for these latter can provoke severe allergies.

Masters and Johnson's studies, completed in 1963, added to the puzzlement over why some good investigators got poor results with the new aerosol foam. The St. Louis sex researchers wanted to see which vaginal spermicides disperse most efficiently. By studying women volunteers using a clear plastic penis for artificial coitus, they were able to photograph the action of various contraceptives—creams, jellies, suppositories, aerosol foam, and foam tablets.

Only two products, vaginal cream and aerosol foam, achieved immediate widespread distribution. The foam, in addition to giving immediate coverage to the vaginal wall and cervical os, was well distributed in the folds and creases of the vagina. Little slipped outside of the vagina, either from penis friction or liquefaction.

The cream provided protection for a matter of hours, even with repeated coitus, but some of the material was drawn out by the penile shaft during thrusting. There were also minor complaints of postcoital dripping.

Vaginal jelly provided very poor distribution, collecting more in some areas than in others. Drainage occurred due to body heat, vaginal secretions, and friction. The drainage sometimes produced irritation. Virginia Johnson has suggested that since proper distribution of jelly does not occur until active coitus, premature ejaculation may contribute to jelly failures.

Foam tablets often caused discomfort, itching, and heat, and when vaginal lubrication was lacking they did not dissolve adequately.

Suppositories dissolved slowly and did not distribute spermicide as well as foam and cream. Dripping and drainage reduced user satisfaction.

Recent studies show that among current spermicides, foams are most reliable, easiest to use, and least displeasing. Creams are in second place. Foam gets to work immediately, while cream takes several minutes to distribute. Both are said to stay safely active for an hour or more, but a repeat application seems advisable if further intercourse occurs, in cost per dose, foam is a fairly expensive method, averaging 35 or 40 cents per use when purchased retail, and more if the user adds an extra half-applicator full, as many women do. (And many satisfied foam users live by the rule of "better safe than sorry," and *double* the standard amount.) However, unlike, for example, the pill, one only pays for foam when one is having intercourse, *not* on a day-in-day-out basis. One also saves on doctors' fees—you don't need such frequent visits to your doctor for checkups. Thus, the overall cost of foam remains in the ball park with other methods, unless a woman is exceptionally active sexually—in which case foam can be expensive.

Recent Studies of Foam

Drs. Howard and Joy Osofsky, authorities on abortion and birth control, have expressed their confidence in foam. They have suggested that the explanation for the poor results shown in some studies of foam is that they were done on non–English-speaking women, teen-agers, or others who were not properly instructed in its use. Some of these women reported jumping up and douching immediately after intercourse. Others applied the foam to the external vulva. Some used it *after* intercourse, not before. In one study, whose point was to see if less than the standard dose would be effective, the women were instructed to use only half the recommended amount. *Many* of them got pregnant. (Recommended amounts may be a bit on the low side, in our opinion, possibly because the manufacturers may be trying to keep down costs so as not to price the product beyond the range of population programs and clinics.)

Another problem was that in the 1960s many family planners pinned all their hopes on the pill and IUD. They often told patients that foam was chancy. Under such circumstances, patients are apt to use a method carelessly because they don't trust it anyhow. They figure: "Why bother, if I'm probably going to get pregnant anyway?"

In 1971, the reliability of foam was clarified in a

definitive study directed by Dr. Gerald Bernstein of Los Angeles which included almost 3,000 women, most of them "medically indigent" and chronically unsuccessful at birth control. Bernstein's clinic staff came from backgrounds similar to those of the patients, understood their problems and life-styles and spoke their language. They maintained regular contact and encouraged their patients to trust the foam.

Over half dropped from the study, but of the remainder, the *pregnancy rate was 4 per 100 woman years*, including patients who admitted they were sometimes careless. Among careful users, the rate was 3. The clients were told they could insert the foam as long as three hours before intercourse, perhaps because some of them had impatient husbands or lovers. Three hours is a rather chancy interval, so this probably kept the figures from being even better. In any case, these were remarkably low pregnancy rates for clinic patients who have chaotic lives and more than their share of health and contraceptive problems. The pill, in such populations, rarely succeeds so well. The success of the study has been attributed to the counseling approach used by the staff. The patients had no serious side effects, but 117 of the dropouts found the foam irritating and 17 said that their husbands had such a reaction.

Another surprise concerning foam was contained in the National Fertility Study of 1970. This report showed generally poor contraceptive results among couples who had not yet completed their families. Americans, it has been suggested, often fail to use birth control conscientiously *until we have all the children we want*. Many women are apparently ambivalent about preventing pregnancy, up until that point.

Some younger couples could not even get the pill to work although ideally this is an almost certain method in the laboratory, if not in life. The actual pill-failure rate in this study was around 6 percent and for foam it was much higher.

Yet when older couples who firmly wanted no more children were interviewed, it was found that they used foam more successfully than the diaphragm or condom. Toward the end of the reproductive lifespan, the failure rate for the pill was 1 percent, foam 2, the diaphragm 6, and the condom 7. The IUD was the most effective method for this subgroup of older women, even more effective than the pill—a reversal of the situation at younger ages.

By 1970, as many U.S. women were using foam as were using the IUD, although they rarely spoke of it. Like the condom, the other good over-the-counter method, it suffered from a poor image, a much worse image than it deserved. Foam's reliability, when *optimally used* with no slip-ups, is no less than 97 percent, which places it below the optimally used combined pill or a well-fitted diaphragm with jelly, about on a par with the condom, the IUD, and the recently banned sequential pill, and a little above the all-progestin mini-pill.

On the whole, the clinical track record of foam supports our contention that it is a rather good method *that has been downgraded because it's not doctor-controlled.*

We have some recommendations for women who use foam—and we think that if manufacturers would include these points on their labels or with their directions, the reliability of foam would be even higher:

• Insert foam no more than an hour before intercourse—it's a better safety margin than the two or three hours manufacturers now recommend.

• Don't douche after intercourse.

• After childbirth or abortion, use more than usual because the cervical opening has been stretched.

• And since *all spermicides*—foams, creams, and jellies—*deteriorate* in time, we also think it would be beneficial if all the makers printed expiration dates on their labels; some have started to.

We would not recommend foam to women for whom abortion is unthinkable, nor to those who find it diminishes sexual pleasure. Such a woman should take the risk of the combined pill or use a carefully fitted diaphragm, or be sterilized (or her husband should be)—or prepare herself to have one or two unplanned children.

Repeated abortions may have their dangers, such as reduction of fertility, but one in a lifetime (or even several) is a *far better health bet* than continuous use of the pill or the IUD. There's just no comparison in safety.

With foam, as with many methods, the experiences

of the first year or two are predictive of long-term results. Women for whom a given method is apt to fail tend to have the failures early. Thanks to mysterious differences in personal anatomy, foam may disperse better in some women than in others, or secretions of the individual vagina may help or hinder it. A majority of failures are in early users who, understandably, switch then to a different contraceptive. A veteran user of foam, of three years standing or longer with no pregnancies, can view it as a 99 percent sure method *for her.*

One in 30 female users, and 1 in 150 men exposed to it, complain that foam makes them itch. Some couples find the product messy. It need not inhibit oral sex, for insertion, which is much like using a tampon, can be accomplished in a matter of seconds without getting up. Since foam disperses immediately, application can be delayed until the moment before intromission.

The lubrication provided by foam is regarded as a benefit by some women. Its popularity with women over 40 may be due to a reduction in their own vaginal secretions.

The Effects of Spermicides

In the early part of the century it was thought that both the skin and the vagina were impermeable by drugs. Now we know better. Some vaginal medications are systematically absorbed. Thus, manufacturers are being cautioned by the FDA to make sure that no potentially toxic ingredients remain in any vaginal products.

The chemicals must be safe for a fetus as well as mother, in case the contraceptive user is unknowingly pregnant. It has been found, for example, that a single injection of pure mercury on the tenth day of gestation produces malformations in mice. (The pill and the IUD have, of course, been *proven* unsafe to pregnant women and to human fetuses, while the barrier methods, thus far, have a clean bill of health.)

A final concern focuses on the teratogenic (birth-defect) potential of damaged sperm. If a foam-treated sperm should retain its capacity to fertilize, the conceptus, or fetus, might be abnormal. Animal studies indicate that this is unlikely and there are no reports of human birth defects attributed to any vaginal contraceptives.

Attention was focused on possible side effects of spermicides when the Japanese discovered that Koromex, a popular diaphragm jelly, contained undesirable levels of mercury. The news was circulated by the women's health movement in the United States and England, where Koromex already had a poor standing because it sometimes blackened diaphragms, underpants, and fingers. Many birth control clinics continued to stock and prescribe Koromex, despite the Japanese report and the complaints of users who found it esthetically unpleasing.

The Koromex incident provoked a much-needed review, by the FDA, of the ingredients in vaginal products that are sold without prescription. The FDA chose as chairman of their Advisory Committee Dr. Elizabeth Connell, who is a puzzle to both feminist and consumer observers. Connell, who has served on Planned Parenthood's Medical Advisory Board since 1963, is a staunch defender of the pill, which she tested on clinic patients in Spanish Harlem in New York. She opposes giving women full information on the risks as well as the advantages of a product which is being prescribed for them. ("Tell a hundred women about headaches and you'll get ninety-nine phone calls with imaginary complaints," she has stated.) Connell has performed research for the following drug companies: Lilly, Syntex, Mead Johnson, Organon, Ortho, and Searle.

On February 24, 1970, at Senator Gaylord Nelson's hearings on the pill, the following dialogue ensued between Connell and Senator Robert Dole:

Senator Dole: "I think it might be well to clarify something, since the quotes will be part of the record. You do state that you had obtained grants, and [your] clinic has been sustained in part by grants from pharmaceutical companies. . . ."

Dr. Connell: "I think one has to look at this fact in context. . . . We have never had sufficient funding. It has been the practice of medicine to accept funds from the private sector in order to run programs. . . . This is how medical technology has been advanced in this country."

Connell has little regard for vaginal methods of contraception, for at the Nelson hearings she lamented that, in response to publicity on the dangers of the pill, more Planned Parenthood clients were requesting diaphragms.

In January 1975 we attended a meeting of Connell's FDA Advisory Committee. She repeatedly spoke of *banning* over-the-counter contraceptives, a move unlikely to be successful but which may, if she is able to demonstrate *any* inherent dangers of foam, get the products moved to a "prescription only" category. Once again: There has never been any report of death or serious injury due to foam (or any modern spermicide), so the dangers under discussion are purely theoretical.

Foam, VD, and Vaginitis

In developed countries today, gonorrhea is reaching epidemic proportions, while syphilis has also risen well above its 1950s rates. Urbanites 24 years old and under seem most at risk. Initially gonorrhea does not show symptoms in 60 to 80 percent of the women who contract it, but if it remains untreated it often progresses to PID (pelvic inflammatory disease) and gonorrheal arthritis.

VD is usually transmitted by direct contact from an infected person to another's mucous membrane. Antibiotics, especially penicillin, brought a dramatic reduction after World War II. Many strains of gonorrhea have grown resistant, however, so that the necessary injection dosage must now be 150 times as great for men (2.4 million units) and 200 times as great for women (4.8 million units) as it used to be. The present procaine penicillin treatment for women can *hurt*.

The pill neutralizes the normal vaginal acids, making women who use it more susceptible to gonorrhea. Pill takers also have an increase in vaginal carbohydrates that encourage bacterial growth. VD and other infections, as well as common vaginitis, are twice as frequent among pill users as in the general female population.

It isn't clear whether IUDs make women more susceptible to VD. What *is* established is that once VD is contracted, an IUD makes it more likely to evolve into serious disease.

In addition to gonorrhea and syphilis, nearly thirty

other infections are transmitted through sexual contact by spirochetes, bacteria, viruses, protozoa and fungi. Common vaginal spermicides, including both major brands of foam, Delfen and Emko, and numerous jellies and creams used with diaphragms, have been shown to be powerful killers of VD organisms—syphilis as well as gonorrhea—as well as the bugs that carry herpes, trichomonas, and monilia infections.

Many years ago, in the 1930s, a physician at Bellevue Hospital in New York City, Evan Thomas, reported to the medical profession convincing evidence that spermicides had a preventive effect against venereal disease and common vaginitis. For whatever reason—maybe because his brother was the anti-Establishment socialist Norman Thomas, maybe because spermicides weren't doctor-controlled—Thomas's finding were greeted with thundering silence from his colleagues.

Not until many years later, at the University of Pittsburgh, did researchers Balwant Singh, John Cutler, and their associates pick up the trail where Thomas left off. Singh and Cutler have now published dozens of papers, which are at last being heeded in the public health community. In 1977 we asked Dr. Singh if he was ready to mention brand names. Which products, we wondered, give women the best all-around protection against VD and other vaginal infections?

Refreshingly, for a medical researcher, Singh pointed out immediately that some of his investigations are sponsored by the Ortho Pharmaceutical Corp., so he is most familiar with their products and perhaps more partial toward them. But in addition, his group has also tested twenty other vaginal preparations with both contraceptive and prophylactic properties. Various brands are "a little more effective against some infections, a little less effective against others," Singh explains.

Recently, Singh's research has taken a still more serious turn. Herpes infections may be a precursor of cancer, and Singh has been delighted to find, and report in the *American Journal of Obstetrics and Gynecology*, that spermicides have a protective effect against herpes virus.

We were pleased when Singh declared to us that he

"supports" the women's self-help movement. He has developed a new self-screening method for genital infections, and would like to hear from women's health centers willing to work with him on testing. His address is:

School of Public Health
University of Pittsburgh,
Pittsburgh, Pennsylvania 15261

Finally, we put to Singh one question that has been troubling us: "In doctors' families," we said to him, "who are successful long-term foam contraceptors, it seems that they often use more than the recommended amount; they use two applicators, or an applicator and-a-half. Does this make any difference from your perspective, the lack of infections and vaginal health?"

"Well, yes, my wife and I would go along with that," Singh responded candidly. "You can add us to that group . . . Of course," he continued, "some people find extra foam too messy, or too expensive. Even at the recommended amounts it's still effective against infections. . . . But more may be better."

— *Delfen Foam* and *Emko Foam* help protect against a spectrum of infections; Singh gives the edge to Delfen for the time being.

— Numerous creams and jellies are effective including Cooper Creme, Ortho Creme, and Preceptin Gel. Lorophyn Suppositories also protect vaginal health. (As with creams and jellies, we could not recommend suppositories for solo employment, but some diaphragm users find them a convenient backup when having serial intercourse.)

Despite the growing optimism of venereologists, it will be some time before the manufacturers are allowed to make any definite claims. In the meantine, many women have personally observed that when they switch to foam spermicides, or to the diaphragm, their vaginitis or "nuisance" infections disappear.

Since so many contraceptives take a toll on our health, it's nice to know there are some that may actually *improve it*. But good as it is already, foam could surely be more convenient. Wouldn't it be grand if they developed longer-acting base materials that would last all day or all night, instead of just a few hours?

CHAPTER 16

Working with Nature: Organic Birth Control

New Art would be better than Nature's best,
But Nature knows a thing or two.
Sir Owen Seaman (1861–1936)
Battle of the Bays

In the West today we tend to think of the human body as a machine. When our body breaks down, we fix it up with surgery or drugs. When we want to prevent some of its functions (i.e., fertility), we do it the same way we would cut off an engine.

But machines do not repair themselves, while living things can and usually do. Some of us are developing a new respect for natural healing, and for the powers of the mind. We are starting to remember that the mind and the body are not easily separable. We are learning to control pain, for example, and high blood pressure through biofeedback. Some day perhaps we will control conception, too.

Early in this century, Bronislaw Malinowski, the great anthropologist, visited the Trobriand Islands, near New Guinea. In his book *The Sexual Life of Savages*, he reported that premarital pregnancy was extremely rare, even though Trobrianders have an active premarital sex life. Women who wished *not* to get pregnant believed that they didn't because, as the Trobrianders visualize pregnancy, the mother must "invite" the spirit of the child into her body.

"It is the unmarried girls who should have children since they lead a much more intensive sexual life than the married ones . . . [yet] the girls seem to remain sterile throughout their period of license, which begins when they are small children and continues until they marry. When they are married they conceive and breed, sometimes quite prolifically. . . .

" . . . I was able to find roughly a dozen illegitimate children . . . in the Trobriands, or about 1 percent. . . . Why are there so few illegitimate children? One thing I can say with complete confidence: No preventive means of any description are known, nor the slightest idea of them entertained. . . ." Malinowski was amazed that they had no recognition of the role of the father in conception. "Very remarkable is their entire ignorance of the physiological function of the testes. They are not aware that anything is produced in this organ. . . . This part of the male body is said to be only an ornamental appendage. 'Indeed, how ugly would a penis look without the testes,' a native aesthete will exclaim. The testes serve 'to make it look proper.' "

How we visualize the workings of our bodies in illness and in health may be crucial to many functions, including reproduction. In his book *The Healing Mind*, Dr. Irving Oyle comments:

"The one great source of healing energy that is utilized less and less as the medical arsenal escalates is the vital factor of the doctor-patient relationship. I learned early in practice that . . . in order for me to be an effective physician, I first had to be convinced from my own experience that my reality structure and its healing system were valid and effective. I made a mental image which I tried to convey convincingly to the patient. For example, in the case of pneumonia, I would give the patient penicillin and create an image of the destructive organisms in the lung absorbing the antibiotic. . . . If the patient believes that I know what I am doing, and I firmly believe in my therapeutic ritual, healing usually takes place. On the other hand . . . if a patient chooses not to recover from an illness, there is very little that can be done to alter the course."

Statistics have proved that the best treatment for habitual miscarriage, a treatment far more effective than any drug, is frequent visits with and reassurance from one's doctor. Similarly, perhaps time will show that the mind can control conception in as-yet-unexplained ways. For now, we do not suggest Westerners practice the inviting or rejection of the child spirit as a form of birth control! Our total environment is not right for it, although it seems to have worked for the Trobrianders.

There would be little profit for drug companies and physicians in mental birth control or improvements in "rhythm" methods—which work simply by identifying the fertile period. There is no research money for the former, and but a trickle for the latter, for who would finance such efforts? Nonetheless, astonishing breakthroughs in rhythm have been occurring, and *right now*, almost in secret, millions of modern women are successfully practicing natural fertility control, which is totally free of side effects.

Making Rhythm Work

From early times human beings have associated fertility with menstruation, but the precise relationship was poorly understood. In the 2nd century A.D., Soranus, a Greek physician, concluded that the menstrual flow prevented male seed from attaching itself to the uterine wall. Soranus concluded that conception occurred just after menstruation, when the uterus was purified. He recommended abstinence to prevent pregnancy in the last days of the menses and immediately afterward.

The belief that woman is most fertile right after her period persisted until about 1930. Medical advice on abstinence was totally wrong, the *opposite* of what would have worked. Then, independent studies by K. Ogino in Japan and H. Knaus in Austria proved conclusively that ovulation occurs *between* the periods of menstrual bleeding.

The formulas of Ogino and Knaus for determining the fertile period were widely circulated and led to the development of calendar rhythm methods, especially in Catholic countries. The Church did not formally endorse rhythm birth control until 1951 (in an address by the Pope to Italian midwives), but had refrained at least from condemning it.

The word rhythm was first used in 1932 in a book by Dr. Leo J. Latz entitled *The Rhythm of Sterility and Fertility in Women.*

Rhythm has several obvious drawbacks, but one is most crucial: *Ovulation normally occurs about fourteen days prior to each menstrual period, but not necessarily fourteen days after the previous one.* Sperm may occasionally live up to seventy-two hours or longer after being deposited in the vagina. Thus, ovulation must be identified in *advance* if rhythm is to work without long periods of abstinence. When the abstinent period is reduced to only four or five days at mid-cycle, rhythm grows much more attractive as a method.

The Calendar Method

If all women had regular menstrual cycles, the calendar method would be glorious, for it is simple enough to calculate the safe days before ovulation, the fertile days surrounding it, and the safe days after. Alas, cycles vary by an *average of seven to thirteen days* (over a year's time) during a woman's twenties and thirties, and by even greater amounts both in her teens and later on, as she approaches menopause. The totally predictable twenty-eight-day cycle is rare.

Calendar rhythm, the grandmother of all "natural" contraceptives, was first advocated in the 1930s. To use this method, a woman records her menstrual history for six to twelve months to determine the intervals between her periods. Ovulation is assumed to occur fourteen or fifteen days before the onset of menstrual flow, and the woman who finds that her cycles are exceptionally regular need abstain from intercourse for only six days—three before predicted ovulation, and three afterward. However, over the course of a year, no more than 5 to 15 percent of women remain entirely regular. To be at all safe, the majority must assume a nine-day fertile period—the tenth through eighteenth days of the cycle—during which they need to abstain. This calculation assumes three fertile days before ovulation, one to two afterward, and four more to allow for cycle variability. The point, of course, is to refrain from unprotected intercourse at least seventy-two hours in advance of ovulation, *whenever* that may occur. For women who have highly irregular cycles, calendar rhythm is no use at all.

This method was highly popular until about 1960, when the Catholic women who subscribed to it started switching to the pill. More than one-fifth of American women were practitioners of rhythm, but by 1970 it had dropped to one-twentieth.

Today, rhythm in its new variations is making a comeback, as the methods that assault the body are being found more and more toxic. Thus it's advisable for all women to keep menstrual histories and have a sense of their fertile times.

The Temperature Method, or BBT (Basal Body Temperature)

In the year 1868, long before the time of ovulation was clarified, a British physician named Squire noted that a small but sustained rise in basal body temperature marks the latter part of a woman's menstrual cycle. Later it came to be understood that this is an effect of the progesterone increase that accompanies release of the egg. (Progesterone, it will be remembered, helps prepare the uterus to nourish a conceptus.)

In the 1930s, the noting of temperature rise was recommended for women who had trouble conceiving, and in 1947 a Belgian doctor suggested that women practicing rhythm record their daily temperatures. The temperature method is now proven to be more reliable (although much more troublesome) than the calendar method alone. A rise of about .5 to 1.0 degrees Fahrenheit usually accompanies ovulation. By avoiding intercourse until three days after the temperature rise, and permitting it only in the remaining days before menstruation, a woman can prevent pregnancy with high reliability. A German study showed that strongly motivated women using BBT avoid pregnancy as successfully as women using the pill.

It is the *shift* in temperature, not the number of degrees, that indicates ovulation. Thus, the readings must be taken daily in the morning, while still in bed, after at least five hours of uninterrupted sleep, and prior to eating, drinking, smoking, or conversation. *Any activity* can increase BBT. Readings may be taken either orally or rectally, as long as the same method is always used. The rectal method is faster.

Temperatures do not rise during cycles where ovulation fails to occur. Thus when no increase is recorded, a woman cannot be sure whether she is having delayed ovulation or a cycle with none at all. The temperature method's greatest drawback is that it does not predict ovulation in advance, and hence requires a long period of abstinence. However, some experienced women combine the calendar and ovulation methods. They record their menstrual cycles to estimate the preovulatory safe days, while using a thermometer to establish precisely when ovulation occurs.

Sometimes, a fever due to infection may lead a woman to *think* she's ovulated when she hasn't.

As women proceed through their menstrual cycles, striking chemical changes occur. These can be charted with exquisite precision in lab tests of urine, blood plasma, cervical mucus, or vaginal and endometrial cells. Such tests have been developed for subfertile couples to help them conceive. Most are too complicated for a woman to try at home.

Until recently, calendar and temperature birth control were the only natural methods most women had. The former is not sufficiently reliable, while the latter requires abstinence for the first half of the cycle. Quietly, however, unheralded and unannounced, a new era of natural birth control is opening, right now. Some innovations are due to scientific advances, and others to women's greater heeding of their own body functions.

The Cervical Mucus (Billings) Method

Not surprisingly, the element in a woman's body that changes most drastically during her monthly cycle is her cervical mucus—it is altered in quantity, structure, and water content, as well as chemical composition.

Early in the cycle, mucus is thick and pasty. It cannot be penetrated by sperm. At mid-cycle, in tandem with ovulation, the mucus becomes fluid, supportive of sperm, easy for the male cells to negotiate. Normally ovulating women who have unusually fluid mucus have longer fertile periods and are more likely to conceive. The opposite is true as well. Mucus is often the key to heightened or lowered fertility.

When couples have trouble conceiving, doctors perform a battery of lab tests that pinpoint the optimum hours for intercourse. Obviously, the same knowledge can be used to by-pass conception.

The tracking of cervical mucus was first suggested, in 1964, by a husband-and-wife team of Australian doctors called John and Evelyn Billings.

The mucus method is predicated on the dividing of a woman's monthly cycle into five phases:

Phase One—Menstruation. The flow continues for some three to seven days.

Phase Two—The Dry Days. Although the interior of the vagina is always moist, there will be little discharge, and sometimes there is a distinct sensation of dryness.

Phase Three—The Preovulation Mucus. A discharge begins that is whitish or cloudy in color and pasty or sticky in consistency. This marks the beginning of a favorable environment for the survival of sperm. The woman's body is preparing itself for her monthly ovulation. Rising estrogen levels influence the development of this mucus, which lasts for an average of six days. Conception *may* occur if a woman has unprotected intercourse during this time.

Phase Four—The Wet, or Peak, Days, immediately before and after ovulation. Estrogen levels are highest now. Cervical discharge increases in volume, becoming clear and highly lubricative, with the consistency of egg white. In appearance it is stringy and stretchy, as opposed to its pastiness during Phase Three. This is the point of maximum fertility, which usually lasts for only one day but sometimes persists for two or three. Conception is *likely* to occur at this time. *On the fourth day after the mucus peaks, a woman may safely resume unprotected intercourse*. If she has an extended (two- or three-day) wet period, she must calculate her safe period from the *last* day of maximum wetness, not the first.

Phase Five—The End of the Cycle. Mucus flow may become clear and watery, or may resume its preovulation stickiness. Patterns are fairly unpredictable, but have no practical significance once ovulation is passed. Any mucus is apt to be cloudy, sticky, or gritty, but *no longer stretchy in the manner of raw egg white*.

A woman is potentially fertile during Phase Three (her Preovulation Mucus) and highly fertile during Phase Four (her Wet, or Peak, Days). She can safely have intercourse during Phases One, Two, and Five.

Many women—30 percent according to one English study—are not suitable candidates for the Billings method. Their mucus flow patterns simply do not lend themselves to it.

Only a woman who (a) falls into the 70 percent with highly discernible mucus patterns and (b) is willing to keep daily track of her secretions can make the Billings method work. Naturally, her sex partner(s) must be cooperative and willing to abstain. Still, with all its limitations, the Billings method has a great potential: Like swimming downstream, it works with nature, not against it, and requires no mechanical aids, not even a thermometer. A woman can do it herself in the wilderness, with only her eye and her fingertips.

A "symptothermic" method is also taught by the "Couple to Couple League," a national organization, in the United States. Essentially, it combines the BBT and cervical mucus procedures, as well as encouraging the search for other body signs of ovulation. The "Couple to Couple League" claims that symptothermic contraception is 95–97% effective. However, a recent field trial in England brought disappointing results. Twenty-two out of eighty-four women eventually got pregnant. The women were trained by the Catholic Marriage Advisory Council, whose methods and teachings may have been somewhat different, with less emphasis on husband participation.

Not for the Squeamish

Proponents of *unnatural* birth control methods point out that rhythm contraceptives do not work for everyone. True, but neither does the diaphragm, pill, condom, or any other method. Doctors and manufacturers may disapprove of the Billings technique because it is totally noncommercial, and in the woman's hands.

Women who dislike touching themselves are not good candidates, however. The practitioner *might* check her underpants but, more reliably should learn to insert her finger, a swab, or toilet paper into her vagina. She must study her own *sensations* of wetness and dryness, as well as become expert in observing the appearance of her discharge.

Mucus readings should be taken late in the day, rather than early.

Leah Jackson, a Boston-based teacher of the method, suggests that her students keep a daily calendar or chart on which they note their cyclical changes. She also cautions that the average period of abstinence (ten days all told— six before ovulation, one during, and three after) is rather demanding.

"Many people feel that a period of abstinence is too great a sacrifice to make, and this facet of the method would keep them from adopting it," Jackson says. "One way to help them make the adjustment would be to use mechanical contraception [condom or diaphragm] during the fertile time, and thus still maintain a high degree of effectiveness. It should be noted, though, that abstinence is ultimately preferable to mechanical methods, because it is easier to distinguish the mucus pattern when there is no interference from diaphragm jellies or creams, seminal fluid, and so on. Also, abstinence doesn't appear as drastic considering that all it represents is a shift in emphasis to forms of affection or sexual activity other than intercourse that the couple enjoys."

Kosasky's Ovutimer

Harold Kosasky, a stocky, ebullient fertility specialist from Boston, fairly glows when you ask him to describe his Ovutimer. He's entitled. If the Ovutimer lives up to its early trials, it could revolutionize organic birth control. The beauty of the Ovutimer is that the woman who uses it, according to Kosasky, can determine her own fertility so closely that she need be abstinent only sixty hours in most cases. It was originally devised to help women who *want to conceive* identify the time of ovulation. Its remarkable accuracy as an ovulation predictor was established when, of 11 Kosasky patients who had been infertile for many years, 9 quickly became pregnant with the instrument's help.

The Ovutimer is a small device into which a woman inserts tiny samples of her cervical mucus each day as she approaches ovulation. It measures the viscosity (thickness) of the mucus; when the arm of the Ovutimer drops, it means that the woman is close to ovulation, and she's got to be careful. The dropped arm indicates that the mucus has reached a cutoff point in fluidity and sperm can now penetrate the cervical canal.

The Ovutimer is presently undergoing field trials as a contraceptive. An expensive version, costing around $500, will soon be available to doctors for their offices. A model for home use, costing about $10.50, may be available to women (if all goes well at the FDA) in the late 1970s.

Curiously, there is talk that the FDA may approve the Ovutimer as a prescription item. Since there is no way it could possibly do physical damage, this seems like a mere political effort to keep good birth control in the hands of physicians.

One drawback to the BBT, or basal body temperature rhythm method, is that many or most women are believed to have what are called *anovulatory* cycles from time to time, and women who are not ovulating never have the temperature increase that tells them they can safely resume sex relations. With the Ovutimer, as Kosasky puts it, "if she's not ovulating the reading will never drop. . . . In other words, it's a go or no-go type of thing—if it doesn't drop, she can't get pregnant no matter what the cause.

"Let's say," Kosasky continues, "the woman has a twenty-eight-day cycle. She knows she ovulates more or less around day fourteen. So the first time she uses the instrument, she'll start at day eight, taking mucus. And then she'll run right through till she's past ovulation. Then she puts the instrument away; she doesn't need it the rest of the month. The following month, since she knows that she ovulates around day fourteen, and the instrument doesn't start changing until day eleven she probably won't start using it till day nine." Kosasky, it should be noted, is here counting back to the start of prior menstruation, not forward to the next menstrual period. Almost all women, as observed earlier in this chapter, ovulate about fourteen days *before* their next menses. Much more variation lies in the interim between prior menstruation and ovulation. A woman with a twenty-three-day cycle has probably ovulated only nine days after the onset of her *last* period, while, in a thirty-one-day cycle, she has probably ovulated seventeen days after.

In its present design, the Ovutimer comes with a disposable part that is thrown away after each use. Cost of each replacement is estimated at about three cents. "It will cost a woman with regular cycles around thirty cents a month to use, but we hope it won't be any big deal even for the irregulars," says Kosasky.

The Ovutimer looks very good indeed—so good that when Kosasky reported it to his colleagues at the Thirty-second Annual Meeting of the American Fertility Society, *Medical Tribune* featured the information as front-page news. Its headline stated: "Ovulation predictable to within one hour in office and home." The article went on to state that despite its simplicity, the Ovutimer may be *more accurate* than basal body temperature or elaborate biochemical assays.

The Ovutimer can be used by virtually all women, though there are some rare exceptions. In eleven years of testing on some 1,000 women, there was one who confounded it—a fertility patient who, it was found, ovulated *during* menstruation. In addition, Kosasky cautions, women who are "having problems with their cervical mucus" would not be good candidates. "For example," he explains, "a woman with active gonorrhea who has an inflamed cervix would have so much pus coming out that the instrument wouldn't work. It also wouldn't work on a woman who has had an operation on the cervix we call a conization [for cancer or for precancer], where the cervical glands are destroyed. It wouldn't work on a woman who has cystic fibrosis—such a patient has thickening of all her body secretions including mucus. It certainly doesn't work on anybody taking birth control pills or any hormone product. That's what the instrument really registers, the relative proportions of hormones in the body. In the case of cortisone [a chemical cousin of steroid hormones] it depends on the dose."

What of the women who, as the Billingses and their disciples discovered, have longer periods of "Prime Time" or more water mucus than is the norm—three days instead of one? Can they use the Ovutimer successfully? Apparently yes, although they will have to abstain for about two days longer than the optimum sixty-hour "no-go" period that a woman with fairly regular cycles and an average one-day duration of fluid or watery mucus may enjoy.

Kosasky explains: "We can set the instrument as far ahead of time as we wish. At the moment, we have it set to warn her three and a half days ahead of ovulation." She is then instructed to continue checking her mucus through what the Billingses call her peak days. When the arm of the Ovutimer stops dropping, she can "go" again.

Margaret Sanger argued that women, as opposed to men, should make decisions concerning pregnancy. She pushed the diaphragm and pill which, while partly in the hands of women, remain unavailable (in our culture) except through physicians. While Sanger urged women no longer to be dependent on their own lovers or husbands where contraception was concerned, she counseled them to look to their gynecologists instead—who, in turn, are likely to be influenced by economics, their moral beliefs, and the prevailing public or government policies. Sanger took what might have been woman-controlled methods and helped turn them over to middlemen or doctors. Kosasky is trying to do the opposite. He is trying to refine a doctor-controlled method and turn it back to women. He is, perhaps, more of a "populist" or feminist than Sanger.

Lunaception

It was a typical pill story. She took it for years. Then, when she developed a fibroid mass in her breast, her surgeon advised her to stop. She, a woman in her thirties, was appalled to notice physical and emotional symptoms typical of menopause: "I was more restless and aggressive . . . I had flashes of moods that would leave me crying from despair or laughing when there was little cause for either." Her eyesight changed. Doctors wanted to put her back on hormones, but she resisted. Then a nutritionist friend suggested she get her own inhouse glandular system functioning again with extra doses of vitamins B and E.

It worked. Inside a month she was back in condition, but when she stopped the vitamins, the problems returned. "I am resigned now to the necessity of boosting my glands indefinitely . . . I can't help but think that my metabolism was permanently altered by the pill. . . ."

Louise Lacey was determined to find an organic method of birth control that would suit her, and be safe. She passed hour after hour in a medical library, reading about ovulation and the reproductive cycle.

Lacey was influenced by René Dubos's book *Man Adapting*, in which the great scientist expounds his concept of health as living *in harmony* with one's environment. She grew interested in biological time, circadian rhythms, and balance; she studied the works of modern physicists, botanists, and cell biologists. "Balance," she concluded, "that's the key word. All life is balance. . . . Rhythms cannot be *controlled*—one can only come into balance with them. I had finally found the concept I had been seeking."

Lunaception rests on the work of Edmund Dewan, a theoretical physicist, who conducted tests demonstrating that when women sleep with a light on for the fourteenth through sixteenth nights of their cycles, it regulates their periods. Dewan's research was expanded and clarified at the Rock Reproductive Clinic in Brookline, Massachusetts.

Exposure to light, visible light from the sun and the moon, and even ultraviolet light invisible to humans, all have critical effects on living things, on "body time," as science writer Gay Gaer Luce has named it. Through the pineal gland in the brain, light seems to influence the reproductive system, and moonlight (when people slept under it) may once have had a special effect on menstrual regularity. The majority of the world's languages have a common root word for moon and menstruation.

Now Lacey started to experiment on herself. "Beginning in October 1971 I used a variation on the Dewan experiment. I kept a daily oral temperature chart, recording it each day immediately upon awakening, and between midnight and 1 A.M., when I normally went to bed. I measured my temperature both times because I wondered which time would be more accurate. I also experimented with various brands of thermometers, finding that cheap ones, in spite of their guarantees, would give different readings within a period of minutes. The more expensive models—around $4.00—didn't do that. At this time I was still sexually abstinent.

"For the first two months I just kept a record of my temperature, charting it on a piece of graph paper. On the fourteenth, fifteenth, and sixteenth nights of the third month, I slept with a light on, a 25-watt night light. In later months, I used a 75-watt bulb in the closet across the room, the door half shut.

"All the other nights of the month I slept in a completely dark room. That wasn't so easy to accomplish, because there was a streetlight right outside my window, and the headlights of cars flashed in on me intermittently. I put up some heavy dark drapes and stuffed a bath towel in the crack under my door. Sometimes I felt rather foolish about the whole thing and considered abandoning my plan. But my lack of alternatives, and a growing interest in one particular man, kept me going.

"At first I could find no pattern in the ups and downs on the chart. I didn't know what it was supposed to look like, so I didn't know what I was accomplishing, if anything. I just kept doing it. . . .

"My chart began to make some sense to me after the fourth month. [When] my periods and ovulations kept perfect step with new and full moons, respectively, for nearly a year, until a series of severe emotional stresses apparently threw me out of step. After six months I returned . . . to a match with the universe. . . .

"Each month, my temperature chart followed roughly the same pattern. From the beginning of my menstrual period until the night before I first slept with the light on, the temperature would remain about the same, within a range of two- to five-tenths of a degree. Within the next day or two, my temperature would show a marked fall and then a steep rise the following day. Sometimes the rise would exceed an entire degree. Then the temperature would stay at the higher level, varying as much as half a degree up or down, until the next menstrual period started, when it would abruptly fall back to its original place. I learned to read my chart like a piece of music and *feel* the rhythm of my body.

"The light triggers ovulation. . . . Since March of 1972 I have used light-entrained ovulation and concomitant abstinence as my only pregnancy-avoidance measure. I don't take my temperature any more except to re-establish the cycle when other factors throw it off. I am not now nor have I been pregnant."

Lacey concludes her book *Lunaception* (now available in paperback and essential reading for women who wish to try her method) with an important question:

"How do I know what I am doing to my body is good for me? . . . Like most other animals, human beings evolved in a consistently light and dark world, day and night always alternating. Yet there are certain times when night is not dark: around the full moon. I've come to believe that the human species evolved a genetic response to the moon, nearly all women ovulating at the full moon and menstruating at the new moon."

Cosmic Birth Control

Eugen Jonas is a Catholic psychiatrist-gynecologist who lives in Czechoslovakia. In the 1950s, searching for more effective methods of rhythm, he advanced the idea that angles of the moon and sun correlate with a woman's fertility periods. Since astrology is viewed as a pseudoscience, Jonas was greeted with skepticism by his colleagues. But some years later, a highly respected Budapest gynecology professor named Kurt Rechnitz claimed to have verified Jonas's laws. In 1970, Rechnitz and others published a study of 1,252 women for whom the method of judging fertility by the sun and moon had proven 97.7 percent effective. It is now fairly popular in Eastern Europe and Germany, and in Czechoslovakia has been officially sanctioned by the Catholic Church.

The method requires discipline. Proponents believe that a woman has *two* fertile periods—her "cosmic fertility time" requiring four days' abstention, and her "ovulation fertility time," requiring ten. Often, but not always, the periods coincide.

Cosmic birth control was described in the United States by Sheila Ostrander and Lynn Schroeder in *Psychic Discoveries Behind the Iron Curtain*. A manual for the practice of this method, *The Natural Birth Control Book* by Art Rosenblum and Leah Jackson, is available from Tao Publications, 31 Farnsworth St., Boston, Mass. 02210; or Aquarian Research Foundation, 5620 Morton Street, Philadelphia, Pa. 19144.

Self-Observation

When a woman is not on the pill, her cervix goes through a monthly cycle of its own: tight and firm at the outset to loose and droopy, to soft and moist, and then back again. There are color changes of the cervix as well: usually light pink at ovulation, dark pink as menstruation approaches (and purplish at pregnancy). Some women are already practicing natural birth control just through daily observation of their cervix.

The techniques for this self-examination have been devised and promoted by two pairs of American health workers, Carol Downer and Lorraine Rothman, who met each other through the Girl Scouts and who operate the Feminist Women's Health Center in Los Angeles, and, in Connecticut, the mother-and-daughter team of Lolly and Jean Hirsch, who publish a newsletter called *The Monthly Extract*. These four pioneers have taught self-examination to thousands of other women who, in turn, give demonstrations in their own communities.

At first the idea was greeted with horror, but it has rapidly grown more respectable. Some family planning clinics and medical centers are now teaching it. Men, after all, see their reproductive organs. Why shouldn't women, too, especially if it can help them to spot infections early and to practice natural birth control?

This technique requires an inexpensive plastic speculum, which can be obtained at most Women's Health Centers. For information on such centers, consult *The New Women's Survival Sourcebook*, or write to Healthright, Inc., at 175 Fifth Avenue, New York, N.Y. 10010.

Here is a woman called Marion describing self-examination in the publication *Country Woman:*

"To examine yourself, you'll need a mirror (I use a magnifying mirror), a strong light source—high-intensity lamp, flashlight, or bright sunlight—and possibly a lubricant such as K-Y jelly (*not* Vaseline), or simply warm water to dip the clean speculum in before insertion. Most women find it easy to use the standard, medium size, but smaller, narrow-bladed speculums are available, as well as longer ones.

"Be comfortable and relaxed; lying back on a pillow, legs apart is probably easiest, but I knew one woman who used her speculum standing up! Breathing deeply will release any tension. . . . I insert my speculum straight, handle up; others do it sideways, then turn it. Hold the blades together and slide them in following the slope of your vagina till they touch bottom (that's your cervix; looking at a sideview diagram of the pelvis will help make this clear). Now press the handle together and lock it by pushing down on the outer part in the groove meant for your thumb (there are different types of speculums, so it's a good idea to practice locking and unlocking yours before using it). Once you've arranged your light and mirror at the proper angle—the speculum should stay in place by itself—the historic moment has arrived: You're gazing at your own lovely round cervix! [The cervix is the neck or lower part of the uterus.] If all you see is vaginal wall, don't get frustrated; though I've been doing this regularly for a couple of years, sometimes I have to start over at a different angle. The uterus is not fixed. You may get the cervix to pop into view by pushing down with your pelvic muscles, or by moving the speculum out a bit, then in again. But to remove it, unlock it and pull out gently at the same angle, allowing the blades to close gradually to avoid pinching yourself. . . ."

It's important to keep a clear, detailed record of your exam findings. Note cervix and vaginal color, position and condition of the os (opening of the cervix), consistency and amount of mucus. . . . Soon you'll learn what changes accompany your personal ovulation cycle and the discharges or the lesions that are the early symptoms of infection. Most important, you'll notice the differences in the secretions of your cervix that are your most important clues to your ovulation cycle.

Body Aware

Gerald Oster is a basic researcher in reproductive science; his wife, Selmaree, a strikingly beautiful black woman, has been a health worker in third-world countries. Modestly supported by the Ford Foundation and working out of a small laboratory in New York's Mt. Sinai Hospital, the Osters are developing simple saliva and urine tests that women can use to predict ovulation.

At the time the cervical mucus grows most permeable to sperm, when body estrogen is at its highest, the chemistry of urine and saliva changes as well. A sheet of paper or matchstick dipped into these fluids will warn the woman (through color changes) that ovulation is at hand.

Selmaree has visited Afghanistan, Haiti, and Kenya among other countries, and says the women are beginning to reject Western contraception. The Osters state that since such women may have poor health to start with (95 percent are anemic in some areas), the pill and devices causing further malnutrition are particularly dangerous.

Women can learn to be "body aware," the Osters claim. They are teaching women to observe their preovulation signs, including breast tenderness. Some women "feel heavy." Others have discomfort in the abdomen specifically, or throughout the midsection and back. The couple is working with 15 women who have "learned to pick up nuances they were never aware of before." Each subject has "different peculiarities."

The Osters hope that their color test, which detects the surge of LH—the pituitary hormone that marks the second half of the cycle—will be ready for distribution by the end of the 1970s. To use the test, a woman must menstruate normally but need not be regular. Medications such as tranquilizers may inhibit ovulation and throw it off. Vitamins change the color of the urine but, according to the Osters, can still be taken while practicing "body awareness."

As the litany of pill and IUD catastrophes grows longer and louder, interest in "organic" birth control is rising. Dependable contraception is an urgent goal, but it need not, and should not, endanger the user's health. The argument that the pill is safer than pregnancy was finally buried by Valerie Beral in the issue of *Lancet* for November 13, 1976. The "excess mortality" from cardiovascular and circulatory diseases associated with the pill appears to be *twenty* per 100,000 women aged 15 to 44. The mortality from "all causes associated with childbearing" is only about *one* or *two* per 100,000 women in developed countries. There's simply no comparison in risk. Eleven months later, on October 11, 1977, *Lancet* published a yet more chilling analysis by Beral and Dr. Clifford Kay, of the Royal College of General Practioners. The death risks from the pill increase with duration of use—substantially after the five-year mark is passed. Equally tragic, the risks remain somewhat elevated (contrary to what had previously been hoped) even after the drug is discontinued. All told, the pill appears to be the leading single killer of reproductive-age women, ranking well above accidents as well as pregnancy.

Important new studies by Dr. Howard Ory, of the Center for Disease Control in Atlanta, and Dr. Anrudh Jain of the Population Council have further clarified how pill use interacts with other coronary risk factors. The factors that may be especially pertinent include high cholesterol, high blood pressure, diabetes, obesity and smoking. Dr. Ory believes like Spellacy, Wessler and others that pill users should be "profiled" (by means of lab tests) on their risk factors. He also says that short of this "women who smoke and take oral contraceptives should decide which they want to do more and eliminate the other—especially if they are over 30."

However, the time draws near when most women will be able to pinpoint ovulation so precisely that abstinence, the surest and safest of all contraceptives, will be no burden. Couples will have the further option of using barrier methods, such as the diaphragm or condom, in the brief interval when pregnancy can occur. Most of the time they will need no method at all! It is toward these healthy and desirable goals that research into "organic" contraception is directed. Such research clearly deserves a much higher priority and more generous financing than it gets.

CHAPTER 17

Sterilization: The Ultimate Control

> *. . . The principle that sustains compulsory vaccination is broad enough to cover cutting the Fallopian tubes. Three generations of imbeciles are enough.*
>
> Justice Oliver Wendell Holmes

Female sterilization was mentioned by Hippocrates, but was not fully described until 1834. Essentially, it involves cutting, blocking, crushing, or cauterizing both Fallopian tubes so that sperm is barred from reaching egg.

Traditionally, sterilization was performed through a large abdominal incision called laparotomy. Today, so-called Band-Aid or "belly-button" surgery—developed experimentally in the 1930s and '40s—is very much in vogue.

Laparoscopic sterilization is the formal name for these new procedures. The laparoscope is a lighted, pipelike instrument through which the surgeon can peer into the abdominal cavity and operate, making only one or two small incisions. Originally laparoscopy was a diagnostic procedure, and is still widely employed as such. When a woman who has, say, pelvic inflammatory disease (see chap. 12) is laparoscoped by her doctor, it just means that he wants to view the condition of her organs. Laparoscopic sterilization *combines two procedures*, laparoscopy and closing of the tubes. When sterilization is performed, the tubes are, as a rule, blocked with electric current, a process called coagulation.

Before her laparoscopy, the patient is given either a local or general anesthetic, then about two quarts of carbon dioxide are pumped into her abdominal cavity. The gas helps to push away the intestines, giving the surgeon better access to her tubes. Laparoscopists have a motto: "An eye in the pelvis is worth two fingers in the vagina."

But not all doctors agree. In Bombay, India, at a 1973 meeting of International Planned Parenthood, vaginal sterilization was endorsed: ". . . the vaginal route . . . involves less postoperative pain and is, in many cultures, not regarded with the same apprehension as a procedure involving an abdominal incision." Indian women are said to accept sterilization more readily if the word "operation" is not used. It is described to them as merely "a stitch in the vagina" that will protect against pregnancy.

Vaginal sterilization is technically called "colpotomy" and was first performed in 1895 by a German obstetrician. It did not grow popular until the 1960s and '70s.

Some major complications, such as damage to other organs, are thought to occur less often with vaginal techniques. On the other side, vaginal procedures have a higher failure rate. Most people are surprised to learn that sterilization has a failure rate at all. *Subsequent pregnancies occur in 1 to 2 percent of patients.* Three reasons are given. Sometimes the pregnancy is not "subsequent" at all. It was merely undiagnosed at the time of the surgery. In other instances the doctor occludes the wrong structure —round ligaments, for example, instead of the tubes. Finally, the severed or crushed tubes may just heal themselves over time—grow back together through natural processes. Unexpected pregnancies can occur *as long as ten or twelve years after sterilization*. These pregnancies are often ectopic, for the tube has healed enough to permit sperm and egg to meet, but not to allow the fertilized ovum to proceed on its normal course into the uterus. Ectopic pregnancies are medical emergencies, which sometimes result in death.

Deaths also occur at the time of the procedure. For conventional tubal ligation, the estimated mortality rate is 25 per 100,000. With laparoscopy, the rate ranges from 20 to 30 per 100,000. Thus, while "Band-Aid" sterilization offers a quicker recovery (if all goes well), it cannot truthfully be called a "safe" operation. The skill and training of the surgeon are of paramount importance. Some doctors attempt the procedure precipitously, after watching a colleague do it once or twice. In Philadelphia, a novice laparoscopist tried the "Band-Aid" operation on 5 successive patients using the cauterization method, burned the bowels (intestines) of all 5 with his coagulation instrument, and is now embroiled in 5 malpractice lawsuits.

To avoid the hazards of electric burns, some doctors prefer to shut off the tubes with a band or clip ring or chemical plug. There is a great interest, for example, in the work of Dr. Jaroslav Hulka of Chapel Hill, North Carolina, who, with bioengineer George Clemens, has developed a potentially reversible spring clip for sterilization. Clinical trials of the Hulka clip were begun in 1972, and over 1,000 women in nine countries have been clip-sterilized.

Since this method avoids the use of electrical current, complications resulting from serious burns to the bowel or other organs have been eliminated. Local anesthesia can be used for the majority of patients. An error in the manufacture of the applicator, now corrected, caused tubal tears in a number of cases. One patient, who had heart trouble to start with, died of massive myocardial infarction in the course of the operation.

The Hulka procedure is speedy. Five patients can be sterilized in an hour. When no long-acting medication is used, recovery time is only three hours. A day or two of postoperative menstrual-like cramping is reported by about one quarter of the patients. Often the procedure is done at the same time as an abortion. In four such instances, the broad ligament or other organs in the area were mistakenly clipped in place of a tube.

Hulka anticipates that the failure rate for his method will be 2 to 6 pregnancies per 1,000. He arrives at this after eliminating the manufacturing or surgical errors just discussed—the errors that caused tears in the tubes or led to the clipping of the wrong female structures. We need to be "more attentive to detail in these instances," Hulka confesses.

In an animal study, 10 mature female swine of proven fertility were sterilized by the clip technique, and then were mated for three consecutive months. No pregnancies occurred. The clips were removed, and the severed ends of the Fallopian tubes were rejoined in 8 of the animals. In 2 of them, rejoining was impossible because of "massive adhesions." Of the 8 swine whose tubes were reunited, 6 had subsequent pregnancies. Thus, for 6 out of 10 swine the clips did prove to be a reversible method after three months' use. To date, no clip-sterilized woman has requested a reversal, so the outcome for human females is still uncertain.

Hulka comments that "women need it—potential fertility—for security. It's a psychological thing for women." But he is the first to caution that his spring clip, now widely promoted as "reversible," has not yet proved so in humans.

Serious physical complications short of death occur in about 5 percent of female sterilizations. The nature of these, varying with the procedure, includes cardiac arrest, hemorrhage, infection, perforation or burning of the uterus, bowel, or intestines, pulmonary embolism, emphysema or respiratory difficulties. With laparoscopic sterilizations, occasional emergencies or even deaths also occur from carbon dioxide embolism.

In general, the most effective sterilizing procedures are associated with a higher frequency of medical side effects, while the more benign procedures have higher pregnancy rates.

After sterilization, women suffer a threefold increase in menstrual complaints. Five percent of nonsterilized women have severe menstruation, in contrast to 16 percent of the sterilized. (The reasons for this have never been fully clarified.)

A few patients continue to have pelvic pain for months or years following surgery. This is usually localized in the area of the tubes, and is described as a "tugging," "drawing," or "pricking" sensation. Sometimes such pain is associated with intercourse or any sudden change in position which stretches the pelvic mucles.

Fifteen percent of sterilized women say they are delighted with the outcome, while another 15 percent regret the surgery. The rest, more than two-thirds, are moderately satisfied. Those who express disappointment include (not surprisingly) the ones who get pregnant.

Other reasons for dissatisfaction are: pelvic symptoms, marriage difficulties or divorce, wish for more children, and psychological or religious distress. In a follow-up study of

1,000 sterilized women, 2 became embittered because a child died subsequently, and they were unable to get pregnant and replace the lost child.

Psychologically, sterilization is more of a wrench than many women anticipate. Some depression is apt to follow, for, as one psychiatrist explains it: ". . . the childbearing function is an integral part of the body image. The loss of this function needs to be worked through in a manner analogous to the mechanism of phantom limb appearance following amputation."

Most women, the great majority, recover within weeks or months. A few stay depressed and mournful. They may develop pseudocyesis (false pregnancy with abdominal enlargement, such as is sometimes observed in household pets), or overprotect the children they already have. Sleep disturbances and nightmares are not uncommon. Now and then, sterilization precipitates psychosis. One disoriented woman—in Louisville, Kentucky—wandered through the halls of a maternity hospital, looking for "her baby."

In a review of deaths following laparoscopic sterilization, 2, a suicide and a homicide, were attributed to "abnormal psychological adjustment by the patient or spouse."

With all these drawbacks, sterilization of either wife or husband *has become the most popular form of birth control for American couples past 30*. Among the group aged 30 to 34, a total of 33.7 percent favored sterilization, compared to 21.4 percent who favored the pill. There is also a striking increase in sterilizations among younger women.

Since 1970, according to Judith Herman, M.D., "female sterilizations in the United States have increased almost threefold. Between 600,000 and 1 million procedures are now performed on women each year. Poor women and women of color are heavily overrepresented; 20 percent of married black women have been sterilized, compared to about 7 percent of married white women. Fourteen percent of native American women have been sterilized."

But affluent women are "tying their tubes" also, for the newer procedures make it seem much more attractive. In the *New York Times*, reporter Jane Brody described her own experience:

The operation [laparoscopic tubal sterilization with bands] was done on a Tuesday on an outpatient basis [no overnight hospitalization] under local anesthesia. Before the operation I was given an injection of the sedative Demerol with the tranquilizer Valium, in the arm, and an injection of Xylocaine [a drug like Novocain] in the naval area. During the surgery, I was half asleep and dimly aware of tugging sensations in my abdomen, but felt no pain. I was in and out of the operating room in twenty minutes.

Four hours after the surgery, I went out and bought three pairs of shoes. That night I ate a big dinner, taking two aspirin before bed to relieve what felt like mild menstrual cramps. I took it easy on Wednesday, staying home from work, napping twice and taking four more aspirin. On Thursday I returned to work using no painkiller.

The third postoperative day—not seventy-two hours after surgery—I played my usual Friday morning tennis game. During the first set, my partner kept asking me how I was feeling. During the second, she didn't bother. We won.

White women who want to be sterilized may have trouble persuading a doctor, especially if they are single or have no children at all. But doctors are weakening in their reluctance to do it for private patients. Average fees for tubal ligation begin at $150–$300, and ascend to $750 or more. (Hysterectomies—which should not be performed just for sterilization, but frequently are—come even higher.)

"Band-Aid" surgery sounds safe and simple, and for Ms. Brody it was. But it isn't always. One study showed 1,594 serious complications and 19 deaths out of 63,845 operations surveyed. Noting this, feminist Claudia Dreifus has warned: ". . . the same medical practice that sells tubals to the poor under the stress of labor, sells my affluent friends the lie of Band-Aid simplicity for a dangerous operation."

With a grant from the Fund for Investigative Journalism, Ms. Dreifus spent many months studying the conditions under which poor women are sterilized. She visited Los Angeles where 11 Chicanas are suing USC-LA County Medical Center, certain doctors, the State of California, and the U.S. Department of Health, Education, and Welfare for performing sterilizations they did not want. "Consent forms were pushed at women in the throes of labor—

women who were drugged, women who were under anesthesia. Sometimes, the physicians even disposed of the minimal legal nicety of a signed consent form; they simply cut without permission . . . the L.A. County obstetrics staff, in its zeal to sterilize, was dispensing medical misinformation as if it were aspirin . . . an unusual number of Chicanas were told that they would die if they did not submit. Some patients were misled into thinking their tubes could be 'untied' at some time in the future."

"It would be a mistake to think of the situation at L.A. County as an isolated fluke," cautions Dr. Bernard Rosenfeld, co-author of a Ralph Nader–sponsored health research group study on forced sterilization.

For example, a medical student at a Boston hospital admits: "The name of the game is surgery—bring the patient in, cut her open and practice, and move her out. While she is there she is an object, treated coldly, patronizingly. Backs are turned on patients, questions are unanswered, operation permit forms are not explained. It is jokingly said that the only needed prerequisite for a hysterectomy is not to speak English. It isn't much of a joke."

An intern at a Detroit hospital comments: "Most of our patient population was black, inner city. We had a lot of young girls come in . . . thirteen and sixteen and they'd have two or three children. In those cases, we'd ask 'em, often when they were in labor, if they wanted tubal ligations."

"You mean you sterilized *16-year-olds?*"

"Well, yeah . . . if they had two kids. But we didn't do many abortions. . . . The residents didn't like to do them. You know, you look at a fetus and you see it is a formed human being so we didn't do many."

"In 1973," Dr. Judith Herman, of the Somerville, Mass. Women's Health Collective, recalls, "two black sisters in Alabama, aged 12 and 14, were sterilized in a federally funded family planning program. Their mother had been persuaded to give her consent by making an X on a form which she could not read. She did not know that the operation was permanent. . . . As a result of the case, HEW was ordered to set up guidelines for sterilizations supported by federal funds. The guidelines were minimal, but they did include a requirement that the patient be told that sterilization is permanent, and that she be assured that she would not lose any benefits such as welfare if she refused. A seventy-two-hour waiting period was required . . . to allow the woman to change her mind if she had signed under duress. Almost a year after the court order, the ACLU reported that most of the hospitals they surveyed did not bother to comply with even these minimal guidelines."

Finally, women are organizing to stop forced sterilizations. In New York City, Dr. Helen Rodriguez-Trias and her colleagues organized CESA (the Committee to End Sterilization Abuse), which has developed model guidelines, including a thirty-day waiting period and a "rigorous" definition of informed consent. Citizens' groups have got these guidelines adopted in New York after a long struggle.

In Boston, a coalition from the Women's Union, Women's Law Collective, Women's Community Health Center, and several other organizations are collecting information on the practices in local hospitals. Similar groups are active in Minneapolis and Chicago. In Los Angeles the Chicanas have gotten a court order halting the use of federal funds for sterilizing women under 21. The judge also ordered the state to rewrite its Spanish-language consent form so that "ordinary people can understand it."

Judith Herman reminds us that "The increase in female sterilization has come about not in response to women's demands [as in the case of abortion] but as the result of government policy and pressure from hospitals and doctors."

If women want the operation, and really understand its limitations and dangers, they should have it, of course. Today in the United States, more women are having it than want it, especially if they are "colored," poor, or unfamiliar with the many safe alternatives. In Puerto Rico *one-third of all women of child-bearing age* have already been sterilized, often as "guests" of the U.S. government.

AID, the Agency for International Development, maintains that world population must be controlled in order to end poverty and hunger. One of its endeavors, PIEGO (Program for International Education in Gynecology and Obstetrics), trains 150 doctors a year in the technique of laparoscopic tubal ligation. Three U.S. medical centers are involved: Washington University in St. Louis, the University of Pittsburgh, and Johns Hopkins.

PIEGO trainees are physicians from third-world countries. Their room and board is paid, according to an exposé in *Off Our Backs*, and they are lectured on "the importance of population control for preserving social stability in the home." At the end of his two-week-to-one-month training period, each doctor is presented with a free laparoscope, worth thousands of dollars.

A major drawback of the program is that these foreign doctors lack the formal credentials to practice surgery on humans while in the United States. Thus, their actual training is confined to rabbits.

The director of the PIEGO program at Washington University has defended such training as adequate, pointing out that the reproductive organs of rabbits are smaller. If the surgeon can successfully sterilize a rabbit, his argument goes, surely he can sterilize a woman, too.

Other doctors disagree, and so does the Brazilian government, which has lodged official protests against PIEGO with the U.S. State Department. The State Department was forced to ask that PIEGO and AID stop paying the expenses of Brazilian trainees.

In St. Louis, students, faculty, hospital workers, and community members have formed an ad hoc committee to end the PIEGO program at Washington University. Fifty people picketed outside the university hospital. In response, a PIEGO trainee from Bolivia boasted that back home he had already sterilized up to 80 women per week without their knowledge.

But built into Spanish cultures, as Claudia Dreifus explains, "is the idea of *machismo*, a value that says a man's masculinity is measured by the number of children his wife produces. Given the reality of *machismo*, a sterile woman is considered worthless—useless."

Guadalupe Acosta, a large, somber-looking woman of 35, is one of the Chicanas in the Los Angeles lawsuit. She did not wish to be sterilized, and does not recall giving written or oral consent. The infant to whom she gave birth in L.A. County Hospital, just prior to her imposed sterilization, died.

The relationship between Guadalupe Acosta and her common-law husband of eight years quickly deteriorated. On a smoggy day in the autumn of 1974—a year after Guadalupe Acosta's sterilization—her husband abandoned her and their two living children. She was, as a result, forced on welfare. Then the tubal ligation hemorrhaged and she was hospitalized.

Ms. Dreifus alleges that middle-class women are also being tricked into tubal sterilization, with false assurances of its Band-Aid safety and simplicity. According to the Association for Voluntary Sterilization, more women than men (600,000 vs. 500,000) were sterilized in 1975.

This makes little sense, for in the United States there have been *no recorded medical deaths associated with vasectomy in many years*. The sterilized woman does face the possibility of dying, not only during the operation, but afterward, should he tubes spontaneously rejoin and should she then get pregnant. She must also cope with the risk of greatly enhanced menstrual distress and some residual pain (possibly from adhesions) for the rest of her life. The male vas, located *outside of the main body*, is easier to get to, and uncrowded by other vital organs.

Then there is the issue of reversibility. Some measurable percentage of vasectomies, probably no more than a quarter, can be effectively reversed. The patient is counseled to regard his operation as permanent, but on occasion, surgery has restored male fertility. Success in reversing female sterilization is minuscule. (A few super-specialists, such as Dr. Jordan Phillips of the University of California at Irvine are starting to report better results due to painstaking procedures in which they reattach the severed tubes, layer by layer, under a microscope. Phillips acknowledges that few gynecologists have the patience to do this kind of surgery. The sort of surgeon who enjoys intricate, microscopic detail is much more attracted to such delicate specialties as ophthalmology.)

What is more, surgical reconstruction poses the same risk as spontaneous healing of the tubes. Chances are that the repair will be less than perfect, and ectopic pregnancy, if any, may therefore ensue.

Then there are sperm banks which, while not yet

perfected, hold *some* hope for the sterilized male who changes his mind. We have no banks for ova.

All in all, the woman must regard her sterilization as almost surely permanent; the male (especially if he banks his sperm) still has an outside chance of fathering more children. *Her* situation is more absolute.

Guadalupe Acosta's ligation hemorrhaged more than a year later. Chances are that the surgery was done by an intern or resident. Teaching hospitals push sterilization— and hysterectomy—as much to train beginning doctors as to serve ZPG (Zero Population Growth). They need bodies on which to practice, and their training is not deemed complete until they have fulfilled a "quota" on a range of procedures.

It's dangerous to be a "service" (i.e., nonpaying patient) on a gynecology-obstetrics floor in April, May, or June, as the academic year at teaching hospitals draws to a close. If there's any excuse to operate, they may. (Conversely, if you're really sick, it's better to come to an *emergency room* during the same season, when all of the house staff has had at least a year's experience.) To sum up, doctors in training are more skillful in the spring, but are also (if surgeons) more itchy to operate.

Thus, private patients may face fewer risks of sterilization than public ones, especially if they check around and choose a surgeon who is experienced and careful. Public patients, like Guadalupe Acosta, are a training ground, an intermediate step, between the corpses student doctors first cut into and the paying patients they hope to attract one day.

At public hospitals, the staff doctors, teachers, or professors may be equally indifferent to the health and feelings of the Guadalupe Acostas. In a recent survey, 94 percent of the gynecologists polled in four major cities admitted that they favored *compulsory sterilization* for welfare mothers with three or more "illegitimate" children. Guadalupe Acosta was not, in fact, on welfare, but how could they tell? Dr. Curtis Wood, president of the Association for Voluntary Sterilization, reflects the thinking of many of his colleagues when he states:

"People pollute and too many people crowded too

close together cause many of our social and economic problems. . . . As physicians we have obligations to the society."

Did Guadalupe Acosta break any law? Indeed not. She was punished for being Chicana and poor. Her doctor, whoever he was, placed his perceived obligations to society —or, his need to train on "service patients"—well above any Hippocratic obligation to her. The baby she delivered was dying or dead when he blocked her tubes.

Is any woman safe? Some doctors don't like "hippies" or feminists or Jews or Baptists or Catholics. Some are punitive toward *any* unmarried woman who indulges in sex. Another breed believes that *no woman*, be she as affluent as Ethel Kennedy, has the right to "pollute" this crowded planet with more children than two. When doctors claim the prerogative of deciding whom to sterilize, they cross a Rubicon that many thoughtful people view with alarm. (Justice Holmes, as noted at the start of this chapter, was a disappointing exception.)

In the absence of strict guidelines and, above all, *informed consent*, any doctor becomes free to sterilize any woman at his whim.

It happens to males too. In India, for example, millions of illiterates are bribed or tricked into vasectomies not knowing them to be irreversible.

And even women who volunteer for sterilization, who seek it, often learn afterward that it was all more complex than they thought.

Kathy B., a health-conscious woman of 32, selected her doctor most carefully. Indeed she interviewed three surgeons before deciding which to entrust with her tubes. Medically, the operation was a success, although Kathy admits: "I didn't feel myself again, physically, for several months. I was dragged out and tired. The propaganda doesn't really warn you about that, although Eli [her doctor] tried to. He was totally honest and straight."

But Kathy says she "isn't certain" she would do it over, and she doesn't go around recommending it to others. Kathy now believes "I really should have talked to a therapist first. My motives were twisted, because I've never had trouble with birth control, never needed an abortion.

But you see, I have four stepchildren, my husband and his wife had three sons and a daughter. The boys don't need me or pay too much attention to me. They are in high school or college and we get along so-so. But that little Backy, my 9-year-old stepdaughter, I'm closer to her than her own mother is. I thought the operation would show her how much I love her, show her that she is the only daughter I'll ever have. I did it for her. It didn't work, of course. It only confused her. Maybe I wanted her to feel guilty and more 'bound' to me. It was a dumb idea, all things considered, but at the time it seemed to make perfect sense. Yes, I do like the freedom it gives me from using contraception, but not my worsened menstrual cramps. Anyhow, I now believe I did it for neurotic purposes."

Jennifer L. admits: "My tied tubes are the outcome of a power struggle between me and my husband. We have a picturebook family, an ideal marriage (people think) but our erotic life leaves much to be desired. Hal was gay, actually, before he met me, and I converted him, somewhat. After our kids were born I used a Lippes Loop for five years. It was fine, but then I got a series of infections. The doctor said it had to come out. I would have gone back to the diaphragm, but as a married woman who does have other 'friends' it wasn't practical. Hal would have noticed. He offered to get a vasectomy, and I thought, 'Good grief, that's all I need. What a hideous situation, if I got pregnant!' So I had to rush quickly to get sterilized before he did. My regular doctor wouldn't do it so fast. He said that it was an irreversible decision I should think over carefully, etcetera, etcetera, and so forth. Frankly, I was furious at him—Big Daddy—he treated me like a child.

"I heard about this guy who does it, no questions asked. In fact, he winked at me and said, 'Playing around, eh honey?' He got a little sexy with me also. A revolting person, but a good technician, I guess. I was a little gassy for a week or two after surgery, and a little too bloated to wear my jeans.

"I love the operation, really, but Hal's never been convinced that my motives were innocent. I keep pointing out how some of our male friends were so *sore* after vasectomy, and he says 'baloney.' My laparoscopy cost us $1,000, and his vasectomy would have been $150.

"He watches my whereabouts more carefully now. I don't blame him."

Peggy G., five feet two inches tall, weighed 182 pounds when we met her, three months after her laparoscopy. Her eyes were like slits, her face like a balloon with a face painted on it.

"The doctor punctured something," she explained. "My kidneys or my bladder. I can't move out my wastes. They don't really know what's going to happen to me."

Peggy is 40 years old. "I didn't want the operation," she said. "My doctor took me off the pill on account of my age, and he told me that he would 'just put this little plug' in my tubes. . . . 'Jack and I could just use condoms like we did at college,' I explained to him. Truthfully, we don't have *that much* sex any more.

" 'Posh,' said the doctor. 'Why should you do that to old Jack? It's not really surgery. Be at the hospital at ten Wednesday morning, and you'll be out by three. You don't even have to pack a nightie.'

"And so I did what he said."

CHAPTER 18

Abortion: Relief if Not Pleasure

I would think that this priest, instead of flailing at a Baptist like Carter, would instead be standing outside of an abortion clinic, shouting his wrath at any Catholic woman he sees coming and going. They are the ones who are defying the Catholic Church. . . .

Mike Royko, in the *Chicago Daily News*

Whose Right to Life?

Men make abortion laws and women have abortions, whether the law allows them or not. Abortion is a "woman's secret," so statistics on its frequency are not fully reliable.

It is estimated that, worldwide, there are 1 to 2 induced abortions for every 4 live births. It is thought that in "illegal" countries, such as most of Latin America, abortions are *almost* as frequent as in legal ones. The notable difference between illegal and legal countries is in the maternal death rate, and the health of women who are sexually active, especially the poor. From 1958 to 1962, according to the National Center for Health Statistics, the average number of U.S. women who died from abortion was 292 a year. In 1973, when abortion became legal, the figure dropped to 36, a reduction of 88 percent.

Reporting in *Hospital Practice*, in 1975, Dr. David Fisher made telephone calls to a dozen large public hospitals around the country: "Some striking facts emerged. At Los Angeles County Hospital, where 10 to 15 septic abortion deaths a year were once the rule, there have been no such deaths in at least three years. In 1974, the entire city of Baltimore, a community that certainly has its share of urban problems, did not have a single maternal death from any cause. At Jefferson Davis Hospital, in Houston, where septic abortion formerly claimed 4 or 5 women's lives a year, there have been no fatalities over the last two years. Similarly, at Yale–New Haven Medical Center, where septic abortion deaths ranged between 3 and 8 a year in the mid-sixties, the mortality reduction has been absolute."

Dr. Fisher is speaking here of *death*, no lesser complications, such as near-death or permanent sterility. Until the early 1970s, many urban hospitals had entire wards set aside for the management of septic abortion. The chief of obstetrics and gynecology at one such center confided to Fisher, almost regretfully: "Septic abortion is so rare that I have serious doubts about the ability of our emergency staff to recognize and manage it."

Definitions

Abortion denotes the termination of pregnancy, before the fetus is "viable" or capable of surviving on its own. Twenty-eight weeks, counting from the first day of the last normal menstrual period, has been the standard estimate of when *viability* occurs. Advances in the care of premature infants are leading scientists to revise the estimate downward to twenty-four weeks. Few if any infants born before the twenty-fourth week have survived under any circumstances.

Viability is not the same thing as *quickening*, the moment when the mother starts to feel the fetus move within her. Quickening occurs earlier, usually by the twentieth week, but not before the sixteenth.

Quickening is a crucial event to the mother, if not to the baby. It is at quickening that most mothers start to perceive their child as human and alive. Miscarriage after quickening is usually more distressing to the mother than miscarriage before, and so, we are learning, is abortion.

Until the 19th century, the European, British, and American common law was generally tolerant toward abortion before quickening. Even the fathers of the Catholic Church held that the fetus was animated by the entrance of the soul, which occurred at forty days after conception for a boy, and eighty days after for a girl.

This discrepancy might seem puzzling now, but the church philosophers believed that the female soul was lower and weaker than the male, falling somewhere "between" man and beast. In any case, early abortion was viewed loosely by most clerics, and it was not until 1869 that Pope Pius IX declared all abortion to be murder.

The prohibitive abortion laws of the 19th century were also influenced by a prevailing fear of surgery and surgeons. In many areas, regulations against abortion were tacked on to legislation limiting surgery in general.

It's of some interest, but more a source of sorrow and puzzlement, that abortion rates are especially high in Catholic countries, where the laws remain prohibitive. In most of South America, every grown woman knows about "la sonda," or the tube, a catheter which passes from hand to hand, to be inserted in the uterus.

Also, in New York City, where, since legalization in March of 1970, exceptionally reliable records have been maintained, department of health studies have established that Catholic women get abortions at a slightly higher rate than non-Catholics.

Every laywoman knows the difference between *miscarriage* and *abortion*. Doctors, however, tend not to use the former word. Instead they make a distinction between *spontaneous abortion* (i.e., miscarriage) and *induced abortion*. Throughout this chapter we will use *abortion* in the lay sense, meaning deliberate interruption of pregnancy.

Incomplete abortion is an abortion (or miscarriage) in progress. In illegal countries, women who perform their own abortions often seek medical aftercare for bleeding caused by the retention of placental tissue. "A knowledgeable woman," in the words of Dr. Christopher Tietze and Marjorie Cooper Murstein of the Population Council, "will wait until she feels sure that the process is irreversible." Then, frequently, she pretends she is having a miscarriage. The doctor may have his own suspicions, but in fact he usually cannot tell for sure unless she has badly injured her cervix or perforated her uterus.

Septic abortion is a serious infection, complicated by fever, inflammation of the endometrium, and inflammation of the tissue adjacent to the uterus. Most septic abortions are induced—in unsanitary circumstances—but on rare occasions a bona fide miscarriage may engender such infections.

Abortion Methods

Most abortions fall into one of four categories. These are: (1) *surgical or mechanical*. The principle behind them is evacuation of the uterus, through insertion of a foreign body, and then scraping out, or suction. This can be accomplished by medical instruments and under hygienic circumstances, or by the woman herself with twigs, roots, metal rods, clothes hangers, or catheters. Infusions of soapy water, or common household disinfectants, are widely "self-employed" to evacuate the uterus by women who lack better means.

On occasion, doctors who get a kick out of cutting use much more extensive surgery than they need to. In England, for example, abortion by hysterotomy (in essence this is an early caesarean section) is still quite popular . . . a curious matter, since the English are generally much more wary of surgery than we. Once a woman has had a hysterotomy abortion, subsequent pregnancies (if carried to term) will often require caesarean section, as her uterine wall may be much weakened by the scar.

Surgical abortion of any sort is most chancy for a woman to do on herself. Untold millions *have*, but optimally it requires the approval and cooperation of others.

(2) *Physical abortions* are well known to the young and the poor, and all of the most desperate. These involve exertion and trauma to the general corpus—violent horseback riding, for example, or throwing oneself down the stairs. In New York City, when midwives were outlawed early in this century, immigrant women lost their folk knowledge (often carried by the midwives) of "menstrual induction" by herbal or other medicinal means. Lacking horses, the stairs in their tenement apartment houses were their court of last resort.

Theresa K. saw her grandmother die from such an abortion.

"It was 1932, the depths of the Depression. I was 5

years old, and my grandma was about 47 or 48. She still had nine children living at home, and she was the baby-sitter for me and my brother, the children of her oldest daughter who had a job. Grandma also had a couple of boarders, young immigrant men who gave her six dollars a month for a cot in the kitchen and meals. They were distant cousins or something from the same little town in Sicily. My grandfather was dead.

"One of the boarders (I never liked him), I guess as they would put it nowadays, he and Grandma got it on. Lord knows where they found the privacy. Well, she was pregnant. I know, because I heard her discussing it with her girlfriends. I watched her standing at the top of the stairs practicing how to fall. I watched her break her neck. It wasn't recorded as an abortion death. I and the neighbors never told anyone, not even my mother."

Raina G.'s recollection was more cheerful:

"My grandmother, she's dead now, but she lived to see abortion legalized and she was so happy. She did it three times by falling, and never hurt herself much. I guess you might call her a premature Chevy Chase."

By the mid-1960s, when anthropologist Steven Polgar and sociologist Ellen Fried studied the abortion attempts of 126 poor women in New York City, only 2 reported "accidents and exertion" as their method of choice. The ingestion of turpentine, Clorox, and massive doses of quinine had become quite popular, as had Lysol "douches" or insertion of "the tube," hangers, knitting needles, and bark (perhaps laminaria) into the uterus.

Polgar and Fried collected information about 322 abortion attempts. In 3.4 percent of those cases the women died. In short, the death rate was more than 1,000 times as high as a few years later when abortion was legalized.

The Polgar and Fried study illustrates that the "official" death figures from clandestine abortion, cited earlier in this chapter, are probably far too low.

About one-half of the respondents had attempted abortion not by any uterine method but by ingestion of potentially toxic substances. Resultant deaths would be mistakenly recorded as suicides or poisonings.

In many cultures, spells and incantations supplied by witch doctors and the like have been traditional means of abortion. We term this (3) *psychogenic abortion*, and we have no doubt that it works on occasion.

In our culture, it's well known and accepted that the opposite can happen. "Habitual aborters" as they are called—i.e., women who have repeat miscarriages with no underlying cause—are best treated by psychotherapy, reassurance, or even hypnosis. In short, *fear* of a miscarriage can produce one, so why not faith?

The fourth and final category, *medicinal or pharmacological abortion*, consists of drugs which dilate the uterus and/or cause contractions.

Many old herbal manuals mention formulas to bring on delayed menstruation. Some of these products are thought to be toxic, while others are of doubtful effectiveness. But some may work quite well very early in pregnancy.

In *The Sexual Life of Savages*, Malinowski, who was satisfied that unmarried Trobriand women did not use birth control (see chap. 16) went on to admit:

". . . I cannot speak with the same conviction about abortion, though probably it is not practised to any large extent. . . . My informants told me that a magic exists to bring about premature birth. . . . Some of the herbs employed in this magic were mentioned to me, but I was certain that none of them possess any physiological properties."

That was written in 1929. Herbal remedies are viewed more respectfully now that modern pharmacologists are finding active substances in so many of them. Of all the drugs used today, it is estimated that a high percentage were known to the ancient Egyptians.

Laminaria, a combined herbal-surgical abortifacient, is a marine plant whose dried stems expand in the presence of moisture. Applied to the cervix or inserted in it, it stretches or dilates the canal. Its action is sufficiently slow and gentle that some modern doctors now advocate laminaria as the best way to open up the cervix without injury.

In the United States, many women believe that very early in pregnancy, 6 g (6,000 mg) daily of vitamin C, taken for five days, *sometimes* produces abortion. In parts of Mexico, the women gather a handful of aniseed and steep it in boiling water for ten minutes. A quart daily may give cramps and, ultimately, abortion. Margaret Fiedler, who has worked as a midwife in Mexico, witnessed its effective use.

At this writing, in the United States, talk of herbal or medical abortion may seem quirky or quaint. It is not. The advantage of such an approach is that it remains in the hands of the woman. She is not dependent on the skill —or the will—of an outside surgeon, nor the winds of political change.

Many feminists—and other supporters of abortion rights—believe that the future lies in medical abortifacients. As a recent report from the Population Council stated:

"The development of an entirely medical, rather than surgical, method of early abortion that would be safe and effective for use in a nonclinical setting, perhaps as a do-it-yourself procedure, remains an important objective."

The most promising new method for the stimulation of uterine contractions is the prostaglandins (PGs), compounds that are found in the tissues of many species of animal, including man.

Naturally occurring prostaglandins from the seminal vesicles of sheep were the first to be used in obstetrics. Recently, prostaglandins have been synthesized.

The most probable route for home use will be the vaginal suppository, which usually initiates bleeding within three to six hours. Research on this method is well advanced in Scandinavia.

Thus far, the suppositories work efficiently and quite safely in the weeks just following the first missed period. Once the second period is missed, they get more chancy.

In a study of 75 patients who were but a few weeks late, all aborted and only 2 had incomplete abortions, calling for follow-up curettage. (The sign of trouble was that their bleeding persisted for more than two weeks.)

By contrast, a study of 42 patients advanced further in pregnancy (although still in the first trimester) brought the following results:

32 women had a complete abortion

2 did not abort

7 required follow-up curettage

Two patients in 5 have no side effects whatever with

suppository abortions. Many get uterine cramps, usually mild, but severe in about 1 in 15 cases, and some have gastrointestinal symptoms such as vomiting and diarrhea.

Prostaglandins are also being used for midtrimester abortion, a more complex and serious matter requiring medical supervision. Some authorities prefer prostaglandins to saline for late abortions, but most consider saline to be safer.

Safety and Current Techniques

Dilatation and curettage (D & C), a surgical procedure, is done for a number of gynecological purposes, including menstrual problems and abortion in the first three months, or trimester.

The surgical canal is stretched, usually by the insertion of a series of dilators, each of a progressively larger size. The contents of the uterus are removed with a small forceps, followed by scraping with a metal curette.

Suction or *uterine aspiration*, developed in China in 1958, is progressively replacing the D & C. After dilatation, a rigid cannula of metal or plastic is inserted into the uterus to dislodge the products of conception from the uterine wall. A flexible tube connects to the cannula on one end and a pump on the other. Most such pumps have an electric motor, but some are operated by foot. In very early pregnancy, a small hand-held syringe may produce sufficient vacuum.

Suction is thought by most authorities to be simpler, quicker, and less traumatic than surgical curettage. Some doctors still like to finish up with a bit of curetting, just to make sure that no placental tissue remains.

D & C or suction can be performed under local anesthesia by paracervical block, or under general. Used skillfully, the paracervical block—a numbing injection of Xylocaine or Novocain—can deliver an almost pain-free abortion, and a minuscule complication rate. Hundreds of women have assured us that they felt little or no discomfort during carefully performed, locally anesthetized abortions.

Women who've gone to abortion mills often tell a different story.

In their rush to meet the hourly quota of four or more patients, some abortionists omit the paracervical block, or they fail to wait until it takes effect.

Aware of the pain endured by outpatients at her clinic in New York City, one with an excellent safety (and profits) record, a former abortion counselor decided, upon facing an abortion herself, to enter a hospital and have general anesthesia.

When the uterus is emptied, cramps may occur for ten to thirty minutes, as it contracts to normal size. Pain-killers such as Tylenol or codeine taken just *before* the procedure, keep discomfort to a minimum. The doctors at the clinic we just mentioned did abortions skillfully but wasted time on such "frills" as Xylocaine or analgesics. Abortion is also one of the special situations where a "minor tranquilizer" such as Valium or Librium may be worth taking an hour in advance. Recently we saw a woman faint before her abortion out of either fear or mixed emotions. Tranquilizers can allay fear or anxiety, but we have doubts as to the wisdom of using such drugs where the problem is ambivalence about having the abortion. Under such circumstances, the doubts should first be resolved with a clear head.

MR, menstrual regulation, is a variant of the suction procedure. Some people call it "minisuction," as it is limited to the first two weeks after a missed period, and does not require that dilation be performed. A small and flexible tube is inserted into the cervix and, again, attached to a vacuum such as a syringe or pump. Complications are minimal, but there is one important drawback. Fairly often—1 time in 25 is the official estimate and the true rate may be higher yet—minisuction fails to terminate the pregnancy. Patients who try this method are advised to have follow-up pregnancy tests a week or two later.

Menstrual extraction is similar to minisuction abortion, but is employed *when the monthly period is due*. At first it was hailed as a great boon to women, a means of avoiding monthly bleeding and birth control all in one.

But many users have been disappointed, and few continue with it as a regular technique. Some deem it painful, for anesthesia is rarely used. Others were distressed to find themselves pregnant afterward, menstrual extraction or not. The most crucial drawback is that we still don't know the long-term effects of such periodic trauma to the uterus. Thus, menstrual extraction on a regular basis must be considered highly experimental.

In the first trimester, legal abortion entails very little risk. In the United States, the mortality rate for abortions performed in the first eight weeks was 0.4 per 100,000 in 1972–73. Since then it has declined substantially as more doctors have developed better abortion skills. Late abortions, at sixteen weeks or more, involved a mortality of 17 per 100,000 in 1973. By 1974 it had dropped to 15 per 100,000 according to the U.S. Center for Disease Control. Nine deaths were associated with 59,368 saline procedures. Late abortion occurs most frequently among poor women who are very young. They are inexperienced about recognizing pregnancy symptoms and afraid to seek help. Birth itself is also dangerous for the 12- or 14-year-old.

Others requesting late abortions include women in their late forties and fifties who interpret their missed periods as menopause, and women who have learned, through a process called amniocentesis, that they are carrying an infant with mongoloidism or other birth defects. Still other applicants for late abortion have medical disorders, such as serious heart or renal conditions, which make full-term pregnancy extremely hazardous. Usually they are women who were planning to have the baby, but did not go in for a checkup early enough to know whether they should. Again, they usually are poor. New improvements in techniques of late abortion are, tentatively, dropping the mortality figures to about 10 per 100,000.

In seeking a late abortion, it's essential to select the facility and doctor most carefully. Applicants should try to find a center that maintains a separate abortion service, for this indicates a high level of expertise and commitment. As Dr. L. S. Burnett and his colleagues at the Fertility Control Unit of Johns Hopkins have stated:

"We found that most of the hospitals [we] surveyed lacked something very basic, in our thinking, to the requirements of a functioning abortion program—the recognition that it should be set up as a unit completely separate from existing delivery or gynecologic operating room facilities. . . . By separating abortion patients from other obstetric and gynecologic patients, one not only affords them a privacy they need, one also concentrates specially trained personnel responsible for and responsive to them."

In the United States the most widely used procedure for late abortion is still the replacement of amniotic fluid by saline solution. The uterus is tapped by means of a needle and catheter through the abdominal wall. Labor usually starts within twenty-four hours, and the fetus and placenta are expelled some hours later.

The installation of saline is not usually painful, but it must be done very slowly and carefully. The patient must let her doctor know immediately if she feels waves of heat, extreme dryness, dizziness, or backache; salt solution injected into a blood vessel by mistake can cause shock and sometimes death.

The contractions are not as strong as full-term delivery, but may be painful nonetheless. General anesthesia is not advised, but painkillers and tranquilizers should be available.

The patient usually stays in the hospital for twenty-four hours after the delivery.

Major and minor complications are many times as frequent for late abortions as for early ones.

Minor complications include vomiting after the anesthesia, or a single day of fever. About 1 woman in 20 has minor complications following a first-trimester abortion, and 1 in 100 develops more serious complaints. *The procedure is safest when abortion is done under local anesthesia before the second missed period.*

After that, with each successive week, the complication rate rises slightly, but does not go up sharply until month four. Many gynecologists hold to a belief that abortion is especially dangerous during the thirteenth through sixteenth weeks. They prefer to skip the fourth month altogether and schedule the abortion at the start of the fifth.

Figures from both the United States and United Kingdom demonstrate that this notion is mistaken. The maternal death rate is notably higher in the fifth month than the fourth. However, fourth-month abortions do require special handling (the amniotic sac is too small for transabdominal saline), while vaginal evacuation requires more extensive dilation of the cervix and general finesse. But saline, prostaglandins, and other suitable chemicals can be introduced vaginally, while some skilled practitioners are comfortable using surgical evacuation methods. Instead of waiting out this "lag period," we suggest you seek a doctor or clinic familiar with fourth-month procedures.

The serious first-trimester complications, which are extremely rare when abortion is legal, include perforation of the uterus, sometimes combined with injury to the intestines or other organs, as well as major hemorrhage and laceration of the cervix.

Delayed complications include the following: retention of fragments of the placenta, causing postabortal bleeding; infection ranging from mild to severe; blood clots. (One source of infection is the inadvertent spread of preexisting and undiagnosed gonorrhea. A cervical culture to check for gonorrhea should always be taken prior to abortion.)

There is one delayed complication that is highly controversial. Some investigators believe that following an abortion, or abortions—especially if the patient is in the early teens—the woman faces an increased risk of miscarriage or premature birth in her subsequent pregnancies. The cause, they believe, is damage to the cervix at the time of dilation, or too vigorous curettage which harms the basal layers of the endometrium.

Other investigators disagree. They claim that with modern techniques and skilled operators, infertility is most unlikely. (Normal delivery, it is pointed out, stretches the cervix more than abortion.)

The issue remains unsettled, but many observers say this: Frequent, repeated abortions may impose sterility on some women. An abortion or two in a lifetime apparently does not. Nobody advocates abortion as a regular method of birth control.

When a woman obtains a legal abortion before her second missed period, her chances of dying from it are 1 in 250,000. Compare that statistic to the pill, where the death rate from blood clots alone is 3 per 100,000 per year and from cardiovascular disease, 20 per 100,000.

Out of every 100,000 careful diaphragm users, 1,000 or 2,000 annually (i.e., 1 or 2 percent) may require an abortion. Thus the combination of diaphragm and early abortion will lead to 1 death per 12.5 to 25 million users per year.

Were these same 12.5 to 25 million women taking the pill instead—and if it worked perfectly (which it does not) and none of them ever required an abortion—there would still be 375 to 750 clotting deaths in the group, as well as 2,500 to 5,000 cardiovascular deaths.

Abortion may precipitate some guilt or depression, anger at the inseminator or men as a class, or a temporary loss of interest in sex. These feelings are short-lived as a rule, and rarely of a serious nature. Most women say that their overriding emotion is—relief.

The World Health Organization concludes that emotional stress—or lack of it—is influenced by the following factors:

- whether the abortion is legal or clandestine
- the length of pregnancy
- the type of procedure and amount of pain
- the attitude of the woman's family and friends
- the attitude of professional and others involved in the abortion

Thus, if a woman can get a legal abortion early and painlessly, if her associates condone it and the personnel are kind, she need not experience it as an ordeal. . . . Unless, of course, she *wanted* the baby. No woman should be pushed into abortion, any more than she should be refused it. Good abortion counseling helps ambivalent women to make a sound choice.

Abortion and M.D. Mismanagement

Whose fault is an abortion? How can the rate be reduced? It is usually assumed that a woman's "carelessness" is to blame, but two recent studies find otherwise:

In Nassau County, a New York suburb, Dr. Joel Robins interviewed 100 women seeking repeated abortions and concluded that "deficiencies in medical management" of birth control were often responsible. For example, 10 women had stopped taking the pill *after* complaining to their doctors about side effects, but in only 1 instance had the doctor offered an alternative. In another 3 cases, doctors removed IUDs and suggested no other method. Seven women were offered no contraceptive advice at all, following delivery or a previous abortion. One was refused contraception after delivering an out-of-wedlock child because she was "still in high school."

"After personally interviewing each of the patients in this study," Robins concludes, "I am not convinced that any one of them was consciously using abortion as her primary method of birth control. Most seem to have been the victims of inadequate or poor advice" from their doctors.

Some of the women in the Robins study were explicitly given incorrect information by physicians; were told, for example, that they could not get pregnant because they were nursing or had retroverted uteri.

In a California report on 692 women seeking abortion at Stanford, many (according to the psychiatrist who evaluated them) showed "a lack of understanding of conception and contraception." Only a small minority of the women depending on rhythm were actually well informed about the facts of ovulation and correct use of this method. Adolescent and menopausal women were especially "vulnerable" to the medical myth that they were unlikely to conceive because of "subfertility."

His Turn? Methods of Contraception for Men

Although it's a well-known fact that it takes two to make a baby, contraception in general is viewed today as a woman's problem. Since *she* has the most to lose (or gain) by becoming pregnant, prevention—and the details of it—rest mainly in her hands.

Partly as a result of today's egalitarian movement, partly because of the economy, perhaps also because of a rising consciousness of population control, men and women are coming to regard contraception as a shared problem.

There seems to be a stumbling block that hinders development of new contraceptives for men. We think it is the belief, conscious or not, on the part of male doctors and researchers, that it is dangerous—if not blasphemous—to fool around with the male reproductive system. And since so much has already been done in the area of contraceptives for women, the argument seems to go, it hardly seems necessary, does it? Also, for men who wish to participate in birth control, there's always the condom.

In spite of the current popularity of the pill and the IUD for women, condom sales have not declined. But as a regular form of birth control among most couples, it seems to be not completely satisfying. Increased availability and a better image might improve the use of this very practical method.

Vasectomy is an increasingly popular method among middle-aged men who have already completed their families, but there is so much confusion and misconception about this operation that it is the exceptional man who will seek this method of birth control. And, also, the operation is not without some risks.

But a pill for men—that seems to be the magic solution that many modern-thinking people of both sexes are waiting for. The surprising thing is that unbeknown to most people, it's already here! It is legal, it is available, it is effective. It has already been used by hundreds of thousands of men—but not as a contraceptive. The pill we are talking about is the combined androgen and estrogen drug that is given for osteoporosis, a common bone disorder among older men and women, and for complaints of "male menopause." It has shown itself, in testing on young males, to be an effective suppressant of sperm. Why hasn't this drug been hailed and rushed into production especially as a contraceptive? After all, as a prescription drug, it would still be doctor-controlled, so that can't be a factor in its poor reception.

Maybe the reason is that the men taking it showed some of the uncomfortable side effects that women on the pill have. Unlike some of the unfortunate women who took the pill, no man has died from taking this male counterpart. But like women who use hormones, some of the men got nausea or temporary changes in sex drive.

On the other hand, some of them, like some pill-using women, felt just fine.

CHAPTER 19

King Condom

Like the lead pencil, the bicycle, and the razor blade, the humble condom is holding its own in a sea of technological wonders—*more than* holding its own. Worldwide, the condom, or sheath, which was invented by an Italian anatomist in 1564, is still the number-one method of birth control, the *preferred* method in such sexually sophisticated, low birth rate nations as Japan, England, and Sweden!

The Japanese, especially, enjoy Japanese-made condoms, which, as we shall see, are only one-third to one-half as thick as ours, and the placing of which, during foreplay, is considered not an interruption but an erotic art.

The Swedes appreciate the condom, for it has helped them reverse a galloping VD epidemic and is now widely advertised and promoted for that purpose. (On U.S. television, by contrast, institutional ads telling viewers to get VD checkups are deemed acceptable, while ads informing them that condoms *prevent* the spread of VD are *not*. One out of 4 high school students does not even know that condoms serve this prophylactic purpose.)

Over the centuries, condoms have been fashioned out of linen, animal skins, sheets of gold, nylon, plastic film, and the intestinal membranes of lambs, calves, and goats. Vulcanization, perfected in the 19th century, led to the mass production of latex rubber condoms, which sold for about fifty cents each (and were reusable) at the turn of the century.

The Advertising Blackout

In the United States, Merry Widows, as they were called, became an under-the-counter item in the 1860s and '70s, when widespread vice laws banned contraceptives as "obscene" articles. Today, in a number of states which continue to restrict their distribution, sale, advertisement and display, condoms are—incredibly—an under-the-counter item still.

But even in states where laws are not prohibitive, condoms are associated with prostitution in many people's minds, and so are regarded as less savory than most other "personal products" and birth control methods. Thus hemorrhoid preparations, vaginal deodorants, and jockey shorts are acceptable for TV advertising, while condoms are not.

A survey of druggists taken in 1972 showed that about half would not sell condoms to minors. As one pharmacist put it, "I tell them, 'Run along, sonny, and come back when you are a man.'"

Playboy magazine refused condom ads until 1970 on the grounds that it was reluctant to "disturb the euphoria of our readers." The *Journal of the American Medical Association* accepted *its* first condom ads in 1954, but the word contraception was notably absent. The ad featured Ramses as a trichomoniasis preventive, and was extremely subtle. The doctor would have to study it quite closely before he grasped what the product in question *was*. The first limited drugstore displays of condoms were granted the Schmid Company, makers of Ramses, in 1955.

After the great *Playboy* breakthrough, some other print media, including a few newspapers such as the *San Francisco Chronicle*, began to accept condom ads in the 1970s.

While the Schmid Company opted to emphasize the contraceptive value of its products, its major competitor, Young's (Trojans), decided to promote the condom's use as a VD prophylactic as well. Here is Lewis R. Brenner, an executive at Young's Drug Products, describing his hardships from 1960 onward:

"Although we were a company with a reputation of almost fifty years for quality products and ethical distribution . . . no one in the media wanted to do business with us. Our advertising agency held a meeting in its offices with the editorial and advertising executives of some of the nation's leading periodicals; during this meeting we literally begged them to accept our hard-earned cash in return for the 'privilege' of using space in their publications to promote greater public awareness of the VD problem. Except that the corporate signature appeared at the bottom, the proposed first ads were not the least bit commercial; and yet, with one exception, no one would take our money—no one would run an ad presenting the facts about venereal disease and its preventability. . . .

"Finally, in June 1969, *Sport* magazine accepted an ad from Young's, the first consumer ad ever run anywhere in the country by any condom manufacturer. The ad simply said, 'VD can be prevented'; it consisted of approximately fifteen lines of type that did not even mention prophylactics or condoms in the body copy. . . . After the first ten insertions, however, *Sport* canceled our series. No one is yet sure why. . . .

"One of the biggest and earliest surprises was the refusal of *Playboy* magazine to take our advertising. *Playboy* finally accepted our VD prevention ads in 1972. . . .

"The reasons for rejection by various magazines and newspapers to our campaigns cover the whole range of human hypocrisy and ignorance.

"The *New York Times*, a leading liberal newspaper, ran a front-page article on venereal disease that included such topics as prevention, use of the condom, etc. It was excellent! Yet, the same week that this article appeared, they flatly rejected our all-copy ads talking about this same disease. . . .

"The list of recognized and 'reputable' publishing institutions that refuse fully paid advertisements of our products—products that would help prevent the leading reported communicable disease in the country—is rather long. Our files contain rejections from the late *Saturday Evening Post* and *Life;* from *Time, Newsweek, Ingenue, Woman's Day, McCall's, Cosmopolitan* (the magazine whose editor is Helen Gurley Brown, author of *Sex and the Single Girl,* and which featured Burt Reynolds in the nude as the first naked male centerfold), *Sports Illustrated, Good Housekeeping, Reader's Digest, Family Circle,* and more.

"The list of newspapers that have refused is equally long and equally ludicrous. The only papers in the United

States that have carried our ads are the *San Francisco Chronicle*, *San Francisco Examiner*, and *Los Angeles Times*. The same publications that refuse these ads gleefully seek and accept ads that promote the consumption of cigarettes and alcohol, products that have been known directly or indirectly to kill millions. Few of these newspapers refuse advertising promoting X-rated movies. Is it not strange that a newspaper would carry advertising for *Deep Throat*, but not for the prevention of venereal disease?"

One sympathizes with Mr. Brenner and with Samuel Baker, his counterpart at Schmid. It's tough to have a good product that's treated with disdain, even by such liberated editors as, say, Hugh Hefner and Helen Gurley Brown. When magazines do accept condom ads they usually isolate them, as if other advertisers would be contaminated by them.

The Matter of Size

American condoms *are* good products for birth control and VD prevention. They are the longest, thickest, and most capacious in the world. On an open market, Japanese products are usually more popular as they are one-half to two-thirds thinner; they come in small, medium, and large and in pretty colors as well. (The Japanese have specialized in condoms and in foam; Japanese women do not use the pill or the IUD.) Since 1938 our FDA has set rigorous condom standards, which apply to goods sold in machines and dispensers in some states as well as drugstores. The thickness of American condoms ranges from .05 to .09 mm.

They are tested electronically for pinholes by the manufacturer, inflated with air and filled with water to check burst and tensile strength by the FDA, and guaranteed to have a shelf life of at least two years. Those condoms that are properly packaged last well, both in dispensing machines and on drugstore shelves.

Some authorities think that American condoms would be more popular if they weren't quite such a barricade. And their size *has* been an embarrassment in some developing countries, as the following editorial translated from a Thailand newspaper reveals:

CONDOMS OF THE WRONG SIZE
[Column of April 1, 1973]

The population problem is becoming big fun, and even America seems to be joining in the fun. . . .

The Agency for International Development sent condoms named "Silvertex" for Thais to try using, and it turned out that these condoms used for birth control were too big and too long for Thai men. Officials of the family planning project in Sara Buri province reported that complaints were received from men who are ordinary members of the public, and who had had "Silvertex" distributed for them to try and use. The complaint indicated that these condoms did not obtain much result because they could not be kept in place, and a string had to be used to tie them to the waist, due to their size not fitting.

Such an incident should have never occurred. It causes suspicions from the start that AID had not realized at all that the "Silvertex" it had been so kind as to send were of the "wrong" size. . . . AID must be a big organization that is very strange, because such a problem is a very preliminary one that should have been fully realized, since it is utterly impossible for "Silvertex" produced for use by American men to be of a size to fit Thai men. . . .

AID might believe that Thai men are not particular, that so long as the thing given can help in birth control that they would be satisfied. . . .

Though Thailand might be behind the fashion to a considerable extent in various other matters, the sexual taste of Thais is most particular and fussy. . . .

The "Silvertex" sent by AID moreover emphasized their excellent quality and flexibility, that they make sexual feeling almost like normal, as when no condoms are used. But when used, it turned out that the extent of their flexibility was minimum, causing hardship to men using them who had to find a string to tie them to their waist for the sake of safety. The use of this string caused considerable inconvenience, while at the same time becoming an obstacle obstructing their sexual feeling in an unnecessary manner. . . .

Since the problem has reached this extent, nothing can be done to remedy it, except to send these "Silvertex" of the "wrong size" back to AID in order that they could be made use of by American men.

Advantages and Disadvantages

American men generally prefer not to use the condom because it interferes with sensation. Few women are troubled on this score—many in truth cannot even guess correctly whether a condom is being worn—although there are some exceptions. Some women report soreness following intercourse with male partners using condoms. If a woman is inadequately lubricated, or the condom improperly fitted to the man, it's possible her vagina could be irritated.

The main objection of women to the condom is that they are *unaware of its reliability*. In a recent study of families having trouble with birth control (each couple had at least four pregnancies in the previous six years), free condoms were distributed first by a social worker, and then by mail. Subsequently, there were only 2.8 pregnancies per 100 women per year, making this a *more reliable* method than most IUDs.

And, it could be more reliable yet!

We interviewed a 76-year-old woman who, in her lifetime, had two pregnancies (both planned) despite an exceptionally active participation in sex.

"I never understood this fuss about birth control," she told us. "I always made my husband or lovers use a condom, and *they had to test it first*—in front of me. I watched them while they filled it with water, or blew it up like a balloon. Maybe that sounds unromantic, but abortion seems a lot worse."

The teen-age VD and out-of-wedlock pregnancy rates are both climbing precipitously. Were the condom readily available and still in fashion with male adolescents, neither of these problems would have reached such proportions. High school boys have difficulty buying condoms. A recent Planned Parenthood study of 421 northeastern high school boys living in a large city turned up the rather startling information that the *mean* age for starting sex relations was only 12.8 years, at which point knowledge of conception and VD prevention was minimal. Sophistication did *not* increase with age, and the oldest group (18 to 19) achieved identical information scores with the 12- to 15-year-olds.

It appears that the 1960s revolution in female contraceptive technology has freed many young American males of any sense of responsibility they may once have had. And it appears that those who *want* to use condoms—

for whatever reason—have trouble getting them and would much prefer that they be dispensed in anonymous machines, while pharmacists and, indeed, most condom manufacturers prefer to restrict them to drugstore sale. Despite what almost seems a conspiracy to keep condoms unavailable to teen-agers, insofar as the youngest age groups use *any* method, this is the one.

Packaging and Selling

Controversy surrounds the reliability of drugstore *vs.* machine-dispensed condoms. Some observers, including Consumers Union, point out that the drugstore brands, especially Schmid and Young's, have the best quality-control records (in terms of avoiding FDA seizures for pinholes and so on) and are therefore preferable. Other authorities argue that machine brands can be and usually are perfectly good, and do not deteriorate faster than drugstore brands *if* they have been hermetically sealed. Pharmacists naturally oppose efforts to place free-standing vending machines in their communities, and so do the condom companies, whose goods enjoy longstanding drugstore distribution. Yet, so long as many pharmacists refuse to service minors, these exclusionary policies contribute to all the social evils that condoms could help prevent.

In the United States, the largest manufacturer of condoms sold by machine and nonpharmacy outlets is Ackwell Industries, which coincidentally is also our largest balloon maker. Schmid's and Young's products are merchandised through 50,000 drugstores and to a smaller extent by mail. A fourth company, Circle Rubber, manufacturer of brands such as Saxon and Prince, is starting to capture a significant share of the market.

Only American-made condoms, or those which meet our standards, are legally available in the United States. Every country has its own, perhaps arbitrary, requirements. Some experts such as Dr. Philip Harvey, director of Population Services at the University of North Carolina, Chapel Hill, urge that thinner, Japanese-style condoms ought to be allowed here too. There might be a very slight loss in reliability, Harvey argues (1 added pregnancy per 2.5 to

5 million acts of love), but this, he believes, would be more than made up for by the greater willingness of users.

Condoms made from natural animal tissue (the sheep cecum, imported mostly from New Zealand and Australia) are said to transmit heat and provide a higher degree of sensitivity than any latex product. Brand names of skin condoms include Schmid's Fourex, Young's Naturalamb, and Crest Skins. These cost a dollar or more each, several times the price of latex condoms. However, some users find that skin condoms actually *enhance the man's pleasure* when the evaporating lubricant creates temperature changes. (Cecum condoms must be lubricated with a wet substance which makes the condom cling to the penis, since the lack of elasticity does not otherwise permit a snug fit.) Many men agree that skin condoms interfere the least with sexual feeling, although some find them "messier" to apply, or they worry more that the condom might slip off. (It doesn't, even though it may *seem* insecure at first to a man who is accustomed to the tighter-fitting latex variety.) Five to 10 percent of American condom users buy skin brands. The figure might well be higher if they were not so costly. Skin condoms may be less likely to burst, especially on men who are generously constructed.

Very recently, U.S. manufacturers have started imitating Japanese condom design, so that our own new products are much more attractive and colorful. Unfortunately, the FDA will still not permit our manufacturers to compete with the Japanese for thinness. The Schmid Company, besides marketing its traditional Sheiks, Ramses and Fourex Skins, is now putting out such brands as Excita, Fiesta, Nuform, and Fetherlite.

The theory of American condom manufacturers that "one size fits all" doesn't seem to hold up any more than it does for, say, women's pantyhose. There are always those persons at both ends of the scale who get poorly fitted. So as not to embarrass men who would have to ask for "small," manufacturers could make condoms in A, B, and C sizes—after all, small-breasted women are not upset by buying A-cup bras. The condom companies could go all out and give their sizes fancy, macho names such as "Ferrari," "Jaguar," and "Rolls Royce." Or perhaps take a tip from the olive companies, who bottle olives in sizes "Jumbo," "Colossal," and "Super-Colossal." Not only comfort, but reliability also is at stake. Just as average-sized condoms slip off men in the smaller range, they break when the user is extra well endowed.

How to Select American Condoms

Condoms are available dry or lubricated. Most users prefer lubricated brands, for lubrication factilitates entry, decreases chances of breaking, and increases sensitivity. Some lubricants have a slight medicinal odor which may be perceived as unpleasant. A dry or "silicone" lubricant is preferred by many, for it is odorless and provides a slippery surface rather than a wet one.

There are several variations in condom shape, which have long been popular in Japan and England but are newer to the United States. Some men, and women, do have personal preferences that can only be learned through trial and error. Preshaped condoms may reduce the chance of slipping, and are also preferred by some as being more sensitive.

Transparent condoms are generally, but not always, preferred to opaque. Color preferences are highly personal and have little bearing on the skin color of the user. The blond Swedes especially like pale green and black models, while in black Kenya, blue and white are the favorites.

While the quality of American condoms is consistently high, according to Harvey, the packaging factor also bears on reliability. Minor damage to the condom between purchase and use is probably a more significant reason for failure than defects in the manufacturing. When condoms are not hermetically sealed, there is an increased chance that dirt or other particles may damage the latex, especially if the contraceptives are carried around in wallets. Harvey suggests that the preferred condoms for clinics to stock should be hermetically sealed, transparent, and silicone-lubricated. There are many brands of this description.

Couples who have never tried skin condoms, or the newer, more sensuous latex brands, might be quite surprised and pleased.

Correct Use

A condom should be placed on the erect penis prior to intercourse, *not just before* ejaculation, for the following reason: Most men, when sexually aroused, secrete several drops of pre-coital fluid. In some, a minority, these contain a sufficient number of live sperm to cause fertilization. If the condom does not have a reservoir tip, a half inch of space should be left at the end to catch the discharge without bursting the rubber.

When dry condoms are used, lubrication of the outside, with a spermicidal cream or jelly, prevents tearing and facilitates entry. *Do not use Vaseline for this purpose as it can deteriorate the rubber.*

Some condom users suggest that a small amount of foam or cream inside the condom enhances the man's pleasure, just as foam or cream applied to the outside of the condoms may heighten the pleasure of the female partner.

After intercourse, when the penis is withdrawn, the rim at the base of the condom should be held secure to avoid spillage.

The ecologically minded should not dispose of their condoms down the toilet. Recently, fish have been found strangled by condoms wrapped round them.

Here is a rundown of the current selection of Schmid products, with descriptions by the manufacturer and wholesale prices. Condoms made by Young's and the other companies are fairly equivalent. A young volunteer named Jonathan tested some of these for us; his comments are included.

FOUREX SKINS CAPSULE PACK
Made from natural animal tissue that has the texture and sensitivity of soft skin. Lubricated inside and out for added comfort and sensitivity. Natural aqueous lubrication. Folded and packed in a blue capsule.
1 doz. $8.50 . . . 3 doz. $22.00 . . . 6 doz. $41.00
Jonathan thought this one would feel really special and was disappointed.

XXXX FOUREX SKINS FOIL PACK

Made of natural animal tissue. Lubricated inside and out for added comfort and sensitivity. Packed in foil for added convenience.

1 doz. $8.50 . . . 3 doz. $22.50 . . . 6 doz. $41.00

Same as above.

EXCITA

Unique flared and combined with ribbed surface, creating a new dimension in stimulation for the female through a gentle massaging action while at the same time providing sensitivity for the male

1 doz. $4.50 . . . 3 doz. $11.00 . . . 6 doz. $19.50

Jonathan rated this one as least objectionable; almost lives up to its name, he says.

FIESTA

Exotic pastels—pink, yellow, blue, green—and black. A change of pace for those who want to try something different. Lubricated with Sensitol for greater sensitivity.

1 doz. $4.50 . . . 3 doz. $11.00 . . . 6 doz. $19.50

Jonathan chose black, then decided it lacked aesthetic appeal.

NUFORM LUBRICATED

Latest development among condom shapes. Flared and provides a loose fit around the male glans (greatest concentration of nerve endings), permitting freedom of movement inside the condom. Greater sensitivity for the male. Attractive coral-colored, lubricated with Sensitol.

1 doz. $4.00 . . . 3 doz. $10.00 . . . 6 doz. $18.50

Jonathan was unimpressed with the shape; overrated, said he.

RAMSES SENSITOL LUBRICATED

The standard for high quality among condoms. Transparent, lubricated with Sensitol for exceptional sensitivity, plain end, packed in gold foil.

1 doz. $4.00 . . . 3 doz. $10.00 . . . 6 doz. $18.50

Jonathan rated this one as okay.

NUFORM NONLUBRICATED
Flared end, provides loose fit around male glans, permitting freedom of movement inside the condom. Great sensitivity. Nonlubricated.
1 doz. $3.75 . . . 3 doz. $9.50 . . . 6 doz. $15.00
Jonathan rated this, and the other nonlubricated models, as most uncomfortable, just as Dr. Harvey says.

RAMSES NONLUBRICATED
Transparent, hardly noticed when worn, plain end, nonlubricated.
1 doz. $3.75 . . . 3 doz. $9.50 . . . 6 doz. $15.00
No again, for lack of lubrication.

FETHERLITE LUBRICATED
Extra thin, coral-colored, lubricated with Sensitol, plain end. Popular price.
1 doz. $3.25 . . . 3 doz. $7.50 . . . 6 doz. $13.50
Jonathan said this seemed no different from Ramses Sensitol Lubricated. The price is lower.

SHEIK SENSI-CREME LUBRICATED
Reservoir end, highly sensitive, lubricated with Sensi-Creme for greater aesthetic appeal. Popular price.
1 doz. $2.75 . . . 3 doz. $7.00 . . . 6 doz. $13.00
Jonathan said the condom is okay but the reservoir end doesn't seem necessary.

SHEIK NONLUBRICATED
Attractively opaque, reservoir end, popular for over forty years. Unsurpassed for functional utility. Very economical.
1 doz. $2.25 . . . 3 doz. $5.75 . . . 6 doz. $10.50
No, again.

To summarize the art of choosing and using condoms:
• Get them in the Orient if you can. They fit better and interfere with sensation less. Japanese condoms made for *import into this country* must still meet the thickness requirements of our FDA.

Some people think that Scandinavian and English condoms are better, too.

• Some people prefer the more expensive models, such as skin condoms, or (in Jonathan's case) the Schmid Company's Excita. But lubrication is the main issue to most users. Thus Jonathan found Sheik Sensi-Creme Lubricated, the second cheapest model in Schmid's entire line, to be as acceptable as most of the higher priced products. He found it *more acceptable* than the expensive products that lacked lubrication.

• Reliability is probably not affected by price, except where the cheaper brands are carelessly packaged. Look for products that are hermetically sealed. If the package shows any evidence of damage, throw the condom out or at least pretest it.

• If the packaging is adequate, condoms sold in dispensing machines are reliable, too. We would like to see such machines in every men's—and women's—public rest room. They would do more to stop the spread of VD, and of teen-age pregnancy, than any other simple change in our social customs.

• Condoms, as we have mentioned, were once considered a reusable contraceptive like the diaphragm. It was the man's responsibility to wash them, test them for leaks, dry them and dust them with powder. We have been able to find no recent research indicating which kinds of contemporary condoms are most durable, and would like to hear from readers who have experience in this matter.

• A reliable brand of contraceptive foam is a good back-up for *immediate* use (several applicators-full) on the rare occasions when condoms tear or slip off. This is a better bet than douching or jumping up and down. The condom, with foam as a fail-safe measure, is as reliable a method as the diaphragm or pill.

CHAPTER 20

Vasectomy: The Myths and the Facts

Vasectomy, or male sterilization, is a procedure by which the vas deferens, the internal tubes that carry sperm from the testicles to the penis, are either cut or blocked. As surgery goes, it is remarkably safe and simple (most of the time) and can be done in a matter of minutes in a doctor's office, or even in an assembly-line situation, such as the railroad station vasectomy booths in India.

The idea for this operation was first conceived about two hundred years ago by the great English anatomist John Hunter. Some years later his student, Sir Astley Cooper, perfected vasectomies on dogs. The first human use was as a means of reducing complications from prostate operations, a practice still observed by some surgeons. Then, at the turn of the 20th century, Harry Sharp, an Indiana physician, reported that he had performed some 500 vasectomies to discourage masturbation or sexual excess (whatever that is!). He helped popularize it also "as a means of preventing procreation in defectives."

Sharp's views did not enhance the operation's image, or endear it to normal men. It was generally reserved for the retarded, the criminal, and the mentally ill. In the 1920s, however, vasectomy grew chic among older men, when a Dr. Eugen Steinach promoted it mistakenly as a sexual rejuvenator.

It was not until after World War II that vasectomy was introduced as a general contraceptive, an event owed largely to the modesty of rural women in India and Bangladesh.

When family planners arrived in these provinces, all the respectable women fled. It was unthinkable, by their standards, to undress before the male physicians in order to have birth control devices prescribed or fitted. This

left the doctors with a need to shift their focus quickly—
to men. Someone remembered vasectomies, and from then
on the operation was vigorously promoted with "incentives"
or (some would say) bribes. Payments of cash, food, and
clothing were offered not only to men who would volunteer for vasectomy, but to canvassers who found them and
doctors who operated as well. Employed men were granted
six days leave with pay following vasectomy—a luxury
compared to the custom in the United States where most
patients resume work the next day.

But even without incentives, vasectomy quickly caught
on in the West. By the end of the 1960s, a quarter of a
million U.S. men were getting sterilized each year. In
1970, as news of the danger of the pill came out, the figure
suddenly tripled.

By 1976 Charles Westoff, director of the Office of
Population Research at Princeton, observed: "The most
dramatic change [in birth control] since 1970 has been
the acceleration of reliance on surgical sterilization." For
the first time, sterilization is, today, more popular than
the pill with all married couples over 25 or 30.

While generally most men who have vasectomies are
in their forties, the age of sterilization has steadily lowered
and, for the first time, many couples and individuals are
seeking it in *their early twenties*. Most doctors are still
reluctant to operate on the childless, but the Association
for Voluntary Sterilization (708 Third Avenue, New York,
N.Y. 10017) sometimes helps such candidates find a willing surgeon.

Reliability and Safety

Vasectomy has chalked up an amazing record. At first it
proved less reliable than expected, for, in a small percent
of cases, the severed sperm tubes mysteriously healed and
unexpected pregnancies occurred. In a landmark malpractice case in Pennsylvania, a patient attempted to sue
his surgeon and lost. The court concluded that the birth of
a normal healthy child was *not* a cause for damages.

Now that the procedure has gotten more sophisticated,
although it is not standardized—there seem to be as many
diverse vasectomy techniques as surgeons. Most prefer

local anesthesia, for example, but some advocate general. Some doctors make one incision in the scrotal midline, while others do one at the site of each vas. After cutting, they may seal the ends by any of a half-dozen ligating or clamping techniques. A few surgeons prefer absorbable materials, such as catgut, for stitches that do not require later removal, but others say silk, Dacron, cotton, or stainless-steel wiring is safer. A physician at the University of California Medical School, Dr. Stanwood Schmidt, employs an electric needle to scar the vas tissue, and claims he has had no failures in 1,500 successive cases.

At first the instruments used for vasectomy were borrowed from older procedures. Now an array of special tools are available, including hooks, clamps, staplers, and electrical spark boxes such as those used by Schmidt. In the 1970s, spontaneous regrowth of the vas has almost been eliminated, and vasectomy approaches perfect reliability, except for human error.

Such error may occur on the patient's part, or the doctor's. The patient *must not abandon other contraception* until his reproductive tract is fully cleared of sperm. This may take from five days to six months. The more ejaculations he has, the faster the clearance of sperm, and most men are sterile after ten to fifteen orgasms. Even so, for absolute safety it is essential to have sperm tests to ensure that sterility is established.

A few men, oddly enough, have an extra vas. If the doctor misses it, the man remains fertile.

Finally, a vas may be difficult to locate, and can easily be confused for an artery, or other structure, by an untrained eye. In one such case, in Cincinnati, the doctor cut an artery by mistake; the patient developed gangrene and his penis sloughed off. Needless to say, the doctor was not an experienced vasectomist.

Thus, however quick and simple the operation may seem, it is important to find a highly experienced surgeon. The candidate for vasectomy should ask his doctor not just how much he charges, or how he does it, but the number of previous vasectomies he or she has performed. (One of the busiest vasectomists in Chicago is a woman, Dr. Lonny Myers.) This is no situation to search out bargains. A report from the Sanger Research Bureau listed 6 failures out of 236 procedures the year its vasectomy service opened. Four of these failures were attributed to physicians in training, and 2 to general surgeons with little experience.

No vasectomy deaths have been reported in the United States, although in India a tragedy occurred in 1971, after 62,000 men were sterilized at a Family Welfare Festival. There were 5 deaths from tetanus infection—probably because the men applied cow dung to their wounds. Vasectomy should always be postponed if *any* infection is present, whether it be local or systemic. Men who have an exceptionally thick, tough scrotum also pose special problems, and should probably bypass this method of contraception, as should men with systemic blood diseases, like hemophilia.

Possible Side Effects

For a fortunate few, or maybe even half of all men, vasectomy is effortless and pain-free. But many men have some discomfort, if the truth be told.

Skin discoloration: This is caused by blood seepage resulting from anesthetic puncture. Usually concentrated in the scrotum, it may spread to the skin of the penis, the groin, inner thighs, or lower abdomen. Scary-looking, it is harmless, requires no treatment, and subsides within weeks.

Swelling: Like bruising and discoloration, this may occur in up to two-thirds of cases. It also subsides.

Pain: Difficult to measure, it may occur when the anesthesia is injected, when the vas is tugged into view, or when the operation is over. These sensations are all distinct. If the anesthetic needle touches the spermatic nerve, acute pain may ensue. The first intercourse following vasectomy is often painful, and some discomfort may persist at ejaculation for a number of months.

There are striking cultural differences in the perception of vasectomy pain. Koreans seem to mind the anesthetic needle most. Indians report pain in the legs, abdomen, or entire body, while Americans and Europeans do not. In a study of traditionally stiff-upper-lipped British patients, only 1 percent felt "excessive pain" or asked for more anesthetic.

Postoperative discomfort is usually relieved with ice packs and aspirin, and avoidance of strenuous exercise for a day or two. Occasionally, when masses of clotted blood form from injured vessels, the scrotum must be reopened and drained.

Infection: Superficial skin infections can occur three or four days after surgery, while deeper infections involving internal tissues may take longer to develop. Most respond well to antibiotics (which are sometimes given routinely) but, on occasion, reopening and drainage are needed.

Swelling and tenderness, which sometimes occur, may be treated with drugs, bed rest, heat, and the wearing of a suspensory. Most such symptoms can be controlled within a week.

Long-range effects and sperm antibodies: Vasectomy has grown so popular that in recent years a great many studies of after effects have been made. Generally the news is reassuring, far more so than the news concerning chemical contraceptives. Metabolism is apparently not affected by vasectomy, nor are there changes in testicular function or pituitary hormones. Spermatogenesis continues as before, although the sperm is prevented from passing into the semen.

There is a theoretical basis for concern, however. When sperm can no longer negotiate the vas, some of them leak into the bloodstream. One-half or more vasectomized males develop an immunity to sperm within their own body. To date, there is no physiological or statistical evidence that the condition causes any harm, or that antibodies attack anything other than wandering sperm. Some researchers maintain that these antibodies have only a beneficial effect (under the circumstances), assisting in the disposal of excess sperm.

Nonetheless, autoimmune responses are but little understood, and are thought to be associated with undesirable conditions such as arthritis. The presence of sperm antibodies *has* provoked controversy, and caution in some quarters. Time will tell whether vasectomized males develop a higher incidence of autoimmune disorders in middle and old age.

With our present knowledge, it seems unfair for the

medical establishment to warn against vasectomy, while endorsing the use of female sterilization, the IUD, and the pill. The dangers of these female methods are undeniable, while the dangers of vasectomy (in the hands, it must be emphasized, of a highly skilled surgeon) are only speculative.

Attitudes Toward Vasectomy

Surgery on the sex organs will undoubtedly have emotional consequences *some* of the time.

Arthur Godfrey, who is delighted with his vasectomy, and has recommended the procedure on television, cautions that it is not an advisable choice for men who have any doubt about their own masculinity. "I enjoy a healthy ego," he explained to us. "But vasectomy can be a real bummer for the insecure guy who is pushed into it by his doctor or his wife."

Most psychiatrists agree with Godfrey and, in Seattle, Dr. Merlin Johnson collected histories of 83 men who had emotional breakdowns following vasectomy. Johnson maintains that the operation has "a unique potential for serving as a focus in the family power struggle."

Outside of marriage, divorced men and bachelors who fantasize vasectomy will lengthen their list of conquests are sometimes disappointed. One explained to us: "The women I go out with just don't trust me. They still put in their diaphragms or take their pills. The doctor should give us tattoos that say, 'This model inoperable for procreation.' "

The vasectomized male must expect a lot of curiosity. Here is what happened to Jim Bouton, the sportscaster, former Yankee pitcher, and father of several children.

"There was an interesting reaction from a good friend of mine. . . . He said: 'My God, Jim. What did you do that for? You're so young.' I explained about not wanting more kids, and he said, 'But you still want sex, don't you?' I didn't know what he meant. 'You can't have an erection any more, right?' I told him a vasectomy has no effect on erection. 'Can you still have a climax? How does it feel when nothing comes out?' I told him that semen comes out and everything feels the same as before; there are just no sperm in the semen. Now, this friend of mine is a bright guy, but he was uninformed."

Bouton had some complications, as he explains, but he would still do it over.

"My own vasectomy took place one evening at my doctor's office. He gave me a choice of a general or a local anesthetic. I chose the latter and asked for a pillow to prop my head up so I could watch the operation. I joked about keeping an eye on him to make sure he didn't slip with the knife. Actually, I was curious. It turned out that the show was more interesting than I'd anticipated, because there were some complications. The doctor was not able to locate one of the two canals that carry the sperms. He probed for about forty-five minutes [the whole operation usually takes only about fifteen minutes], during which time the local anesthetic began to wear off and I had to be re-injected. Fortunately, a local requires only a pinprick in the skin of the scrotum—I didn't even flinch the second time. The reason he couldn't locate one of the canals [vas deferens] was because it had already been severed in an accident when I was a youngster. I suggested to the doctor that since only one canal needed to be tied off, he should be entitled to only half the fee. He didn't see it that way.

"Ordinarily there is no discomfort after a vasectomy, but forty-five minutes of probing for the nonexistent canal caused a hematoma [blood clot]. A swelling developed in the scrotum and became the size of my testicles, so it looked as if I had three testicles. This was sort of interesting, and I think I was a little disappointed when the swelling went away after two weeks.

"At any rate, I wouldn't hesitate to have the operation again—even with my unusual complications. The peace of mind has made sex much more enjoyable for my wife and me. And there seems to be some sex appeal connected, maybe with the freedom from worry about pregnancy. I was on a talk show with Germaine Greer who, when I told her I had had a vasectomy, said, 'That's the sexiest thing a man has said to me in a long time.'"

When asked about doing it over, or recommending it to a friend, most men—upward of 95 percent—express unqualified enthusiasm. Yet, in vasectomy research, there is a continuous hint that some patients may be mentally troubled, and that some marriages may get worse. Husbands may expect more gratitude than their wives wish to give them, or become less considerate in other respects. Hidden fears over masculinity can provoke macho behavior, premature ejaculation, or temporary impotence. An important series of studies from the Scripps Clinic indicated that a period of "decreased marital satisfaction," on the wife's part as well as the husband's, sometimes occurred following vasectomy. These problems were still noticeable two years later, but diminished after four.

Asian males, especially, say they have "body weakness" after vasectomy. This complaint is heard most often from men over 40. Other symptoms reported in Asian studies include insomnia, nervousness, headache, depression, and loss of weight. Western men rarely attribute such symptoms to vasectomy. Half to three-quarters report increased enjoyment of sex and an increase in spontaneity.

Some doctors try to "screen" vasectomy patients, eliminating those who have neurotic attitudes, hypochondriacal fears, or magical expectations. We feel, like Arthur Godfrey, that the *patient can best screen himself*. A man should never allow himself to be bribed or coaxed or bullied into a vasectomy; it's far too personal a matter.

If he wants one, he should screen his doctor carefully for his surgical skills. Patient should interview doctor, not vice versa.

But first, according to sociologist John Gagnon, a former Kinsey researcher, a man considering vasectomy must ask himself the following:

• Do you want more children?

• If your children died, would you want to replace them?

• Were you as rich as, say, the Kennedys, *then* would you want more children?

• If you broke up with your wife and she got custody, would you want more children of your own?

• Does the image of a knife being taken to your testicles give you the creeps?

Gagnon, who had a vasectomy twelve years ago, satisfied himself that his personal answer to all these questions was "no." Like Godfrey, Gagnon counsels that a man who has *any* doubts should pass up vasectomy.

CHAPTER 21

A Pill for Men

I was absolutely astonished when the first oral contraceptive [for women] was approved for sale. It seemed to me that we were just beginning to ask questions, and suddenly it was on the market.
Dr. Sheldon Segal, Biomedical
Director of the Population Council

The human male is a prodigious maker of sperm. In a single ejaculation he releases, to whatever destiny, some 80 million of these tiny life-bearing sex cells. Sperm are manufactured from precursory cells, in a process that takes about seventy days. Spermatogenesis is stimulated by two hormones, FSH and LH, which issue from the pituitary.

Once the female was also a prodigious bearer of eggs. She, or rather her fish and amphibian foremothers, deposited a milky "egg clutch" into sea water and tidal marshes. The male dropped off his sperm in the same neighborhood, and they merged.

Out of the primordial slime, the mammal, the primate, and humankind evolved. Evolution *depended on dramatic advances in female reproduction.* She reduced her cyclical egg release from an enormous quotient to a selected few or one. *She* retained the conceptus—the product of conception—within her own body, developed a placenta, and nourished her babies from her own blood and bones. The advances that make us human rest, as modern embryology explains it, on adaptations that the female of the evolving species made.

Male reproduction—and this is not to minimize its importance—is still much like reproduction in the amphibian and fish. Sperm production is extravagant, not conservative, and the male role is biologically ended when sperm go on their way. The reproductive role of woman is longer, harder, and much more dangerous to her.

Revolution. . . . Often it is sounded to drama, drums, and discussion, but sometimes it just settles over us like mist. While some fortunate women always had access to vaginal spermicides (Cleopatra, for example, used a mixture of honey and dried crocodile dung; see chap. 15) it was *male contraceptive methods*, first withdrawal, and later the condom, that drastically reduced the birth rate in modern times.

Carefully used, these are far more effective than modern people imagine, but each has obvious drawbacks. Although it requires skill and discipline, withdrawal was the sole method of contraception used by two-thirds of the couples in France and Hungary *until 1960!* The birth rate in these countries was admirably low. It shouldn't be overlooked as a method for emergencies.

Margaret Sanger, among other feminists, believed it was essential for birth control to be in women's hands, but, of the new devices, many have proved injurious to health. Senator Gaylord Nelson's hearings on the pill were forced to recess on January 23, 1970, after a raucous demonstration by Alice Wolfson and a group of young, articulate Washington, D.C., health feminists.

"Why are there no patients testifying?" the Wolfson women demanded. "Why is the press whitewashing all the adverse comments against the pill? *Why is there no pill for men?*"

Early Work on a Male Pill

The fear that a pill for men might alter male libido or the sex organs has been a major deterrent to research. *Hormones can have this effect on some users of either sex.* Masters and Johnson have stated that when a woman who was previously orgasmic loses her ability, the first question they must ask is: "Has she been taking the pill?"

Scientists view diminished *male* sex drive more ominously than the female equivalent. After all, they argue, libido is needed to *put sperm into action* but *not* to position the ova in place. Species continuation rests on the libidinous male. One government population official recently put it like this:

"Many women don't have those orgasms you read about, anyway. A lot of that Masters and Johnson and Women's Lib stuff is about the extremes, almost the abnormal. I never heard any hesitation based on whether the pill would affect whether a woman would have an orgasm."

Among the early human subjects to be tested for male fertility control were 8 psychotic mental patients in a Massachusetts state hospital. They received an early form of Enovid in the 1950s. Ten milligrams a day of Enovid had a definite sterilizing effect. However, one young man was found—at the end of the five and one-half months' trial—to have shrunken testicles; his scrotum had become "soft and babyish," according to his doctor's report.

The sex drive of these patients—they can hardly be called volunteers—was not, in general, altered by Enovid. Their psychiatrists kept an eye on them, and they masturbated as much or as little as before.

Therefore, although Enovid was early shown to work for men, the fellow with the shrunken testicles put a damper on follow-up experiments. His side effect was viewed more seriously, we are sorry to report, than the unexplained *deaths* of three Puerto Rican women, during some of the early experiments with the pill.

Sex hormones, whether taken by implant, injection, or mouth, turn off sperm production, just as they do ova production, because they "fool" the pituitary into diminishing its natural output of the pituitary hormones FSH and LH. Within about two months' time (seventy days), sperm will be gone from the semen. Any sex steroid may have this effect, but the pills used for women are too feminizing to be suitable for men. (In fact, it's a little startling to realize that experiments on human males, proving beyond any doubt that *various hormones produce infertility*, date all the way back to 1939.)

Why not use more malish hormones, the androgens? (Both sexes produce male *and* female hormones, actually, but in different proportions.) Testosterone-only contraceptives for men do not cause feminization but may pose other problems, such as heart attacks and an increase of red cells in the blood. (Pills for women also cause heart attacks and blood disturbances, but men fear the former more acutely since they are *normally* at greater risk.)

A logical solution is to find a combination of male and female hormones so balanced that they avoid feminization on the one hand, or immediate overstimulation of the heart, blood cells, and prostate on the other. Such products are being clinically tested by, among others, Dr. C. Alvin Paulsen of the University of Washington, and Dr. Julian Frick from Innsbruck, Austria. Paulsen and Frick are investigating different combinations of drugs, which, inconveniently, involve taking *both* oral pills and monthly injections.

Any contraceptive that works through pituitary suppression is bound to have some long-range effects on the total system. The pituitary mediates *many* body functions, and it is always chancy to tamper with it. Thus, at best, male contraceptives *based on hormones* are unlikely to be safer than the current female pills. They "pool" the risks, but do not eliminate them, and should provide a fine Sincerity Test for men who claim they would die for love.

A Male Pill That's Already Here

The Paulsen and Frick formulations will not reach the market for years—certainly not, it is estimated, until the 1980s. But there are already products on the shelves of every drugstore that promise to be just as suitable.

These are the previously mentioned androgen and estrogen combinations, currently marketed as a treatment for osteoporosis, or bone loss, in aging individuals of both sexes and for the syndrome some people call male menopause. Their effectiveness as a bone treatment is disputed, but *hundreds of thousands of men have taken them, usually for long periods.* Some of the preparations include vitamins and mood brighteners, in addition to their dual sex hormones. *One also contains speed,* and is understandably hard to give up. More than a dozen brands are available, including Ayerst's Mediatric and Formatrix, Lederle's Gevrine, Reid-Provident's Estratest, Schering's Gynetone, Upjohn's Halodrin, and many more.

Far from being feminizing, such products usually contain substantially more androgen than estrogen (up to 500 times as much!) and so—while they are promoted as suitable for men or women—their manufacturers usually issue warnings such as the following:

"Watch female patients closely for signs of virilization. Some effects, such as voice changes, may not be reversible even when the drug is stopped."

Recently, Drs. Michael and Maxine Briggs of the Alfred Hospital, Melbourne, Australia, discovered that elderly men who use these products develop evidence of severely reduced sperm production without any such side effects as developing breasts, shrunken testicles, or grossly abnormal libido changes. They called for younger volunteers and selected 5, who were instructed to take the osteoporosis pills twice daily with their meals.

At the end of the projected seventy days, or sooner, 4 of the 5 had stopped manufacturing sperm. The fifth patient took about twice as long, but finally he stopped also.

The Briggs volunteers stayed on the hormones for thirty-four weeks, during sixteen of which their wives gave up birth control. No pregnancies resulted. Sperm production returned to normal in all cases within five weeks after stopping the drug.

Three of the 5 men had occasional mild nausea, but there were no anatomical effects. Two complained of decreased libido in the first eight weeks, which then returned to normal for the remainder of the trial. Another man had an increased sex drive, which leveled off when he stopped the medication. A fourth reported no changes while he took the hormones, but a decrease in sex drive when he stopped. This outcome might puzzle readers who are unacquainted with the after effects of the female pill (see chap. 10). Any powerful drug suppresses some of our natural functions, which may in turn have some trouble reasserting themselves. As many of us have learned the hard way, we may be all too susceptible to a new infection right after taking an antibiotic.

What are the ethics of giving *an approved drug*, like these osteoporosis or male menopause remedies, *for an unapproved use*, such as contraception? Such questions are hotly debated among doctors, many of whom *do* prescribe hormones for purposes never dreamed of by the FDA or their own manufacturers. Two recent examples are the use of DES and Premarin as a morning-after female contraceptive, and a group of anabolic or "body-building" hormones, frequently prescribed to put flesh on athletes. Anabolic hormones could, in addition to building muscle, cause cancer of the prostate, breast cancer, and blood clots in athletes. They are rumored to have done just that to members of a professional football team.

Should any untoward effects occur, the doctor is in a weak legal position. However, he may get around it by asking the patient to sign a release.

This much can be said for the "new" male pill from Australia, limited as its contraceptive testing has been: A lot more is known about its side effects on men than was known about Enovid when *it* went on the market for women.

His Safety or Hers?

In return for the wonders it may perform, any hormone is bound to have side effects. To pass off such potent pharmaceuticals as "natural" is nothing but fraud. The honorable way to prescribe drugs is to admit the risks, and let the patient decide whether he or she wants to take them. The Rx pad belongs to the doctor—but the *body* is the patient's alone. To prescribe a drug without informed consent is a violation of the Bill of Rights, we think—a kind of chemical assault.

The female pill was approved after little testing (see chap. 7). The side effects of the pill are quite well known now, but 50 million women, worldwide, are willing to take it. The pill is still the preferred method of 1 in 5 fertile women in the United States. Its male "twin," however chancy, will find a market as well, for, contrary to predictions of drug manufacturers and some researchers, men are not unwilling to share the risks. When Dr. Paulsen of Seattle ran a small ad in a college newspaper asking for volunteers, he was overrun with responses. He and others who supervise male programs get letters today by the sackful.

Why has the research only just started? Why was

male contraception ignored for twenty years (the 1950s and '60s) while fortunes were being poured into finding new female products? Only in 1974 did funds for male studies start making any dent in the federal health budget. Nonprofit research groups, like the Population Council, are also supporting male projects, but not as generously as they might. Some $20 million is now being spent annually, the *Wall Street Journal* estimates, which is but one-fifth the amount needed to develop a contraceptive rapidly.

Unfortunately, drug companies have sharply reduced their efforts to develop new contraceptives. Many projects have been abandoned. Executives say they are disenchanted with stringent federal test requirements (making it take longer than formerly to get a new drug on the market) and with costly lawsuits over the pill and the IUD.

A spur to research has been the arrival of a new medical specialty called andrology, concerned with male fertility. Another spur was the feminist charge of discrimination—denied, at first, by scientists who then rallied rather quickly to correct their course. The effort to find a male pill is hardly of crash proportions, but it exists. It is taken seriously. It may bear fruit.

Must a male pill rely on hormones? We hope not. There may be better ways of interrupting male fertility, *without involving the pituitary and higher brain centers.* Theoretically, a *safer* pill for men than for women might be devisable, but no one knows yet for sure. Discussion centers on the greater complexity of the female system. Sheldon Segal estimates that *there are fourteen stages at which a woman's fertility might be interrupted, but only seven in men.*

These male-female differences are looked at two ways. It can be argued, and is in some quarters, that woman's greater complexity affords more chances for interruption. It can be, and is, conversely argued that man's greater simplicity yields more opportunity to intervene *locally*, without widespread bodily effects. In women, reproduction is intertwined with many other functions, more so than in men.

Another debate centers on the natural history of ova and sperm. Unlike woman, whose lifetime supply of eggs is intact at birth, man produces new sperm as he goes along for most or all of his adult time span. It is feared that an imperfect antifertility drug might allow a few damaged sperm to escape, producing defective fetuses. An opposing view is that permanent damage or latent drug effects on the sperm cells are less to be feared in the male. When he stops the pill he is set to manufacture brand-new sperm, whereas a woman's future-ripening ova might be residually influenced by a drug she once took.

Other Sperm Inhibitors

The hypothalamus, a walnut-sized collection of brain cells, might be called the conductor of our endocrine symphony (see chap. 25). In breakthrough research, Andrew Schally of New Orleans has recently isolated the hypothalamic chemicals that trigger the release of LH and FSH from the pituitary. Scientists in many laboratories are seeking hypothalamic suppressants based on his discoveries.

We mention Schally's work for its profound importance, as it much advances our knowledge of reproduction in both female and male. But we think it unlikely that a safe contraceptive will emerge from it. These hormones would affect both the hypothalamus and pituitary, and it is inadvisable to mess with them just for birth control. Local action in the genitals would be safer.

In England, Belgium, and Australia, scientists are working on a protein substance that might be able to block pituitary FSH secretion without altering LH. If the dream materializes, the protein may halt sperm production without at the same time inhibiting natural testosterone, or requiring supplements of the same.

Many drugs inhibit sperm formation in the testes or, if you prefer, testicles (the words are synonymous) without interfering with natural hormones. Thus far, all have exhibited unacceptable side effects, but the search goes on. One group, the nitrofurans, has had wide use as inhibitors of bacterial growth, but dosages high enough to sterilize are extremely toxic. Other sperm suppressants are found among cancer drugs and (at least in mice) in a sugar analogue.

In 1960 a drug to treat intestinal amoebae was tested on prisoners and completely suppressed their sperm. When tried on men enjoying more normal circumstances, it was noted that the drug had the effect of Antabuse, causing dizziness and vomiting when alcohol was consumed. It might still have been marketed for teetotalers, except that during the two-month recovery period, abnormal and bizarre sperm and heart irregularities were reported.

Drugless intervention, such as heat, x-ray, diathermy, and laser beams, may also inhibit sperm and are being investigated.

Heat experiments were initiated, years ago, by Dr. I. Tokuyama of Japan, whose volunteer medical students submerged their scrota in hot water baths for a half hour daily. Elevation of scrotal temperature by just a few degrees proved highly effective in sterilizing some men.

Next, Dr. John Rock, co-developer of the pill, got 75 of his students to either sit in hot water or wear insulated scrotal supporters—Rock's Hot Jock, they were nicknamed around Harvard. Now in retirement, Rock insists that the method *works*, but of course he was also the scientist who declared the pill to be safe.

In any case, Rock says that of his 75 volunteers only 1 complained of a side effect—sweating—and one other failed to show the usual reduction in sperm count. Subsequently, the wives of a number of these students conceived and bore normal children.

There is little question that heat, including fever, reduces fertility some of the time. Hippocrates was aware of this, and today the first thing specialists tell their *infertile* patients is to stop wearing tight jockey shorts and trousers which, by generating heat in the scrotum, inadvertently sterilize some stylish men.

The great promoter of TMS (shorthand for "the thermatic method of temporary male sterilization") has been Martha Voegeli, an indomitable Swiss physician using TMS in India since 1912.

Here is how she describes her method: For three weeks, a man takes a daily forty-five-minute bath in water of 116 degrees Fahrenheit. He then remains sterile for six months, after which normal fertility returns. If desired, the treatment can be repeated. (We suggest that men who try this get a sperm count done afterward to make sure it worked.)

At the University of Missouri, Dr. Mostafa Fahim, chief of Reproductive Biology, has been studying ultrasound for many years and has already designed a chair apparatus to administer ultrasound birth control in doctors' offices. He dreams that an ultrasound machine could become a standard home bathroom fixture. His trials on humans are mired down by requirements that, for the time being, he try ultrasound only on men with prostatic cancer, who (should the ultrasound prove dangerous) are already in line to have their testicles removed. At last report he'd located only one such patient—and he must find ten before he can proceed with healthy humans. Fahim complained: "We inject hundreds of chemicals into the woman's uterus but we never touch the testes." Some of the most militant feminist supporters are men who are trying to do contraceptive research—on their own sex.

What DES Taught Us About Male Fertility

After leaving the testes, sperm move on to the epididymis, a compact two-inch oblong tissue lying within the scrotum, against each testicle, and containing six or more yards of tubing. Here in the epididymis, where sperm remain for about two weeks, maturation and storage take place. The epididymis is highly sensitive to drugs, and in theory could be "selectively" treated without ill effects on other system. When epididymal function is altered, sperm may be produced in normal numbers, but won't be competent to fertilize eggs.

At Cornell University, Dr. C. Michael Bedford, a veterinarian-physiologist, is doing important research into these crucial but long-neglected components of male reproduction. We are still a long way from a safe epididymal suppressant, but if and when it arrives, it might be the ideal method we have all awaited.

Recently, the epididymis has been in the news for a most unfortunate reason. Sons of mothers who were given the hormone DES to strengthen their pregnancies have a 10 to 25 percent incidence of cysts of the epididymis, which impair fertility. The same effect has been observed in laboratory animals.

Most of these DES sons are perfectly normal in other

respects, which reaffirms scientific belief that the epididymis is an especially susceptible target organ (see chap. 4).

Sperm Switches, Sperm Banks

Sperm is formed in the testes, matured in the epididymis, and transported in the vas deferens, the spaghetti-like site where male sterilization—vasectomy—is performed. *Reversible* vasectomies, or "sperm switches," involving clamps, plugs, and faucets, have been so discussed and prematurely publicized that many men ask for them, thinking they are available.

They are not. While research continues at ten universities and private laboratories, many observers are doubtful of success—ever. A narrow living channel like the vas is all too apt to scar over any temporary blockage, making the blockage permanent. No man should agree to be a test subject for one of these devices unless he is prepared to accept final sterility.

If "sperm switching" does not seem imminent, "sperm banking"—that is, preserving live sperm by freezing—prior to vasectomy may have a better chance. Animal sperm banks, especially for cattle, have been highly successful, but, in humans, the resurrection of frozen sperm still remains iffy. It is no more than 70 percent successful, tops. No one yet knows why some sperm can take freezing and others not.

Seminal fluid has an amazing composition, which includes trace metals such as iron, zinc, and magnesium, and carbohydrates that appear to be an important source of energy for sperm. An alcohol which may be oxidized into fructose, a sugar, is also present in the human variety.

Certain oral medications such as sulfonamides may be traced in seminal fluid. Thus it is possible that the right oral drug might so influence the fluid as to keep the sperm from "capacitating." Sperm are not fully competent (capacitated) until they traverse the cervical mucus and womb, on their way up the Fallopian tubes to the ultimate egg. The apparent purpose of seminal fluid, the ejaculate, is to carry the sperm from male to female. Still, its chemical complexity, including so much nourishment, suggests that it also plays a part in the sperm's final development. Products that inhibit capacitation on the sperm's last journey might either be added to the seminal fluid, or given to the woman.

When a woman is fertile, the progress of sperm through her vagina, cervix, and womb has been likened to spinning along on a turnpike; other times in her cycle, the sperm's journey is more like slogging through a swamp. Altering of the chemical environment provided by *her vagina* as well as by *his seminal fluid* both offer possibilities for relatively safe birth control.

Foundations and government bodies say that they want to develop new contraceptives for men. Until the 1970s they merely chortled at the notion, so it appears that genuine progress is afoot.

But, as Dr. Philip Corfman of the National Institutes of Health explains, a lot of research that *sounds* maleish could just result in more new products for women to use. Sperm capacitation is an excellent example; contraceptives ensuing from these studies could well be vaginal suppositories or further female pills.

In the meantime, men who truly want to "participate" could experiment with TMS, according to Martha Voegeli's instructions. They could ask their doctors for one of the male menopause treatments, employed by Michael and Maxine Briggs; or they could buy quality condoms, thin ones, in Japan. They could go to France or Hungary for tutoring in withdrawal and, of course, they can get a vasectomy, too.

ERT: Promise Her Anything, but Give Her . . . Cancer

The human life span is divided into five stages: childhood, puberty, maturity, climacteric, and old age. Climacteric covers a span of fifteen years, from about age 45 to 60, and involves gradual changes in all body tissues. Sometime during a woman's climacteric, usually at around age 50, menopause, or cessation of the menses, occurs. For growing numbers of women, menopause occurs earlier through the intervention of surgery.

At the 1970 census, there were 104 million women in the United States, of whom 1 in 4 was aged 50 or over. The 50-year-old woman has a remaining life expectancy of twenty-eight years. She is told that estrogens may prolong her life, and that estrogens may shorten it. She is understandably confused, and yet in the decade from 1965 to 1975 prescriptions for ERT nearly tripled in this country. ERT, or estrogen replacement therapy, is the term we shall use for all the hormone preparations that are employed to "treat" or "prevent" disorders of aging. These often combine estrogen in various forms with tranquilizers, vitamins, testosterone, and even "speed."

The woman who takes the pill feels doubt and confusion also, but at least the pill works, as claimed, to prevent pregnancy. ERT is an iffier proposition, proven effective for only two of the twenty-six so-called menopausal symptoms for which it is prescribed.

In 1971, when the Herbst studies connecting DES with vaginal cancer were published in the *New England*

Journal of Medicine, cancer experts saw at once that the significance went far beyond DES use in pregnancy, for Herbst had shown that estrogen could be "seed" as well as "fertilizer" to cancer in humans.

Scientists at our National Institutes of Health were deeply concerned. They knew that the use of ERT was rising, and on little sound basis. They called a meeting of international research authorities, which convened in Hot Springs, Arkansas, in May 1971. The results of the conference, called *Menopause and Aging,* were published by the Government Printing Office, and remain available for 85 cents.

The preface pointed out that opinion is polarized on the dangers of ERT, and the benefits uncertain. It deplored "the lack of information and data on the menopause as a total process in the human female."

Despite lack of information and data, *and* the proven carcinogenicity of at least one estrogen, DES, the sales of ERT, especially of Premarin, continued to rise. In 1973, *Medical Letter* sounded an urgen note of caution: ". . . The manufacturer's advice to 'Keep Her on Premarin' seems unwise. . . . References frequently cited in promotions of estrogens . . . present personal opinion . . . or poorly controlled studies . . . or no criteria for defining such vaguely characterized states as melancholy, diminished sense of well-being, and decreased vitality. . . . The *Medical Letter* advises against the routine prescribing of estrogens during and after the menopause because there is no adequate evidence that such treatment is beneficial, and because . . . estrogens may promote or aggravate cancer . . . in some women."

By 1975, when a series of studies established that *ERT increases the risk of endometrial cancer,* the risk accelerating with years of use, *Premarin had become the fourth or fifth most popular drug in the United States.* Six million women were taking it, some of them starting in their thirties just to "prevent aging." Some, incredibly, were taking Premarin and the pill simultaneously.

In the following chapters we will discuss what is currently known—that is, *agreed on* by research scientists and, at long last, the laggard FDA—about the risks and benefits of ERT, including which conditions it works for, which it *may* work for, those in which it is no better than a placebo, and those in which it has now been proven downright dangerous. The different ERT preparations and the controversy concerning their relative safety will be described in detail. And in the section following that, we will present a comprehensive catalogue of all the treatments that are alternatives to ERT—for preserving health, good looks, and vigor generally, and for the special symptoms of menopause that trouble some women.

CHAPTER 22

Menopause, Money, and Depression

*It is no wonder that . . . women become depressed
around the time of menopause; professionals and
society have helped to ensure this reaction. At an
age in life when a man is in the upswing of active
social and professional growth, woman's service to
the species is over. Professionals, including female
experts, define the woman's role as one of mortifica-
tion and uselessness.*

> Howard Osofsky and
> Robert Seidenberg,
> *American Journal of Obstetrics
> and Gynecology,* 1970

If they could see how ERT is advertised to doctors in the
medical journals, many women would be shocked.

The ads assume that the climacteric woman is like a
neurotic child, a nuisance to her husband as well as her
doctor, a kill-joy to her family and friends, and the scourge
of her children.

A recent ad for one ERT product, Ogen, depicts a
woman dressed for travel and clutching Delta Air Lines
tickets, but unable to get up from her chair. Her impatient
husband stands behind her, glaring at his watch. "Bon
Voyage?" says the copy. "Suddenly she'd rather not go.
She's waited thirty years for this trip. Now she just doesn't
have the 'bounce.' She has headaches, hot flashes, and she
feels tired and nervous all the time. And for no reason at
all she cries."

Another ERT ad states, unblushingly: "for the menopausal symptoms that bother *him* most." Again we see a
drab and unattractive woman, with her victimized husband
standing by.

And, in some ads, her children are victimized as well. A current entry from the Ayerst Laboratories, manufacturers of Premarin, depicts a harpy who has just done something awful, possibly hit her teen-aged son in the mouth, for his hand covers the lower part of his face and he appears rather in pain. He, his sister, and father are standing aside and staring at Harpy with loathing and fear. Father is comforting sister, who might be about to cry. Worst of all, father is clutching his *unfinished* newspaper.

The Premarin copy states: "Almost any tranquilizer might calm her down . . . but at her age, estrogen may be what she really needs." As there is no valid medical evidence that estrogen improves mental outlook, the ad cites patient testimonials: "Patients taking Premarin alone often report relief of emotional symptoms due to estrogen deficiency . . . and an improved sense of well-being."

The Ayerst Laboratories reverses the strategy in its promotions to women. Here, testimonials from doctors are offered: "While deep psychological problems often require specialized assistance, many doctors find a restoration of hormonal balance helps promote a sense of physical and emotional peace."

Departed mothers are also invoked in Premarin ads. One, which is captioned "When women outlive their ovaries," depicts a sturdy white-haired woman who is apparently the proprietor of a country general store and gas station. She is not like Harpy. She is smiling. She doesn't need Premarin because she is already on it. "I saw what happened to my mother," she says. "It wasn't just how she looked. There was her back, stiff and bent . . . bladder trouble. I dreaded it."

What are the facts? *Do* women "go crazy" during menopause? Are there true personality changes, real physical disabilities?

Depressed—Or Just Blue?

To answer this question it is necessary to distinguish between *transient blue moods* and *genuine depression*. Climacteric women do complain with slightly greater frequency than either young adults or old women of headaches, irritability, nervousness, and "feeling blue." These complaints understandably come most often from women who have severe hot flashes and sleep loss.

On the other hand, such emotional symptoms occur in *both* sexes, in all age groups, and, in fact, are more pronounced in adolescence than in climacteric. Part of the human condition, these complaints afflict men also.

Senator Gaylord Nelson put his finger on the nature of drug advertising during the hearings he conducted on this subject in 1974. Nelson had seen an ad in *Medical World News* for a potent tranquilizer and antidepressant called Triavil. The ad included a list of questions which, if answered affirmatively by the patient, were supposed to indicate that Triavil was needed.

"Here are some of the questions," said Nelson wrathfully:

" 'Lately, have you often felt . . . sad or unhappy? Pessimistic about the future? Disinterested in others? Disappointed in others? Disappointed with yourself? Easily tired?'

"Now I answered all of these 'yes.'

" 'Have you recently had difficulty making decisions?'

"I changed my vote twice in a month on the same issue."

There were some questions, such as "difficulty working?" which Nelson said he would answer no, but, he concluded, *"I think almost everybody is going to give a 'yes' answer to 70 percent of those questions, so you would end up with everybody on that drug every day."*

The incidence of severe depression, requiring psychiatric treatment, is not significantly higher in climacteric women than in other age groups. There is a 7 percent risk of manifesting an affective disorder (depression or mania) during menopause, and a 6 percent risk at other times. *After* menopause, dramatic improvement occurs in emotional as well as physical well-being. In fact, a new study has indicated that postmenopausal women have the least "psychiatric morbidity" of *any* age group!

Again, this is not to minimize the discomforts which some climacteric women experience. These may include nervousness, insomnia, hot flashes, fatigue, palpitations, and occasional difficulty in concentration and thinking. But, as Nelson said, many other people have some of these symptoms too.

The authors of *Novak's Textbook of Gynecology* maintain that *how* a physician and a patient interpret such symptoms is all-important. "Often the best supportive therapy for the menopausal woman is a sympathetic listener and a doctor who will take the time to explain the normal physiology underlying the menopause. A word of advice, encouragement, or comfort . . . may be more valuable than pills."

Unfortunately, it is easier to write a pill prescription and push it across a desk than to talk to a patient. Indeed, the standard way of terminating medical visits is to write a prescription. Many patients expect it, and fear that they do not get their money's worth if they leave the doctor's office without a piece of paper.

Not a True Antidepressant

Some women may believe that ERT relieves emotional symptoms, but this is not a direct effect of the estrogen. There are four other factors.

First, depression is almost always self-limiting, lasting a few days to a few years, and then lifting spontaneously. If a drug has been introduced during the interim, the patient may attribute her spontaneous recovery to the drug. The woman who goes to her doctor for ERT may also be taking more realistic steps to improve her situation, such as returning to school or taking a job.

Second, by controlling flashes and sweats—which may also produce insomnia—ERT does get at some of the precipitants of nervousness and anxiety. But these "vasomotor symptoms" can usually be controlled by safer remedies, as we shall see.

Third, unknown to the user, many ERT products also include powerful antidepressants, tranquilizers, or sedatives. If these are necessary, they would be better used alone.

Finally, studies of many pharmaceuticals—and especially mood drugs—indicate that inevitably some patients benefit from a placebo effect. To test such effects, patients are divided into three categories: those who are untreated, those who are treated with a placebo, and those who receive an active drug.

In a typical two-month study of an *effective* antidepressant, the results are usually something like this: 30 percent of the untreated patients recover, 40 percent of the placebo patients recover, 70 percent of the treated patients recover. (One amusing study from England revealed that green placebos are better for anxiety and yellow placebos are better for depression.)

So far as mental symptoms are concerned, ERT must be viewed as a placebo, except, perhaps, when the symptoms are an outgrowth of vasomotor complaints. There is even some evidence that estrogens increase the undesirable physical side effects of antidepressants.

Attitudes Toward Menopause

While too little is known about the underlying physiology of menopause, women's adjustment to it has been very thoroughly charted. In contrast to the ads for ERT, and the personal beliefs of doctors who advocate its use, the data run in a different direction.

In a recent study of menopausal women, one respondent stated, sensibly: "Because you have been told you will feel depressed during the menopause, on a day things don't go right, it's tempting to attribute your mood to menopause. If you were 21, it would be because your period was due."

There is one subgroup of women who are apt to suffer depression, real depression requiring treatment, in the climacteric period of their lives. These are devoted mothers who experience "role loss"—the empty-nest syndrome, when their children grow up and leave home. Such depressions seem to be especially characteristic of some Jewish women; sociologist Pauline Bart called her study of this syndrome "Portnoy's Mother's Complaint." However, the essential factor is "an overinvolved or overprotective relationship with one's children," and, adds Bart, "You don't have to be Jewish to be a Jewish Mother."

Portnoy mothers are apt to have busy or neglectful husbands, and not to have been in the labor force themselves. They feel useless and lonely when their children no longer need them. They have been, as it were, forced into early retirement from their only job. They make comments like:

"I'm glad that God gave me . . . the privilege of being a mother . . . and I loved [my children]. In fact, I wrapped my love around them. . . . My whole life was that, because I had no life with my husband. . . . The children should have made me happy . . . but it never worked out."

It is sad that such women live in a society of nuclear families rather than in extended families were mothers-in-law and grandmothers play a more valued role. It is sad that jobs are scarce for the middle-aged, maternally minded woman, for there are many kinds of work at which she might be wonderful, despite a lack of formal training. However, these problems are personal and cultural and merely *coincide* with menopause. They cannot be cured by ERT.

The Menopausal Woman's Image

We think that the climacteric woman is amazingly resilient, considering how poorly she is treated in our society. There has hardly been another culture, past or present, primitive or "advanced," where the climacteric woman, at least the one who is without good job skills and an income of her own, is so much in jeopardy.

In traditional Western society, before industrialization, women worked alongside their husbands in small businesses and farms. Men, because they were around their children much of the day, took a more central role in child rearing than they now do. Until about 1835, sex roles—in terms of work—were more interchangeable than they have been since. The woman whose children were grown did not feel obsolete.

Even until World War II, the older woman, if housebound and isolated, was still an object of some respect. If her husband abandoned or children neglected her, society disapproved of them. It disapproves no longer. The climacteric woman is ridiculed in the contemporary novel and film. As author Marya Mannes has observed, our sex-saturated society enshrines the 16-year-old as woman incarnate. The Goddess is now a teen-ager.

Anthropologist Marsha Flint has studied the role of older women in several diverse societies, such as the Rajput of Rajasthan in India, the Qemant in Ethiopia, the Hutterites in South Dakota, the Bantu of South Africa, and reports that they offer climacteric women new and more prestigious roles as reward for their maturity.

But, in our society, Flint concludes, "there is no reward for attaining menopause. In fact, for many women it is a time of punishment. . . . Fear begins at 40 and it's downhill after that, with death waiting at the end. . . . Today's woman . . . falls prey to such ludicrous fears as the end of her sexual desires or femininity. . . . Much of what we call 'menopausal symptomology' may well be culturally defined and engendered. . . ."

Menopause and Psychotherapy

Does psychotherapy help? Undoubtedly, for many therapists are changing their views of woman's role. Yet as recently as 1970, Howard Osofsky, a gynecologist, and Robert Seidenberg, a psychiatrist, pointed out in an article on menopause: "Some [traditional therapists] have urged as primary treatment that women use the pronoun 'we' rather than 'I,' and that they engage in occupational therapy such as tray painting, baby-sitting, gardening, and bandage rolling."

Not long ago, Seidenberg told a story in his book *Corporate Wives—Corporate Casualties* that illustrates some of the cultural prejudice women must combat as they approach the menopausal years. His true tale concerns a 40-year-old woman in a loveless marriage who became involved with a teaching colleague, aged 24. Her husband, a successful businessman, insisted she see a psychiatrist as a condition of the divorce she sought. The psychiatrist informed her that she "could not accept growing old," was "narcissistic," and "had been taken in by Women's Liberation rhetoric." After eight months of "treatment," he and the husband hospitalized her on a psychiatric ward. Luckily her brother, an attorney, intervened and helped to secure her release and her divorce. She married her lover and left the community.

Osofsky and Seidenberg urge that woman's "social expectation of submissiveness" be changed. The solution to the "menopausal syndrome," they believe, originates in girlhood. "From birth on females must be allowed to view themselves as full individuals with deep cognitive and emotional capacities. The intelligence and creativity of young girls must not be sacrificed at puberty, as they are today."

CHAPTER 23

The Selling of ERT

I think of menopause as a deficiency disease, like diabetes.

> San Francisco gynecologist, in an interview with Jane Brody, in the *New York Times*, December 5, 1975

By 1947, a dazzling array of estrogen products, some combined with thyroid, were competing for a place on the American doctor's prescription pad. DES and other female sex hormones were available, from dozens of companies, by mouth, by vagina, and by long-acting and short-acting injection.

In ads in the medical journals, the early Premarin woman was shown waltzing with Arthur Murray's double, while the patient who liked her nightly "nip" could have Lynoral Elixir, "The Most Potent Oral Estrogen in a Pleasant-tasting Cordial" (and in a 14 percent alcohol base).

Gusberg's Warnings

In the midst of all these cheery advertisements—six full pages of them in the December 1947 issue of the *American Journal of Obstetrics and Gynecology*—an alarm was sounded by S. B. (Saul) Gusberg, who was then a young gynecologist and cancer researcher at the Sloane Hospital and Columbia University in New York. Dr. Gusberg is today the white-haired, acerbic chief of his department at the Mount Sinai Hospital and School of Medicine in the same city.

"Another human experiment has been set up in recent

years by the widespread administration of estrogens to postmenopausal women," Gusberg said. He went on to point out that the relatively low cost of oral estrogens and the ease of administration had made its general use "promiscuous." Uterine bleeding provoked in patients by this medication had become so commonplace that at Gusberg's hospital the expression "stilbestrol bleeding" was employed to describe those cases admitted for diagnostic curettage.

What did all these curettages (uterine scrapings) in ERT patients reveal? The pathology reports showed that ERT overstimulates the endometrium, or lining of the uterus, producing among other effects "crowding of the glands into a lawless pattern."

Gusberg speculated that it was not the dosage of ERT, nor the specific product, but *long-term exposure* that causes harm. (Research completed in 1975 showed Gusberg to be correct on two points out of three: Duration of use and high-dose levels are both significant in producing cancer, while product differences appear to be inconsequential.) Early as it was in the ERT game, by 1947 Gusberg had collected 29 cases of women whose endometria were profoundly disturbed by estrogen therapy— 20 with a possibly premalignant condition called hyperplasia, which often necessitates hysterectomy, and 9 with cancer itself.

The scholarly gynecologists, those who read the articles as well as the ads in their monthly journals, responded swiftly to Gusberg's work. They also collected cancer cases, and the promiscuous use of ERT slowed or at least stabilized . . . that is, until January 1966, when the M. Evans Co. published a book called *Feminine Forever*, by a handsome avuncular Brooklyn physician named Robert Wilson.

Wilson versus Living Decay

Feminine Forever, which was excerpted in *Look* and *Vogue* and sold 100,000 copies in the first seven months, promised that menopause could be averted and aging allayed with ERT.

Wilson was widely dismissed as a quack by his more sober colleagues, but rarely in public and always off the record. Even good friends of estrogen, or at least the pill, were growling among themselves. Sherwood Kaufman of Planned Parenthood fumed, at a medical meeting: "The situation has gotten ridiculous. Women come in asking for the 'Youth Pill,' and they say 'Check my estrogen level.' From what they've read, they think it's as simple as driving into a gasoline station and having their oil checked."

Wilson, in the short space of an article in *Look* magazine, listed twenty-six symptoms that the Youth Pill would avert. These included nervousness, irritability, anxiety, apprehension, hot flashes, night sweats, joint pains, melancholia, palpitations, crying spells, weakness, dizziness, severe headache, poor concentration, loss of memory, chronic indigestion, insomnia, frequent urination, itching of the skin, dryness of the eye, nose and mouth, backache, neuroses, a tendency to take alcohol and sleeping pills, or even to contemplate suicide.

"While not all women are affected by menopause to this extreme degree," Wilson conceded, "no woman can be sure of escaping the horror of this *living decay*."

Reporters at the *New Republic* and the *Washington Post* called attention to the money Wilson received from drug companies. In a 1969 book, *The Pill, An Alarming Report*, Morton Mintz of the *Post* summarized:

". . . the Wilson Research Foundation, headed by Dr. Wilson . . . received, in 1964, $17,000 from the Searle Foundation, . . . $8,700 from Ayerst Laboratories and $5,600 from the Upjohn Company. In his writings Dr. Wilson claimed that the menopause could be prevented with the use of birth control pills. . . . He spoke of norethynodrel, a synthetic progestin found only in Enovid [a Searle product]. He told George Lardner, Jr., of the *Washington Post*, that he personally does not prescribe the pill, favoring instead prescribing 'conjugated estrogens' supplemented by a progestogen. 'Conjugated estrogens' are a specialty of Ayerst Laboratories; the progestogen he named, medroxyprogesterone acetate, is made by Upjohn."

In other words, Wilson publicly recommended Searle's

Enovid for ERT, but indicated that he did not use it for his own patients. While accepting money from Ayerst and Upjohn, whose products he said he personally prescribed, he allowed the Searle Company to be his "research sponsor" for the Youth Pill he was pressing the FDA to okay.

By November 1966, the FDA was on to Wilson. They formally notified the Searle Company that he was unacceptable as an investigator for Enovid in the menopause because he was disseminating promotional material claiming that the drug had been shown to be effective for conditions for which it had never been proved to work. *And to this day, neither the FDA nor any other scientific body has ever approved Premarin or other hormone products as a preventive to aging.*

Wilson seemed to pay less attention to the FDA than to the press, whom he and his family courted. "He and his people, especially his son, were always calling," reflects Barbara Yuncker of the *New York Post*. "They were proselytizing like mad." Satisfied Wilson patients, perhaps at his behest, came after Ms. Yuncker also with testimonials.

Yuncker found Wilson's siege neither amusing nor convincing, but other reporters must have been impressed. The Youth Doctor was eulogized in *Time* and in many newspapers. Over the next decade, ERT sales tripled.

When we interviewed Robert Wilson in 1976, he commented, truthfully enough: "There are some people who don't like me. They say I shouldn't do what I'm doing. They say that menopause is a natural process. We should grow old gracefully and enjoy it."

Then he warmed to his topic: "They say we should do nothing to retard menopause. Just think of that. Isn't that dreadful? The estrogen regimen should start at age 9—9 to 90. It's necessary to begin then, and to check your estrogen level all through life, so that it never leaves you. Don't allow it to."

We asked Wilson to comment on endometrial cancer. "That's the worst lie in the world," he said, "the worst fallacy. I have over forty doctors working all over the world, Switzerland, Czechoslovakia, all over the world, and we haven't seen one case of cancer."

The Service for Media

Other pro-ERT books followed Wilson's, including *After Forty* by Sondra Gorney and Claire Cox, published in 1973:

"Just about everyone—particularly women—has become cancer-conscious, thanks to effective campaigns in the press and broadcasting media and the insistence of many doctors on regular examinations. Some misconceptions that hormones are a potential cause of cancer persist, however, which builds up resistance and anxiety among menopausal women who might otherwise be helped through replacement therapy.

"What are the facts? Dr. Robert A. Wilson of Brooklyn Methodist Hospital, head of the Wilson Research Foundation, has pointed out that the incidence of cancer is low among women during their young and fertile years when natural estrogen levels are high, while the number of cases rises in later life. . . . No tumor in a human has been blamed on estrogen."

On the jacket of *After Forty*, Sondra Gorney is identified as "Executive Director of the Information Center on the Mature Woman." What the cover fails to mention is that the Information Center, formerly located in New York City, and finally closed in 1976, was a "service for media" thoughtfully provided by the Ayerst Laboratories, manufacturers of Premarin.

The Pharmaceutical Manufacturers Association, to which Ayerst belongs, has a code of ethics which maintains that prescription drugs will not be directly promoted to the public. Ayerst, in violation of the code, hired the talented and energetic Ms. Gorney to provide free filler items, lauding ERT, to magazines, newspapers, and other mass media. Gorney's copy was widely picked up and used —rarely, if ever, with any indication that the source was a drug company.

A typical "Background Paper" from Ayerst Information Center states: "It was once believed that the change of life meant every woman had to resign herself to years of anguish and suffering. . . . When ovarian production stops, a woman's endocrine system is thrown into disarrangement. . . . Emotional problems can affect entire families. If not overcome, they can cause lasting harm to a woman's personality."

The mailings to the media seemed perfectly synchronized with medical journal Premarin ads, even to subject matter, copy, and illustrations, except that while the ads in the medical journals cite *patient* testimonials, the propaganda aimed at prospective patients invokes the authority of *doctors* . . . i.e., "many doctors find a restoration of hormonal balance helps promote a sense of physical and emotional peace."

Clouds on the Horizon

Ayerst's slogan, *"Keep Her on Premarin"* succeeded, thanks in large measure to Wilson, to David Reuben and his books, and to Sondra Gorney and her Information Service, and others who played on the fears and hopes of climacteric women.

Millions of normal women were staying on Premarin for an average of a decade or longer. Most stopped only when they had to stop, because of side effects, such as the uterine bleeding so long ago noted by Gusberg.

Others, many others, were taken off Premarin because of changes in the breast tissue, or allergic reactions, or edema, or metabolic disturbances, or gall-bladder disease. A stand-off developed between the physicians who prescribed long-term ERT, most often gynecologists, and those who mopped up after it. One woman, convinced that Premarin had kept her skin from wrinkling, told us she would "do it over"—even though at 48 she developed breast cancer, that had metastasized, which her doctor believed was accelerated by Premarin.

By 1971, when the government conference on menopause and aging convened in Hot Springs, Arkansas, it reached the conclusion that ". . . the association of abnormal and elevated estrogens and abnormalities of the endometrium is very suggestive. . . ."

And by early 1975, *before* the conclusive studies on ERT and cancer had been completed or published, *Novak's Textbook of Gynecology* concluded:

". . . estrogens can be of importance in the development of cancer in those organs and tissues which are normally estrogen dependent, e.g., the genital tract and breasts. . . . Any gynecologist who spends time in the pathology laboratory can be impressed by the large number of postmenopausal endometria in which extreme degrees of hyperplasia and even endometrial adenocarcinoma are observed in women who have a history of prolonged estrogen therapy."

Novak also noted that "a very high incidence of endometrial cancer" was showing up in DES-reared cows, although such cancer is virtually unknown in cows unexposed to hormones.

Even so, in all the years since Gusberg's brilliant early report, no well-controlled studies comparing cancer frequency in human ERT users and refusers had been completed. Thus, defenders of ERT argued that a cause-and-effect association had not been proven, and that the extent of risk, if any, remained unquantified. Cancer specialists knew it was just a matter of time.

The Bubble Bursts

The time came. In the fall of 1975 rumors were flying in the drug industry and among knowledgeable physicians and science reporters. The *New England Journal of Medicine*, it was whispered, was to publish a series of articles comparing ERT users and non-users, and showing that the risks of endometrial cancer in the former increased five- to fourteen-fold!

Numerous doctors and journalists tried to obtain advance proofs of the articles, but were unsuccessful. One worried gynecologist, Marcia Storch, called the Ayerst Laboratories directly and was told by them precisely what the articles contained. However it came to them, Ayerst knew the specific content of the *New England Journal* articles before publication.

This gave Ayerst time to tool up its propaganda machine. On December 16—less than two weeks after publication of the cancer findings in the *New England Journal*—Ayerst sent a "Dear Doctor" letter concerning Premarin to physicians across the United States.

The letter was reassuring, making it appear that the

New England Journal articles were "weak studies," and that the link between ERT and cancer was not really established. Alexander Schmidt, the FDA commissioner, described the Ayerst letter as "misleading and irresponsible."

Meantime, the physicians who advocated the Youth Pill found it hard to retreat. Perhaps fearing lawsuits, they too were inclined to deny the seriousness of the new reports. Some clung, more than ever, to the notion of menopause as illness.

"I think of the menopause as a deficiency disease, like diabetes," a San Francisco gynecologist told the *New York Times* in early December. "Most women develop some symptoms whether they are aware of them or not, so I prescribe estrogens for virtually all menopausal women for an indefinite period."

"Everything in life is a trade-off—there are risks and benefits, and you must weigh one against the other," said another gynecologist.

However, these male physicians, unlike their patients, were not personally at risk. We wonder: Would they take a drug—and for symptoms they were "not aware of"— that greatly increased their chances of cancer of the penis?

CHAPTER 24

The Flash and the Flesh

There is . . . testimonial evidence but there really are no controlled studies or any objective evidence to indicate that estrogens . . . have any benefit in helping women look and feel young.
Dr. J. Richard Crout, director, Bureau of Drugs, FDA, April 1976

When a growing girl reaches the critical weight of 94 to 103 pounds, she is ready to become a woman. Hypothalamus signals pituitary gland, which signals ovaries to start the menstrual cycle. Ovarian hormones, estrogens, and progesterone, which existed before in small quantities, commence their thirty-five-year-long ballet with the gonadotropic hormones of the pituitary.

And then the music stops.

The ovaries, for reasons which still elude scientists but for which most women are grateful, are ready to put aside their procreative function. They rebuff the pituitary.

Most women, today as always, want to become mothers in their season. They view the menstrual cycle as a necessary nuisance. Two out of 3 women responding to a questionnaire on the subject would just as soon not menstruate, *if* the process could be safely averted without impairing fertility.

Menopause Compared to Puberty

At climacteric, the endocrine systems of the male and female undergo changes which are comparable in many respects, but the male only rarely has hot flashes. The period of hormonal-caused discomfort in the male is the pubertal transition, when high levels of androgen course unpredictably through his bloodstream. Sudden growth spurts, physical uncoordination, acne, high-to-low voice register changes, and emotional withdrawal are characteristic of this state. "Adolescent turmoil" (more frequent in males) may sometimes be difficult to distinguish from schizophrenia.

A current endocrinology text explains that while androgen effects on libido and sex drive are much emphasized, its effects on personality are not only sexual. Aggressiveness and the rambunctious behavior of the teen-ager are well-recognized effects of androgen stimulation.

Adolescent girls may also have awkward and emotionally tumultuous phases, but rarely to the same extent as their brothers. As a rule, the transition to adult womanhood is smoother and shorter than to adult manhood.

But at climacteric, some of the sex advantage of puberty is reversed. Here the female has the more uncomfortable transition. Although her underlying health remains good and her mortality rate is lower than that of her male age mates, her hot flashes are comparable to the voice-register changes of the male adolescent, for they are also a temporary response to hormone imbalance.

The Anatomy of Flashes

Flashes are generally believed to be a response to the flooding of pituitary gonadotropins, which seem to be whipping the ovaries to continue egg production.

One woman in 3, or 2 in 3, depending on the study, escapes hot flashes altogether. Some who have them point out that they had them before, especially in connection with pregnancy or extremely hot weather. As Dr. George Molnar has written in *The Journal of Applied Physiology:* "The hot flash . . . is a subjective experience which can occur without noticeable manifestations and can be identified as such only by the person having it. . . . It is not peculiar to menopausal women but . . . they are the ones who most commonly have [it]."

Recurring flashes may last for only a few weeks or months, or up to two years, and occasionally longer. At their peak, they may occur four or five times a day or sometimes more. They are most frequent at night and may cause temporary sleep disturbances.

A hot flash is a sudden sensation of heat in the upper body, sometimes accompanied by a patchy redness of skin, especially of the face. It usually lasts from several seconds to several minutes, and may involve some sweating—or even excess sweating. When it is over, a woman often feels chilly. When accompanied by a flush, hot flashes may be visible to others, but frequently they are not. In this respect they are less of an embarrassment than the voice changes of the adolescent boy.

Most women who have hot flashes maintain that they are not incapacitating. Dr. Bernice Neugarten, author of *Personality in Middle and Later Life* and similar studies, reports that even in America only 4 women in 100 think of menopause as a major source of worry. The authors of *Our Bodies, Ourselves*, who did their own survey, say: ". . . our questionnaire definitely suggests that most women feel positive or neutral about menopause, are untroubled by the loss of fertility, and go through the two years or so with minimal discomfort."

Severe Flashes

There are a few women, the exceptions, for whom hot flashes reach severe proportions. They are sometimes accompanied by numbness of the hands and feet, shortness of breath or feeling of suffocation, heart palpitations, dizziness, and even fainting. One respondent to the *Our Bodies* questionnaire said:

"As a modern liberated woman, the major myth I had to overcome was the one which maintained that menopause was only a problem for neurotic women. I was taught that if a woman was physically active, busy, enjoying life, career-oriented, and fulfilled, she would not experience any special discomfort during menopause, as these symptoms are all neurotic and psychosomatic. I am healthy, very busy, and active, and was amazed to discover that certain physical menopausal symptoms did indeed occur. Night sweats, joint pains, dreadful nervous instability, terrible feelings of anxiety and of impending disaster—these prompted me to talk to my gynecologist, who prescribed estrogen replacement."

A 65-year-old loyal supporter of ERT has testified at FDA hearings that attempts to limit the use of ERT are "irresponsible," like "taking insulin away from a diabetic." She states that her doctor (Robert Wilson) saved her life when he started her on ERT at 50. Her extensive correspondence, she says, attests to the fact that "Premarin has saved families and prevented suicides."

This woman, who has had three breast lumps removed, still uses Premarin when she "cannot cope physically with menopause symptoms."

Her experience illustrates what we consider a hidden drawback to ERT. At 65, and having had three breast lumps, she still depends on it for "menopause" complaints. We believe that, for some women, ERT is physically addictive as well as psychologically habituating.

Hot flashes are, as a rule, self-limited, ceasing within two years or perhaps less. They are apt to occur at around the time menstruation ceases. By 65, or even 55 or sooner, a woman who had menopause at 48 or 50 is usually feeling fine. Margaret Mead and others have proposed the term PMZ—Post-Menopausal Zest—to describe the well-being many women enjoy in later climacteric and early old age. Hormone havoc behind her (menstrually and menopausally), the woman has not yet begun to feel the deterioration of extreme old age. In the Bernice Neugarten studies, when 460 women were divided into five age groups from adolescence to 64, it was the *oldest group* that had the fewest symptoms. Adolescents had the largest number of psychological complaints, such as tension, while the women in menopause had the most physical complaints, such as headaches and hot flashes.

Some women take ERT for a time, and then stop with no aftermath. Others, however, learn the hard way that it only delays hot flashes instead of curing them. Thus, while we have found *no woman* who, having declined to take ERT, was still having hot flashes after 55, we have found many *older* women who developed hot flashes after stopping ERT.

Our interviews also suggest that medical intervention may *increase* both the severity and frequency of hot flashes in contemporary American women.

In most women menopause is a gradual process, occurring over a period of several years. About 15 percent, according to the *Our Bodies, Ourselves* survey, may go a year or longer without menstruating, and then resume. Symptoms are most pronounced when menopause is abrupt.

Among women who have a natural menopause, no more than 10 to 20 percent report extreme discomfort. Other studies place the figure as low as 4 percent, but 20 is the maximum reported by any reliable source.

Among women who, by contrast, have a surgical menopause, *half* undergo a period of substantial discomfort. Thus medical intervention, in the form of oophorectomy (removal of the ovaries) increases the odds of having *severe* menopause, and also the subsequent development of osteoporosis.

Cold Turkey

Severe menopause may also be pharmacologically induced. Those women who were placed on ERT by their doctors at 30, 35, or 40, before menopause, are often most uncomfortable when they stop years later. The Premarin has masked what might have been a gradual menopause adjustment, and instead they are left with withdrawal symptoms. Women who suddenly terminate ERT *often* describe themselves as "climbing the wall" or going through "cold turkey." Few women employ such vivid phrases to describe their discomforts during untreated menopause.

We have not been able to ascertain whether the "cold turkey" phenomenon is due chiefly to estrogen withdrawal or to the lacing of many ERT products with habituating additives such as tranquilizers or "speed." Few of the women we interviewed had been told by their doctors exactly *what* preparations they had been given. As far as they knew, they were just on "Premarin" or "estrogen," and yet, from their descriptions of the pills, it was obvious that many were, in point of fact, receiving combined products.

We suggest that all women who experience gross discomfort on quitting ERT check with their doctors or pharmacists to find out precisely what was in their pills. If they cannot get such information directly, we hope that the product descriptions in chap. 30 will provide a guide.

Early Studies of Flashes

Precisely what happens physiologically when a hot flash occurs? Is it dangerous? As we write this we have before us, on our desk, the complete current literature on this topic. It consists of *one* paper, which is a study of *one* woman over a period of eight hours.

You think we exaggerate?

The *Index Medicus* from 1903 to 1973 reveals that in all those years, with all the pronouncements doctors made about menopause, they only performed five studies that even remotely bore on this most central symptom.

The first study, performed at Johns Hopkins in 1926, recorded the basal metabolism of 12 women following removal of the ovaries. No change was observed.

Fifteen years later, in 1941, a dermatologist recorded the face temperature and finger volume of one woman during a flash.

After that the 1940s brought a great outpouring of research—namely *three* additional studies. In 1944, one researcher measured daily internal body temperatures in 24 menopausal women but, for all his trying, he never caught one during a flash. In 1946, in France, a study was made of a 50-year-old woman who flashed fifteen to twenty times a day with heavy sweating and temperatures of 97.7° to 98.6°. And finally, in 1949, one doctor succeeded in measuring the oxygen consumption, which rose 5 to 15 percent, and the cheek temperature, which also rose slightly, of several women *during* flashes.

And then, nothing—for twenty-five long years. Twenty-five years during which ERT became standard treatment for flashes, even though it was not known what they *were*. (One would hope or think that before prescribing a proven animal carcinogen for people, physicians and researchers would at least try to find out if the symptom really warranted it.)

Molnar's Unique Study

The great breakthrough, the *one* modern paper to which we referred, was published by George Molnar, of the V.A. Hospital in Little Rock in 1975. Molnar is a student of sweating and "thermal comfort" in hypoglycemia as well as menopause. His subject, who was 59 years old, had been on ERT, which she had to discontinue when she developed spotty bleeding. Molnar wrote:

"Shortly thereafter, hot flashing . . . became very annoying and discomforting. . . . She felt so hot that she either partially disrobed or stepped outdoors (41–50°) to cool off. On one occasion, oral temperature was measured. It showed no elevation, so a more complete investigation was decided upon. . . .

"Since her flashes occurred most predictably between 7 P.M. and 9 P.M., the measurements were made during those hours on four days. The subject lay on a nylon mesh bed which was mounted on an underbed scale. In three tests she was nude and in one fully clothed. . . .

"Temperatures were measured . . . internally (rectum, vagina and ear) and on the skin surface (forehead, cheek, neck, chest, abdomen, upper and lower back, leg, finger and toe). . . . Sweating was determined by means of sweat prints . . . by weight changes with the underbed scale . . . and by changes in skin temperatures. . . . The electrocardiogram was recorded continuously . . . blood glucose concentration was determined on finger capillary blood. . . .

"Flashes occurred twice during each test . . . the mean duration was 3.8 minutes; range 2.4 to 4.7 minutes. Within 15 to 30 seconds after the onset, the subject called out that she was having a flash. The termination was sometimes less certain subjectively, ending with 'I think it's over. . . .'

"The sweat prints indicated profuse sweating on the forehead and nose, moderate sweating on the sternum and adjacent areas, and little or none on the cheek or leg . . . the total amount of sweat loss was small.

"The digits [fingers and toes] warmed very rapidly. . . . The only other area that showed a rise in temperature during a flash was the cheek. . . . The forehead temperature always started to fall immediately with the onset of the flash. . . .

"The subject also had remarkably low internal temperature. . . ."

Molnar sums up his findings: "In our subject, the onset of a flash was always sharply demarcated by the . . . occurrence of tachycardia [rapid heart beat], undulations in the ECG base line, detectable sweating and consequent fall in skin temperature and peripheral vasodilation [dilation of the blood vessels] as suggested by rapid warming of the digits and cheeks. . . . There was never any indication . . . that a flash was impending. . . . A hot flash is thus apparently an explosive activation of certain areas of the brain resulting in subjective heat distress . . . [from] sudden discharge of a neurohumor [a chemical substance liberated by a nerve impulse]—possibly gonadotropin. . . .

"Environmental stimuli which may provoke discharges [of neurohumors] . . . may be more prevalent during certain hours . . . [and] . . . may determine the distribution of flashes throughout the day. . . . A finger prick evoked a flash in our subject. . . . She had also found that during the evening hours she often flashed at the sound of a doorbell or telephone or of a person suddenly talking to her. . . . Eating of the evening meal was conducive to flashing, as was also hot weather. On the other hand, in the absence of obvious stimuli during sleep after midnight, she was awakened almost every night by a flash. . . ."

To date, this is the only woman whose flashes of menopause have been so thoroughly studied. During flashes she obtained relief by local cooling of her cheeks and cheekbones, a possible hint for others. (Try applying ice, or a cold cloth, to the *cheeks*, instead of the forehead or chest.)

Assuming his subject is typical, Molnar's study reveals that flashes are physically measurable but not dangerous. She did not run a fever, or "sweat buckets," but her heart speeded up, and the blood vessels in her extremities constricted or narrowed, while those in her face dilated or widened. At the end of the flash she returned to normal.

ERT works to control—or, as in the case of Molnar's subject, *delay*—hot flashes. On this count it is effective, as claimed. But how about its other "flesh" effects? Does it keep the skin more youthful, the breasts firmer, the hair more luxuriant?

Flesh Effects

Most certainly not, for if it did, the manufacturers and the doctors who make such claims for it would have produced some *demonstrable* evidence in all these years. There is none—not one study in which women on ERT and off it were independently rated by dermatologists, beauty experts, or even by the crowd at the corner drugstore.

There are personal testimonials for ERT as a Youth Pill, but that is all. "At 50," according to ERT supporter Dr. Robert Wilson, "women on ERT still look attractive in sleeveless dresses or tennis shorts."

True enough, some *do*. But so do some older women not on ERT. We think the *tennis* is a more likely factor.

Nowhere in their official labeling are the manufacturers of these products allowed to say that they promote either the *feeling* or *appearance* of *youthfulness*. ERT is an accepted treatment for "the menopausal syndrome," meaning flashes and related complaints, but is not an *aging* preventive.

We had an interesting chance recently to do an informal survey on the subject of ERT and youthful appearance. We posted a notice at a gym many affluent middle-aged women attend, asking if we could interview them concerning their experience taking or avoiding ERT.

Prior to the interviews, we privately jotted down our guesses of the women's ages. Our estimates were on the low side (by five years or more), particularly for the *nonusers* of ERT. We were low three times as often for that group as for the others.

The curious thing was that the ERT users *imagined* they looked young for their ages, but in fact did not. On the other hand, the women who did not rely on ERT but instead were very conscientious about exercise and diet were (in our opinion) deceptively young-looking. We concluded that ERT sometimes gives women a false sense of security and prevents them from doing commonsense things for themselves.

According to the beauty editor of a leading women's magazine, many actresses and society women who have face lifts and plastic surgery are reluctant to admit it. When they appear looking somewhat rejuvenated, they are much more apt to hint that they owe their suddenly younger faces to a drug, because this is somehow considered more respectable. On close top-secret interviewing (and this editor knows the *real* beauty secrets of many), she has found that the women of this "set" don't take ERT at all seriously as a youth preservative. Some of them may take it for hot flashes and other *symptoms*, but they have no illusions about its ability to improve their looks. These women, unlike the estrogen users at our gym, can't afford to fool themselves, for their *livings* depend on their looks.

Included in the acknowledged side effects of ERT are edema, increase in body weight, and allergic rash. Women who try ERT for appearance's sake may find that it backfires—cruelly. One such woman, aged 53, developed estrogen blisters on her face, neck, chest, and hands that, although they went away when she stopped ERT (after eight years of use), left her with permanent scars.

Novak's Textbook of Gynecology explains sympathetically that many women are afraid they will become obese during the menopause. "Although most women do put on some weight at this time, the gain is usually moderate and easily controllable. To the thin, angular type of female, the menopause may actually be a physical blessing, in that the figure becomes more rounded and attractive."

The Youth Pill came back to England only recently, according to Dr. William Inman—that country's equivalent of the FDA commissioner—when an American doctor (whose name Inman forgot) appeared on British television to show off a 65-year-old ERT patient who had "youthful breasts." (The British TV codes are more liberal concerning nudity.)

This, according to Inman, started a craze for ERT, and now large numbers of British women are taking it, too. By the close of 1975, when the news of endometrial cancer reached England, *The Lancet* ran an editorial called

"Dangers in Eternal Youth," which concluded that women who really believe in the wonders of ERT and won't give it up are advised to have hysterectomies to protect themselves from cancer. Further news in 1976, however, indicated that even those women who have had hysterectomies and taken ERT face an increased risk of breast cancer, 12 or 15 years later. They can't win!

CHAPTER 25

The Ovary Explained

. . . the average menopausal woman is not truly estrogen-deficient. Estrogen levels necessary for adequate maintenance . . . are much lower than those necessary for . . . reproduction.
            Novak's Textbook of Gynecology,
            9th ed., 1975

The word hormone is derived from the Greek "horman," meaning "I arouse to activity."

Hormones serve as our body "messengers," for they course through our body and *stimulate* many organs, tissues, and functions in very specific ways. When estrogen levels increase at puberty, they promote the growth and development of the vagina, uterus, Fallopian tubes, and breasts, as well as contribute to the shaping of the skeleton, the growth of axillary and pubic hair, and pigmentation of the nipples.

The ovaries, or, in the case of men, testes, are but two of the thirteen glands that produce natural hormones, and comprise our endocrine system.

The hormone-governing gland is the pituitary, which used to be called "the master gland" and even "the conductor of the endocrine symphony." Recently, the pituitary was demoted to concert master when scientists learned that the hypothalamus, a small area of the brain situated near the pituitary, signals *it* when to stop and go.

Our largest gland, the pancreas, weighs nearly 3 ounces while our smallest, the pineal—formerly called our third eye because it is located in the middle of the brain— is no bigger than a large grape seed. Besides pancreas and pineal, the pituitary and our two sex gonads (the ovaries or testes), our remaining glands include the thyroid, the thymus, two adrenals, and four parathyroids.

The function of some glands remains elusive. The pineal, long considered vestigial, is now believed to influence our body cycles, and our circadian (daily) ebb and flow of hormones. In 1971 Martha McClintock showed that college roommates and close friends often come to have menstrual cycles which start and end around the same date. This intriguing phenomenon, called "menstrual synchrony," may be a manifestation of pineal activity.

The thymus is but little understood. It shrivels by childhood's end and may influence early immunities. In some fashion, it helps with adaptation to life, but when it fails to appropriately reduce its function it may be associated with later diseases, such as a neurological disorder called myasthenia gravis (the disease Aristotle Onassis suffered from).

How the Ovary Works

For all the pronouncements about the postmenopausal ovary, only in the past decade has much research into its function been performed. It is fanciful, and possibly insulting, to view the egg-producing ovary as the "control tower" of womankind, for a normal woman ovulates and menstruates during only half of her life span, starting at around age 12 and concluding at 50. Except for her gonads, woman's endocrine structure is identical to the male's, and, in both sexes, the hypothalamus and pituitary are the master switches.

The ovary is better compared to the thymus, endowed with certain time-limited, specific functions. The function of the ovary, besides producing hormones, is to make reproduction possible, by maturing and releasing egg cells and preparing the uterus for a possible conception.

The clitoris, woman's organ of sexual stimulus, has no known reproductive function. Woman's reproductive and excretory organs are also more differentiated than the male's He possesses only one canal for the emission of both seminal fluid and urine, while women have separate orifices for reproduction and excretion.

Biologically, woman is at an advantage, compared to the male, during the climacteric and later years. She has more resistance to stress and fatal illness, and her sexuality need not be placed in jeopardy when reproductive functions decline. Ordinarily, the male must ejaculate in order to reach orgasm, but orgasm in the female is not at all connected with ovulation.

Follicle Stimulating Hormone

We have mentioned that the human life span divides into five inexorable time zones: childhood, puberty, maturity, climacteric, and old age. The ovary is not without function during the first and latter stages, but it is in the second and third—puberty and maturity—that it is "busiest," as it were, and most influential.

As Dr. Rose Frisch discovered in 1973, when an average growing girl reaches a critical weight her hypothalamus signals her pituitary to start production of a gonadotropic hormone (meaning that the target organs are the ovaries or gonads) called FSH.

FSH stands for Follicle Stimulating Hormone, and its job is to ripen, in turn, during one menstrual cycle after another, a total of 400 to 500 of the half-million egg cells with which a newborn girl is provided. The egg cell is contained in a follicle that manufactures estrogen as it develops, stimulated by FSH. Many follicles are stimulated in a given cycle, but only one is "selected" to mature fully and emit an egg.

Why that *one*—or very occasionally more—is selected remains a mystery that researchers have never been able to solve.

"We should always be humbled when we think of what we do not know about the female reproductive cycle. We still have no understanding of the mechanism that makes one follicle in one of the ovaries of a normal woman maturate and ovulate each month. This is a baffling problem. Until we know that mechanism that selects one follicle, out of perhaps hundreds of thousands, to maturate each month, we still have to proceed with caution on any long-term hormonal treatment of the human female," said

Charles Dodds, creator of the first synthetic hormone—
DES.

During the reproductive years, with urging from the
pituitary, the ovaries and their follicles emit three forms
of estrogen, called estrone (E_1), 17B-estradiol (E_2), and
estriol, as well as progesterone. The term estrogen is
derived from the Latin "oestrus," which means frenzy.

Hormone production is patterned throughout the
menstrual cycle. FSH and LH (Luteinizing Hormone,
which also issues from the pituitary) remain essentially
constant at low levels until midcycle, when, stimulated by
a burst in estrogens from the ovaries, there is a large surge
in both FSH and LH, which in turn trigger ovulation and
the production of progesterone. In the first half of the
menstrual cycle estrogens predominate; in the second half,
after ovulation, both estrogens and progesterone are
present.

Later in the cycle, barring pregnancy, estrogen and
progesterone production both reach their nadir, and menstruation begins.

Thus the menstrual cycle—the female reproduction—
rests on a most delicate feedback system of oscillating hormones, pituitary signaling ovary and vice versa, with the
hypothalamus serving as overseer. When the reproductive
years have been negotiated, this "frenzy" of gonadal hormone production is no longer needed. Ovulation declines
and then ceases, after behaving skittishly while winding
down.

At this juncture the pituitary, more than the ovaries,
undergoes a period of adjustment. In an apparent effort
to maintain the old feedback system, or to keep the ball
in play, so to speak, the pituitary increases production of
gonadotropics as much as twenty times over! And thus the
hot flashes of menopause are *not due to estrogen deficiency*
but to pituitary excess. What ERT accomplishes is *not* to
restimulate ovulation *or turn back the clock* but merely to
"fool" the pituitary into calming down.

ERT Proponents

There is a second viewpoint, held by promoters of ERT
such as Robert ("Feminine Forever") Wilson, and a few

other prominent and vocal gynecologists including Robert Greenblatt, Herbert Kupperman, and Helen Jern.

Greenblatt: "Our viewpoint . . . is that endocrine deficiency syndromes require endocrine replacement, and the menopause is no exception."

Kupperman: "One would treat the estrogenic deficient female in much the same way one treats a thyroid deficiency *whether or not there is a presenting symptomatology*."

Jern: "Menopause is an ovarian deficiency disease."

ERT proponents have differences among themselves (see chap. 30). Greenblatt, unlike Kupperman, maintains: "There are many women who, though their menses cease, continue to have adequate endogenous estrogens [produced within the body] to maintain a normal metabolic and autonomic nervous system balance. They do not have flashes; no evidence of estrogen lack is seen on vaginal cytology. . . . Unless other psychodynamic changes are present, they are no different psychophysiologically from premenopausal women. In our view, these women do not need to be treated."

Ziel and Finkle and the Youth Pill Fantasy

In an article published in 1976 in the *American Journal of Obstetrics and Gynecology*, Harry Ziel and William Finkle —who had been among the principal researchers to affirm, the previous year, that ERT causes endometrial cancer (see chap. 28)—stated, with unconcealed relief: "The 'estrogen forever' philosophy has fortunately not dictated the standard of therapy of the menopause, with estrogen use limited to only 23 percent of our postmenopausal population." Ziel and Finkle were referring to "the population" at Kaiser-Permanente Medical Center in California, where they work. Nationally, the figure is estimated at *over 50 percent*.

". . . Yet well-meaning physicians frequently prescribe these hormones, giving some patients estrogen even before the menopause and continuing it in some for the duration of their lives. Adverse effects may become . . . manifest only after years of exposure. . . . By then many patients have become psychologically addicted to estrogen and . . .

object to its discontinuance. These chronically exposed women are uniquely jeopardized."

Ziel and Finkle dismiss the "deficiency" concept of menopause as a fad, and the Youth Pill as medical fantasy. They conclude by saying: "[The] patient is readily deluded by . . . her physician's implication that estrogen promises eternal youth."

Ovaries and Hysterectomy

Women are variously told by their gynecologists that (a) without the ovary's estrogen they suffer from a deficiency disease, and (b) the postmenopausal ovary is useless, so it might as well come out. Most hysterectomies are performed for uterine conditions such as fibroids, but it is quite standard practice to remove the ovaries as well as the uterus in women past 45 who are undergoing hysterectomies. We have interviewed many women whose normal ovaries were removed still earlier—in their thirties and even in their twenties.

At the time of the National Health Survey of 1960–62, about 5 million American women aged 50 to 64—more than one-quarter of the total—reported having had surgical rather than natural menopause. By 1976, an FDA bulletin reported that "the prevalence of hysterectomies has been rising in the past decade." The proportion of American women who now have surgical, not natural, menopause may be creeping up toward one-third. In their 1972 book, *Man and Woman, Boy and Girl,* sex researchers John Money and Anke Ehrhardt were moved to state: "Oophorectomy [removal of the ovaries] has been, and sometimes still is, recklessly included in surgery for hysterectomy. Usually it is unnecessary and undesirable and should be expressly forbidden by the patient when she signs the operation permit." In 1976, Blue Cross–Blue Shield advised subscribers to get a second and third opinion before agreeing to *any* elective surgery—a recommendation based in part on various medical audits showing that in many regions of the United States more than 40 percent of the hysterectomies and oophorectomies have involved removal of *normal* organs.

What *Medical World News* calls "the most sophisticated study of unnecessary surgery" was completed in New York State in 1971. Three common operations were reviewed: hysterectomies, appendectomies, and prostatectomies. The examiners concluded that "Overall, the prostatectomies and appendectomies were justified and well handled, but the track record for hysterectomies was dismal. Of 148 procedures reviewed, 64, or 43 percent, were deemed unjustified."

The legitimate reasons for removal of the ovaries include: ovarian cancer, which is a relatively rare disease; certain hormone-dependent cancers of the breast or other organs; and highly cystic or otherwise benignly diseased ovaries. In the last instance, however, there is rarely need to remove *both* ovaries.

Healthy ovaries are often excised as a preventive against cancer. The logic of this is elusive, for the patient is then given ERT, which is apparently *more* carcinogenic than naturally occurring ovarian hormones.

Hysterectomy, like any surgery, always entails risk. The chances of dying from a surgical complication are 1 in 500. Some hysterectomies are necessary, and even lifesaving, but it makes no sense to accept unnecessary surgery, followed by an unnecessary drug.

David Reuben's Old Tune

In his 1969 best-seller, *Everything You Always Wanted to Know About Sex*, psychiatrist David Reuben states:

"As the estrogen is shut off, a woman comes as close as she can to being a man. Increased facial hair, deepened voice, obesity, and the decline of breasts and female genitalia all contribute to a masculine appearance. Coarsened features, enlargement of the clitoris, and gradual baldness complete the tragic picture. Not really a man but no longer a functional woman, these individuals live in the world of intersex."

By 1974 a good deal more was known about the postmenopausal ovary—and endocrine profile—yet Reuben never shut off his hard sell of ERT. Even Greenblatt, a major advocate, had acknowledged that "many women" don't need it, but Reuben's third best-seller, *How to Get More Out of Sex*, states picturesquely:

"A woman's unique femininity is a precious and fragile flower. Unless it is nurtured, it quickly wilts. Ten doses of estrogen at the beginning of the 'change of life' are worth a thousand doses six months later."

Mixing flowers and fruits, Reuben also suggests that women who eschew ERT get to look like "cooked apples," and that doctors who won't prescribe it are chauvinists and puritans.

Reuben was not keeping up with the research indicating that androgens, not estrogens, are the principal libido-stimulators in women. Reuben speaks, in *How to Get More Out of Sex*, of failing "sex glands" and "libido" which, he says, are prevented by ERT.

In contrast to Reuben's description of estrogen "shutoff" and its leading to hermaphroditism, Ziel and Finkle, Novak, and many other authorities maintain that the postmenopausal woman does not suffer "an absence of estrogen." Who is right?

For centuries, the *reproductive* ovary has fascinated scientists. In contrast, much less is known about the *pre- and post-reproductive* ovary. Significant studies of the ovary after menopause hardly number more than 25. Like the pineal gland, it has falsely been seen as a vestigial organ, until recently. Even today, research is minimal, and what we are about to tell you is tentative.

Vermeulen's Research

At the University of Ghent in Belgium, Dr. A. Vermeulen has been comparing three groups of women:

- 52- to 65-year-olds who have their ovaries
- women of the same age who do not
- 18- to 25-year-old nurses and medical students who have their ovaries

Vermeulen is interested in "nycterohemeral" (daily and nightly) rhythms and is careful to note the time when he takes hormone measurements. There is a "significant variation" in levels, the highest being at 8:00 A.M. and the lowest at 11:00 P.M. or midnight.

Vermeulen's most striking finding, which has been confirmed in many other laboratories, is that one of the estrogens, estrone, or E_1, remains at rather high levels in postmenopausal women. Estrone levels were almost as high in Vermeulen's older women as the younger ones. But the source apparently is *not* the ovaries, for the *older women without ovaries* had about the same estrone levels as those women who retained these organs. Vermeulen believes, as do many researchers, that other substances are converted to estrone by "peripheral processes" elsewhere in the body. Adipose (fatty) tissue is a factor in this conversion, so heavier women appear to maintain higher estrogen levels than thin ones. Estrone is the only estrogen that remains prominent after menopause. Levels of the others decline.

The older ovary is not inactive, however. It secretes testosterone and androstenedione, both androgens, in significant amounts. Researchers P. K. Siiteri and P. C. MacDonald had earlier demonstrated, in highly technical studies, that androgens, especially androstenedione, are the substances that are converted into estrone in the older woman. What this leaves unexplained is where the older women who lack ovaries get the androstenedione to convert into estrone.

Another project of Vermeulen's is to compare women and men of the same age groups. He reports not surprisingly that the adrenals and other endocrine glands reveal parallel changes in both sexes as they progress through the life cycle.

Further confirmation that the postmenopausal ovary remains productive has been issuing from Dr. Howard Judd and his associates at the University of California. First Judd showed a "marked fall of testosterone" and a "significant decrease of androstenedione" in older women following surgical removal of their ovaries. Next he took blood samples from the ovarian veins and arm veins, respectively, of another series of women beyond menopause. These samples were compared. Higher ovarian than arm-vein concentrations were found for all of the hormones studied. Ovarian concentrations of testosterone were 15 times as high, of androstenedione 4 times as high, and of estrone and 17B-estradiol, twice as high.

Their ovarian veins would not have been accessible had not the Judd patients, of whom the oldest was 69 and 20 years beyond her menopause, been undergoing surgery for conditions that ranged from endometrial polyps to metastatic breast cancer. It is possible that the hormone profile of these women was not entirely typical. Nonetheless, the Judd studies showing high hormone concentrations in the ovarian vein do lend a new dimension to the older ovary.

CHAPTER 26

The Vagina and Sexuality

*. . . sexual dysfunction in older women is often di-
rectly related to the psychosexual problems of their
sex partners. . . .*

Saul Kent in *Geriatrics*, May 1975

The climacteric vagina, like the woman who comes with it,
is often in its prime. Many women, especially those who
maintain a regular pattern of sexual intercourse once or
twice a week, sustain a healthy vaginal condition into advanced old age. Orgasm dramatically increases the vascular
supply to the vagina. With regular usage, say Masters and
Johnson, the aging vagina does not constrict significantly
in size, and continues to lubricate well.

Lubrication is the first physiological sign that a woman
is responding to sexual stimulation. In young adulthood it
occurs within fifteen to thirty seconds, but in old age may
be delayed for as long as five minutes. This is thought to
be because the vagina has become smaller, while the lining
may become thinner, noncorrugated, and lighter in color.
Consequently, it is stated, there is no longer enough tissue
for the lubricating fluid to develop so rapidly.

The young vagina is a highly expansive organ, not for
sexual reasons but to allow the passage of babies. Capacity
to expand diminishes after menopause, but given the difference in size between an infant's head and the average
phallus, this is hardly a problem.

After menopause, the outer vaginal lips (labia majora)
may become flatter, the inner lips (labia minora) may
color less brightly just before orgasm; and the hood of the
clitoris may decrease slightly in size. The woman may find
intercourse uncomfortable or painful, *if she has not first*

been gently aroused. Rough pawing may irritate her clitoris more than ever.

If the vaginal mucosa has thinned substantially, overly vigorous penile thrusting can produce infection. The older woman may occasionally find that intercourse irritates her bladder and urethra.

ERT is effective in combating these conditions. The vagina—target organ for estrogen—laps up ERT and *does* become more "youthful." The hot flashes of menopause and the vaginal discomforts of advancing age—occurring, on the average, ten years or longer *after* menopause—are the only conditions for which ERT is established to work. Labeling of ERT preparations, including a package insert for the consumer, will indicate this, as well as the cancer risks.

Absorption Through the Vagina

But even if ERT works to allay signs of vaginal aging, is it necessary? Do women want to die for their vaginas, or do men only think so?

Most of the problems of vaginal aging can be circumvented without ERT by the following means:
- tender and imaginative love-making
- regular orgasms
- harmless local lubricants such as KY Jelly or cocoa butter

When these do not suffice, local creams and suppositories containing estrogen are the next logical step. Some hormones from the cream are absorbed into the system, but not, it is thought, to the same extent as with oral preparations or injections. The target organ, which benefits from ERT, receives it. The mucosa, or superficial layer of the vagina, is "very sensitive to hormones, particularly estrogen."

However, our knowledge of the extent to which drugs might be systematically absorbed through the vagina is only tentative. There is little data on most of the vaginal drugs in current use, and also little information on the mechanisms and dynamics of absorption in the vaginal mucosa. It has been demonstrated that *some* hormones, for example the progestins contained in an experimental diaphragm called the "silastic ring," may be absorbed sufficiently to prevent ovulation.

Some compounds whose progress through the body can be easily traced have been shown to be stored in the kidney, liver, lungs, stomach, spleen, ovaries, and uterus after tablets are inserted in the vagina. A 1974 study showed that hexachlorophene, a prescription antibacterial cleanser readily absorbed through the outer skin, is also absorbed through the vaginas of rats.

Thus, although it seems likely that vaginally applied hormone creams are "safer" than ERT, it is possible theoretically that some organs such as the kidneys may be *more* affected by local treatments (see chap. 28).

Better Sex After Menopause

Sexuality is as personal as one's fingerprints . . . and as variable. In general, menopause doesn't alter it much. Married couples who have a good adjustment sustain it, and when there is a poor adjustment, it rarely improves.

But there are some exceptions. It is not too unusual to hear: "I feel better and freer since menopause. I threw that diaphragm away. I love being free of possible pregnancy and the nuisance of birth control. Menopause has made my sex life better."

Or: "I feel in better shape physically—in my prime, unencumbered by the cycle of pain, swelling, discomfort, nuisance, etc."

One happily married woman described her middle-aged sexuality this way: "I thought I would die of lonesomeness when the twins went off to college, and I lost both my chickadees the same week. I miss them of course, but—Marty and I are having a second honeymoon. We pull the drapes and chase each other nude around the house, like a satyr and nymph. I guess we look foolish, but in a way that makes it all the more delicious. Marty is 56 years old, and I am 52."

In a poll of 100 climacteric women—all in good health, married, and living with their husbands—on the effect of menopause on their sexuality, 65 percent maintained that there was no change. Of the remainder, half thought sexual activity became less important, and half thought sexual relations become more enjoyable because menstruation and fear of pregnancy were removed.

Through the research of Kinsey—and then of Masters and Johnson and their successors such as Mary Jane Sherfey—we have come to recognize that sexual desire or libido peaks at a later age in the female than the male. Male potency declines after late adolescence, but in the female, according to Sherfey, sexual experience, and also pregnancy, "increase her venous bed capacity," an essential part of the woman's internal sexual system, of which the clitoris is the visible tip. Provided she is sexually active, a woman's hidden sexual tissues expand and grow throughout much of her adult life.

In general, modern sex research tells us, the more orgasms a woman has, the more she is capable of having and the more she wants. On the other hand, many women can live comfortably, even joyously, with abstinence.

The Older Woman as Sexual Leader

Other anthropologists inform us that in many primitive societies the sexual energy and erotic skills of the mature woman are highly prized. Among the Amatanango Maya, according to June Nash:

"After menopause, women become ceremonial leaders along with men. They act as intermediaries of the gods, and as sexual initiators of young men. Freed from the deference and modesty required of younger women, their personalities expand dramatically."

Donald Marshall, who studied the sexual customs of the Mangaians in Polynesia, writes about the education of the adolescent male: "The period of formal instruction is followed by a practical exercise in copulation. The intercourse . . . must be with an experienced woman. . . . Of significance to the youth is the coaching he receives in . . . techniques. . . . The woman teaches him to hold back until he can achieve orgasm in unison with his partner; she teaches him the positions involved in carrying out various acts. . . . The last day . . . is marked by a feast . . . the signal for the boy to be called a man by his people."

The Mangaians have a reverence for the female

sexual organs, according to Marshall. Their language has many different terms for the clitoris, depending on its size and shape. Clitorises are classified by their degree of sharpness or bluntness, and are also described as "projecting," "erecting," or "protruding."

The languages of Western culture show a much higher regard for the male reproductive anatomy than for that of the female. We speak of *seminal* ideas; we solemnly *testify* (swear by our testicles) even if we have none; and we may hear said of a courageous person that he or she has balls. There are no equivalent metaphors for the female organs. We never say: "That woman has ovaries!" or "She had a clitoral (i.e., exquisitely sensitive) idea."

The Menopausal Husband

More than about menopause itself, the American woman apparently worries about cancer, just getting older, and losing her husband. The average husband is 2.4 years older than his wife, and has a life expectancy of eight fewer years.

With some exceptions, the husband's sexuality declines more rapidly than hers. One study of the sex lives of a large population of aging persons has revealed that having an interested partner is a major factor in the persistence of regular sex relations into old age. When sex relations cease in a marriage, it is generally the husband who is responsible for ending them.

In his late forties, a man's gonadal hormones start to decline. While not marked by a specific event like cessation of menstruation, he may feel the difference, sexually, much more than a climacteric woman does. The interval from ejaculation to the next erection, brief during adolescence and stabilized in adulthood, now grows noticeably longer.

During the "male menopause," frequency of ejaculation as well as erection decrease. "Each illness, emotional upset, or major interruption in sexual outlet seems to leave the aging man a little less potent," says Dr. Sheldon Cherry, a gynecologist.

He relates a case that he says illustrates what might be called the male menopause syndrome:

"Paul M., 57 years old, was a busy accountant. After a particularly busy tax season, his wife reported that he was drinking alcohol in greater quantities and not coming home as often after work. His business trips became more frequent and longer.

"One day Paul suddenly announced to his wife that he was leaving her. He took off with his 25-year-old secretary, cross-country in a Volkswagen camper. Fortunately, his associates continued to maintain his business.

"After three weeks he suddenly reappeared home, without the girlfriend or camper, very distraught, and seeking psychiatric help.

". . . He responded well to therapy and antidepressant drugs, and eventually settled down again to a happy life with his wife who, by the way, was only 39—nearly twenty years his junior."

Instead of estrogen deficiency, Cherry maintains that the trouble with some women is . . . menopausal men.

CHAPTER 27

Osteoporosis: Another ERT Target

We are also evaluating the research on osteoporosis to see whether there is really evidence that estrogens are effective for that use.
Dr. J. Richard Crout, director, Bureau of Drugs, FDA, April 1976

Osteoporosis is a reduction in the density of the skeleton, a loss of bone mass, and increase in fragility. The bones become more porous and brittle. It is a disease of aging, due to the inability of new bone formation to keep pace with bone resorption. Children grow and old people shrink. When old people fall, they may have disproportionately severe fractures, which are slow to heal.

Peak bone mass is attained at around age 35. A plateau may now occur, varying with the individual, or a downward slope may begin. The rate of loss in women is initially greater than in men, and this appears to hold generally true for all bones of the skeleton. Spinal osteoporosis is four times as common and hip fractures are two-and-a-half times as common. Even forearm fractures occur more frequently. But by age 80, these sex-linked differences wash out. Osteoporosis is not separable from the general aging process, but some persons are more susceptible, while others seem protected. Blacks, males, tall women, and obese women have reduced risks of sustaining osteoporotic fracture. These same persons have above-average peak bone mass; whereas small, delicately built women have both a smaller adult bone mass and an increased risk of developing osteoporosis.

Possible Causes and Cures

Dr. Jennifer Jowsey, director of orthopedic research at the Mayo Clinic, has written: "In a way not completely understood [physical] stress stimulates an increase in bone mass. This is not to say that jogging an hour a day will prevent osteoporosis. A full day of [physical] work or exercise is probably necessary if stress is to have any meaningful effect upon the skeleton. Conversely, bed rest or presumably even the relative inactivity of a sedentary life contributes to development of the disease."

In a study of geographical variations in osteoporosis and their association with physical activity, it was learned that the most serious outcome of osteoporosis, hip fractures in elderly women, occurrs much less frequently in cultures where such women maintain high levels of physical activity. In our sedentary culture, hip fractures in the eighth and ninth decade of life have serious effects, for 1 patient in 6 dies within three months of the injury.

An insufficient intake of calcium accelerates bone loss—but phosphorus levels are important also. It appears that, as age creeps up and metabolism changes, excess phosphorus overstimulates the parathyroid, which, in turn, leads to diminished bone formation.

The incidence of osteoporosis is also mysteriously influenced by fluorides. The condition is less frequent in areas that have high fluoride concentrations in the water. On the other hand, direct treatment with fluorides, like direct treatment with estrogens, produces mixed results as well as a host of side effects, such as gastrointestinal disturbances.

At an international symposium on Nutritional Disorders of Women, held in 1975 at Columbia University, Dr. Louis V. Avioli of Washington University School of Medicine in St. Louis gave a paper on osteoporosis which revealed that the stage of our understanding is still embryonic.

Avioli pointed out that although the ravages of the unrelenting decrease in bone mass are all too familiar, the reasons for it are still incompletely understood. Dietary indiscretion, inactivity, decrease in muscle mass, hormonal imbalance, kidney dysfunction, and inability to absorb the nutrients essential for "bone health" are all thought to be contributors. And so doctors have recommended high-calcium diets, exercise, dietary vitamins D and C, or even sunbathing, estrogens, and other agents, such as sodium fluoride, to strengthen bones. These therapeutic measures have only relieved some of the symptoms of osteoporosis.

Osteoporosis is not necessarily "serious." Some older persons show substantial bone loss on x-rays but do not suffer from it in any way. They have no backaches or unexplained fractures. They lead normal lives. Others are much handicapped or pained by the condition. Every nursing home attendant can tell you horror stories of bedridden patients whose bones seem to crumble to the touch.

Albright's Theory

In the 1930s it was proposed by Dr. Fuller Albright of Massachusetts General Hospital that medical intervention in the form of ERT might help prevent or cure osteoporosis.

Albright, like George Smith (see chap. 1) was a leading scholar and researcher of his era (as well as the father of Tenley Albright, the skating star turned surgeon). Albright's Harvard faculty credentials were impeccable. He and his associates were familiar with the animal research as well as the clinical problems of bone loss in humans.

Albright's creative mind got hooked on two apparently related findings. The first was that in preparation for egg laying, pigeons and other fowl show an increase in "osteoblastic activity," or bone formation. Their bones get stronger and less breakable, for the time being. The second point that interested Albright was that women whose ovaries are surgically removed in their twenties or early thirties occasionally develop osteoporosis as early as age 40, much earlier than it is usually seen.

Albright was a painstaking recorder of osteoporosis patients' case histories, including their intake of milk and cottage cheese. He duly reported how each, in turn, was injured by a slip on a rug, a fall from a streetcar, or an unpleasant trauma while driving.

"Essentially," said Albright, "the same story keeps repeating itself. A woman about ten years past natural or surgical menopause receives a minor jolt by going over a bump in an automobile, for example: she experiences a pain in the back; finally she has an x-ray which reveals the condition."

Based on bird research, as well as his findings about early osteoporosis in castrated women, Albright decided to treat osteoporosis with *estrogen*, specifically—when it became available—oral DES. Albright proposed that estrogen might be a specific stimulus to bone formation.

In 1941 he, with Patricia Smith and Anna Richardson, published the first important paper which mentioned estrogen as an aging preventive. Two other papers—one by L. F. Hawkinson and the other by Hans Weisbader and Raphael Kurzork—had been published in 1938 on the benefits of estrogen as a reliever of hot flashes, but both papers warned that long-term use of the drug might be carcinogenic. Neither paper suggested in any way that estrogen could delay aging. In the course of Albright's paper, which appeared in *JAMA* in 1941, he and his colleagues Smith and Richardson reviewed the cases of 42 osteoporosis patients. Estrogen therapy was only mentioned in passing, for it was then considered so daring. The title, which nowhere suggested estrogen, was simply, "Postmenopausal Osteoporosis, Its Clinical Features."

Though they focused on bone problems, the authors hinted in passing that victims of early osteoporosis may also show their age, unduly, in other bodily systems. "There is considerable evidence," they state with an uncharacteristic lack of documentation, "that patients with postmenopausal osteoporosis have a tendency to atrophy of other tissues, notably the skin."

It was a long and circuitous route from laying pigeon hens to women with backaches or hip fractures. During the late 1960s and early 1970s, when ERT finally came into widespread use as an aging preventive, or Youth Pill, the osteoporosis rate in women continued to rise.

Efficacy Still Uncertain

Several years ago, the National Academy of Sciences–National Research Council rated ERT as "probably effective" for some kinds of osteoporosis, but "only when used in conjunction with other important therapeutic measures such as diet, calcium, physiotherapy, and good general health-promoting measures. . . . Final classification of this indication requires further investigation," NAS–NRC admitted.

On the other hand, *Medical Letter*, a publication for physicians that evaluates safety and effectiveness of drugs, which, like NAS–NRC, relies on a distinguished panel of consultants, is frankly unconvinced. *Medical Letter* has said:

"Routine use of estrogens in menopausal patients for prevention or treatment of osteoporosis continues to be recommended by some experienced clinicians, but in the opinion of a majority of *Medical Letter* consultants there is no convincing evidence that estrogen administration reduces the loss of bone mass in aging women. . . . Calcium balance often becomes positive early in the course of estrogen administration in osteoporotic patients, but long-term treatment is accompanied by a less positive, or return to a negative, calcium balance, and it is possible that long-term estrogen treatment may ultimately result in decreased bone formation."

Two new studies from England seem to indicate that ERT prevents bone loss in some women whose menopause is surgically induced and who may be especially susceptible to early osteoporosis.

In the United States, New York University's Lila Nachtigall, an endocrinologist, has identified a second subgroup of osteoporosis-prone women whose bone condition benefits from ERT. Dr. Nachtigall's ten year double-blind study was of women confined in a chronic disease hospital. These patients had very low activity levels, probably a less than optimum diet, as well as little exposure to D-producing sunlight which helps calcium to work.

Understandably, Ayerst is eager to have ERT rated as definitely effective for osteoporosis. So is the entire American Home Products Corporation, because as noted in a recent report from Merrill, Lynch, Pierce, Fenner and Smith: "Premarin [is] one of American Home Products' major [drugs]. . . . We estimate that domestic sales [represent] about 75 to 80% of the total market for estrogen replacement therapy. . . . The company's profit margin on Premarin is extraordinarily high—we estimate 80% pretax—as a result of its market dominance and the low cost of goods . . . the urine of pregnant mares. . . . Thus, domestic sales of Premarin could have accounted for about . . . 10% of American Home Products' 1975 reported earnings of $1.58." *If* Premarin prevents osteoporosis, then, once again, some physicians may be reindoctrinated to "Keep Her on Premarin" after menopause symptoms subside.

An FDA Advisory Committee met to weigh the research on February 18, 1977. The Committee concluded:

There is evidence that estrogen is effective in controlling loss of bone mass in post-menopausal women, but lack of evidence that it prevents fractures.

This leaves the question still unresolved for, as we have noted, fracture, rather than bone loss per se is the crucial issue. Many persons who show bone loss on x-rays remain in vigorous health, without fractures or any discomforts, perhaps because exercise and sensible nutrition keep their supporting ligaments in good condition.

A defense of estrogen for healthy women was given by Dr. Robert Recker, an osteoporosis researcher from Omaha. Recker states that, with aging, the "efficiency" of calcium absorption from the diet appears to decrease. He argues that "estrogens protect against suboptimal calcium intake by forcing better utilization of diet calcium." But, he explains further, postmenopausal women who are treated with calcium supplements and no estrogen (Recker recommends a form called calcium carbonate, 0.6 gm daily) also retain better than average bone mass. Recker postulates that the true calcium requirement for postmenopausal women is 1.4 gm a day, which is higher than the standard recommended allowance, and difficult to obtain from diet alone.

A member of the FDA Committee observed that Recker's research, presumably in support of ERT, was really a better case for moderate calcium therapy. Neither calcium nor ERT are proved to stop fractures once they occur, but insofar as bone loss is a predisposing condition, they seem equally effective in allaying it.

Meanwhile at a nutrition symposium, Dr. E. Neige Todhunter, visiting professor at Vanderbilt University School of Medicine, presented further evidence that dietary supplements of calcium may be advisable for most women after menopause. Older women also use some B vitamins "inefficiently," and may demonstrate abnormally low levels of trace elements, including chromium. The need for other vitamins and minerals is related to the problems of the specific patient, Todhunter emphasized, but "Calcium should be watched carefully."

Besides being safer than estrogen, calcium is cheaper. A year's supply of the supplement Dr. Recker suggests costs five dollars, and requires no prescription.

After the meetings, another FDA employee mused, "I wish they could see my mother, and I wish her old G.P. was still around to hear all this. It would give him a good laugh. Mother is 82 years old, grows all her own vegetables, and still goes horseback riding every weekend. When she started her 'change' her doctor advised her to stay active, and take a calcium pill every day for the rest of her life.

"And she has."

CHAPTER 28

The Reckoning

We live in a society which is becoming one vast hospital. More and more women are being told that they—and their children—have been damaged by previous medication, and that new treatment is required [because of] the consequences of the previous treatment.

> Dr. Mary Daly, National Women's
> Health Network Demonstration at
> FDA, 1975

Nineteen seventy-five was a year of reckoning for the American doctor.

Health was the most inflationary segment of the economy, even beyond food and shelter. The President's Council on Wage and Price Stability warned that the passive and uninformed role of patients gave doctors and hospitals a dangerous monopoly. Patients were struggling to break the monopoly, petitioning the federal government to include consumer labeling on prescription drugs, as well as monitoring hospitals and physicians in their communities. Patients were refusing to sign "anything goes" consent forms when they went into the hospital for surgery. Patients were even suing to obtain their own medical records.

Nineteen seventy-five was also a year when the ERT patient, most particularly, discovered she was getting less than she thought, and more than she bargained for.

Hooked on ERT

The first question to ask about any drug is, Does it work? Does it do what it is supposed to? A standard method of testing this is to try out the drug against a placebo.

Placebo trials are notably missing from most ERT research. In 1975, however, the *British Medical Journal* reported one careful placebo study, performed in England by Dr. Jean Coope on patients with menopausal symptoms. All of Coope's patients were monitored for the following complaints: insomnia, nervousness, depressions, dizziness, weakness, joint pain, headaches, palpitations, prickling sensations, and hot flashes. Half of the patients received pills of conjugated estrogens, while the other half got lactose (milk-sugar) pills.

The first ninety days of the study brought *dramatic improvement* for both groups. There was no significant difference in any symptom, except that the placebo did not relieve hot flashes as completely.

Then, midway in the six-month study, the products were switched, with interesting results. The real ERT maintained the favorable response first brought about by the dummy medication, but the group that had first been treated with estrogen experienced a pronounced return of symptoms when the placebo was substituted.

Coope's study provides confirmation that taking the first estrogen pill is a major decision and, contrary to assurances that it can be used for a few months and then terminated, many women, like Coope's patients, undergo a kind of cold turkey.

The good news, then, from Dr. Coope is that most ERT-treated symptoms can be cured with a placebo. This does not mean that the symptoms were imaginary, but that faith and optimism (that relief is at hand) wield an enormous power over bodily responses.

The bad news from Dr. Coope is that once you've had real ERT, a placebo no longer works.

Linda W., who describes herself as "glad to be 50," is the mother of five grown children, and a busy, prominent figure in the women's movement. At the age of 40, Linda had a hysterectomy, sparing her ovaries, from which she recovered in weeks. She was fine for almost a decade, but in the fall of 1974 Linda began to get an occasional hot flash.

"They were no big problem at first," she explains. "They usually happened at the opera, or in an overheated room. I did not have the kind of flashes that leave the pillow drenched."

By Christmas, however, Linda felt "terribly tired," an uncharacteristic state, and she also experienced "floating back pains—shoulder pains in the morning, waist pains in the afternoon, and so on."

She had only "an hour's worth of energy right after eating," could barely sit up in bed, felt "wiped out," had insomnia, and more flashes.

"Even Betty Friedan, who breezed through her own menopause, and who doesn't really believe in it, commented that I didn't seem myself physically," Linda recalls. After a consultation with her energetic 80-year-old mother in San Antonio, who had been helped by ERT during a severe menopause thirty years earlier, Linda decided to try it, too.

For a year she took it for three weeks a month, followed by one week's rest. Then she tried stopping for two weeks. She felt a drop in her energy level, a loss of interest in sex, and her floating backaches returned. So she resumed her three-weeks-a-month schedule, and is planning to stay with it for the time being. She points out correctly that she need not fear endometrial cancer as she has no uterus.

Linda was not depressed by the loss of her fertility, which she'd relinquished most cheerfully years earlier when her uterus was removed. Neither did she miss her menstrual periods, or go through the typical menopause anxiety of having them come and go unpredictably. Like all women who have uterine hysterectomies, her menses had ceased but not the monthly cycle of her ovaries.

Nonetheless, when in her late forties, Linda's ovarian (and therefore pituitary) output altered, she had a difficult adjustment physiologically, starting with mild hot flashes and progressing, over two or three months, to a state of feeling "wiped out." Because her mother also had an especially uncomfortable menopause, Linda suggests that there may be hereditary factors.

ERT brought Linda speedy relief. Now she is reconciled to staying on it for years, a prospect that would be especially dangerous if she still had her uterus. Even without her uterus, she is altering her metabolism unfavorably, and increasing her risk of gall-bladder disease and breast cancer, as well as other serious illnesses. We feel that safer remedies (see section entitled *Menopause: Wholesome Remedies*) might have seen Linda through her difficult months without ERT.

Warnings to Doctors

On reading the full list of possible ERT complications and side effects in the package insert, many women give it up on the spot. Here is how one company, Syntex, before the great risk of endometrial cancer was clarified in December 1975, described its ERT preparation Evex, in its information for doctors, which women don't see (we have simplified, amplified or omitted some of the technical terminology):

- Evex is recommended for the treatment of menopausal syndrome, as well as the further conditions for which most estrogen products are also employed: senile vaginitis, amenorrhea, inoperable prostatic cancer, and so on.
- Dosage should be carefully adjusted to the individual needs of the patient, and maintained at the smallest effective dose. Cyclic therapy is recommended—three weeks with one week rest period.

IMPORTANT NOTES:
- An increased risk of thromboembolic disease [blood clotting] associated with the use of certain estrogen preparations has now been shown. It has been estimated that users of the estrogen-containing preparations studied are 4 to 7 times as likely as non-users to develop thromboembolic disease without evident cause.
- Further risks, such as elevated blood pressure, liver dysfunction, and reduced tolerance to carbohydrates have not yet been quantified.
- Long-term administration of both natural and synthetic estrogens in animals increases the frequency for some carcinomas. Close clinical surveillance of all women taking estrogens must be continued. It has been reported that the maternal ingestion of diethylstilbestrol during pregnancy appears to increase the risk of vaginal adenocarcinoma developing years later in the offspring.

CONTRAINDICATIONS:

- Estrogen is not recommended for persons with:
  - —markedly impaired liver function, as in hepatitis
  - —known or suspected breast cancer, except under special conditions
  - —known or suspected cancer of the endometrium
  - —undiagnosed genital bleeding
  - —persons who have ever had blood clots, stroke, or pulmonary embolism
- Estrogens should not be prescribed for any woman who might possibly be pregnant.

WARNINGS:

- Estrogens should be stopped immediately if the following symptoms of clotting disorders occur:
  - —severe chest pains or shortness of breath
  - —coughing up blood
  - —sudden migraine, double vision, or protrusion of the eyeball
- Estrogens are excreted in the milk of nursing mothers, and have estrogenic effects on the infant.
- Estrogens should be discontinued if hypercalcemia [abnormally high concentrations of calcium in the blood] occurs.
- Estrogen may cause liver tumors involving serious or fatal hemorrhage, and may also be linked to cancer of the liver. Symptoms are acute abdominal pain, or an abdominal mass.

PRECAUTIONS:

- Signs of excessive estrogen stimulation include abnormal uterine bleeding, breast pain, or edema.
- Conditions influenced by fluid retention, such as epilepsy, migraine, asthma, heart or kidney dysfunction, may be adversely affected by estrogen and should be carefully monitored.
- Patients with a history of depression should be carefully observed. Estrogen should be discontinued if serious depression recurs.
- Under the stimulation, pre-existing fibroid tumors may increase in size.
- Women with a strong family history of cancer, chronic breast cysts, or abnormal mammograms should be administered estrogen with caution.
- A decrease in glucose tolerance has been observed in a significant percentage of patients on estrogen-containing preparations. Diabetic patients should be carefully observed.
- Because they alter the metabolism of calcium and

phosphorus, estrogens should be used with caution by patients who have metabolic bone disease with hypercalcemia, or impaired kidney function.

• Estrogens should be used judiciously in young patients, in whom bone growth is not complete, for they cause epiphyseal closure.

• Since estrogens have been known to cause tumors, some of them malignant, in five species of animals, physical examinations before and during estrogen therapy should include special reference to breast and pelvic organs as well as Pap smears.

• Prolonged high doses of estrogens inhibit pituitary function. This should be borne in mind in treating patients who wish to have children, for fertility may be impaired.

• Continued use of estrogens results in prolonged stimulation of the endometrium and breasts. Cyclic administration may diminish the effects.

• Treatment with estrogens may mask the beginning of menopause.

• Certain endocrine and liver function tests may be affected by treatment with estrogens. If such tests are abnormal it is recommended that they be repeated after the drug has been withdrawn for two months.

• The possible influence of prolonged estrogen therapy on pituitary, ovarian, adrenal, liver, or uterine function awaits further study.

ADVERSE REACTIONS:

• A statistically significant association has been demonstrated between the use of certain estrogen products and the following serious disorders:
 —thrombophlebitis
 —pulmonary embolism
 —cerebral thrombosis

• Evidence is suggestive of an association between estrogen preparations and eye disorders such as retinal thrombosis [a clot in the eye causing blindness] and optic neuritis [nerve inflammation which can also cause blindness].

• The following adverse reactions are known to occur in patients receiving estrogen:
 —nausea
 —vomiting
 —gastrointestinal symptoms (such as abdominal cramps or bloating
 —edema
 —breakthrough bleeding, spotting, or withdrawal bleeding
 —chloasma [skin discolorations]
 —breast tenderness and enlargement

—melasma
—change in body weight (increase or decrease)
—changes in cervical erosion and cervical secretions
—allergic rash
—loss of libido and enlargement of the breasts in the male
—reactivation of endometriosis
—migraine
—hepatic porphyria becoming manifest
—cholestatic jaundice
—rise in blood pressure in susceptible individuals
—mental depression
—possible diminution in lactation when given immediately postpartum

- The following adverse reactions may occur in patients receiving estrogen:
  —headache
  —cystitis-like syndrome
  —loss of scalp hair
  —erythema nodosum
  —hemorrhagic eruption
  —premenstrual-like syndrome
  —changes in libido
  —changes in appetite
  —nervousness
  —dizziness
  —fatigue
  —backache
  —erythema multiforme
  —itching

- In addition [the Evex labeling concludes], lab tests of many functions including thyroid, liver and blood coagulation may be altered by ERT.

This, then, was the Youth Pill before the news got worse, the ERT that many doctors were giving, and continue to give today—*even to women who do not have menopausal symptoms*. Although the Evex labeling runs to several thousand words, it omits some further side effects which were strongly suggested in the scientific literature, even before 1975. These "hidden bonuses" include:

GALL-BLADDER DISEASE

In the city of Boston in 1972, in a vast study involving 24 participating hospitals, 157 otherwise healthy women, aged

45 to 69 and undergoing gall-bladder surgery, were interviewed concerning ERT use. The report, published in the *New England Journal of Medicine* on January 3, 1974, concluded that ERT increases the risk of gall-bladder disease *two-and-one-half times*.

Since then, the mechanism by which estrogen saturates bile with cholesterol has come to be better understood. (See section on the pill.)

DEPLETION OF VITAMINS

Much more work has been done on the pill's effect on nutrition than on the effect of ERT. (This work is elaborated on in the section on the pill.) However, in those studies that included ERT users, the effects were found to be similar, as would be expected.

HEART ATTACKS

It is known that heart attacks increase in middle-aged males given estrogen, and in women, especially those over 40, who take the birth control pill. The situation concerning women who take estrogen alone has not been clarified, but progestins (the second hormone in the pill) have *not* been implicated in heart attacks.

POSTPONEMENT OF FLASHES

Women who take ERT to control the flashes of menopause may simply get them later when the ERT is stopped. Flashes are a relatively "normal" occurrence to women in their late forties and early fifties, but were not intended by nature to occur in *older* women. They may be more severe or troublesome when they occur later. The differences have not been studied, but the reality should be borne in mind by prospective ERT patients: Delaying a symptom is not the same as curing it.

FACIAL SCARS

A serious metabolic condition of middle age called porphyria is sometimes hereditary, and sometimes a reaction to drugs including estrogen. It may involve the excessive growth of facial hair, abnormalities of pigment metabolism, and large skin swellings that form scar tissue as they heal.

HYSTERECTOMY RISKS

The fact that ERT promotes several serious conditions that are apt to precipitate hysterectomy is not really clarified in the labeling. These conditions include:

1. *Hyperplasia*, or an increase in the cellular bulk of the endometrium, shown by Gusberg in 1947 to be stimulated by ERT. Some hyperplasia is considered precancerous, or even the equivalent of early-stage cancer, by some pathologists. When hyperplasia occurs, the uterus, as a rule, *must go*, or cancer is apt to follow.

2. *Rapid growth of fibroids* or fibrous tissue in the uterus, which sometimes can be surgically excised without hysterectomy, but for which hysterectomy is usually performed, especially in women who are finished with childbearing. Left alone with no ERT stimulation, fibroids usually "regress to unimportance" in the years following menopause. Small fibroids are extremely common, occurring in perhaps one-third of women. To feed a fibroid with estrogen is begging for a hysterectomy.

Fibroids are *not* considered precancerous, and may be safely ignored when small.

3. *Endometriosis*, or the presence of endometrial tissue in abnormal locations such as the uterus wall or the bladder wall. Endometrial cells, usually found only in the lining of the uterus, are exquisitely sensitive to estrogen stimulation. It is this tissue of the human body that has now been shown most commonly to turn cancerous when overdosed with estrogen. Endometriosis is extremely difficult to control, and may cause hemorrhaging and severe pain. Like fibroids, mild or moderate endometriosis usually clears up when menopause takes place. But certain supplemental estrogens make endometriosis worse. Some authorities, such as Somers Sturgis, maintain that a history of endometriosis should be a contraindication to ERT. Many physicians do not even ask their patients if they have any such history.

4. *Hematometra*, a condition in which the uterus fills up with blood. When the uterus of a woman in her seventies or eighties is suddenly stimulated with high levels of estrogen, it is not surprising that trouble may follow. Some foolish doctors may suddenly start an older woman on ERT, to treat osteoporosis or spruce up the

vagina. Hematometra can be life-threatening to women of this age. Emergency hysterectomies usually result, which many of these women do not survive.

Another reason surgery may be especially dangerous for the ERT user is that blood clotting factors are affected adversely. In the Coope double-blind study from England, the researchers couldn't usually tell which women were getting the real ERT from the amount of improvement they had in their symptoms. Sadly, however, they *could* tell by blood tests, which revealed abnormalities in the women on real estrogen. Subsequent research, performed at New York Medical College, confirmed that the blood coagulability of some ERT users increases 300 percent!

In the latest (1977) package insert many changes have been made, updating the 1975 information. A long section, prominently set off in a box, describes the risk of endometrial cancer and of birth defects, suggesting abortion if a woman on estrogen becomes pregnant. The recommended use is further restricted to "moderate to severe *vasomotor* symptoms [hot flashes] associated with the menopause. (There is no evidence that estrogens are effective for nervous symptoms or depression . . . and they should not be used to treat these conditions.)" The lowest dose should be used, and "medication should be discontinued as soon as possible."

In addition, new warnings are given about breast cancer, gall-bladder disease, the possibility of the occurrence of the same serious side effects as the birth control pill, high blood pressure, increased risk of jaundice especially in women who had jaundice during pregnancy, decreased folic acid and increased fats in the blood, painful menstruation, monilial vaginitis, breast secretion, growth of facial and body hair, intolerance to contact lenses, changes in the cornea of the eyes, involuntary jerking movements, and amenorrhea during and after treatment.

What new side effects will there be in the next revision, or the one after that?

CHAPTER 29

ERT and Cancer

The conclusions of the California Tumor Registry are that the increase [in endometrial cancer] is . . . due to the . . . introduction of potent carcinogens . . . to the population group involved, and represents one of the most dramatic and significant increases in cancer incidence ever recorded.

Dr. Donald Austin,
December 15, 1975

In the United States, 15 to 20 million women take estrogen products—mainly the pill and ERT—on a regular basis. Others take them sporadically, to treat menstrual problems, say, or to dry up breast milk. Nearly all of us, male, female, and household pet, get estrogens in our meat.

Slowly, inevitably, the users of estrogens are learning that these unnecessary drugs do cause human cancer in one or another or several target organs.

The 1971 findings concerning cancer and DES came from Arthur Herbst and his colleagues at Massachusetts General Hospital. By contrast, the 1975 ERT studies were the work of *many* investigators, which all coalesced, or came together, in December. So many scientists dot the cast of characters that a summary of the contributions of each seems the clearest way to tell the story.

Pentti Siiteri, University of California Medical School in San Francisco, and Paul MacDonald, University of Texas Southwestern Medical School:

Since cancer is more prevalent in older than younger women, it was formerly argued that high levels of natural estrogen might *protect* against it. As we have said (see chap. 25) Siiteri and MacDonald, with various associates, were first to demonstrate that postmenopausal women continue to manifest high levels of estrone (a type of estrogen) which is synthesized in body fats from precursors formed in the ovaries and adrenal glands. They later demonstrated that women with cancer produce twice as much natural estrone as healthy women.

The amount of estrone formed naturally is proportional to body weight, which explains why obesity is one risk factor in cancer, and why a diet high in animal fats may be another. The low incidence of cancer in Japanese women *living in Japan* does not hold for those living in Hawaii or mainland United States.

Premarin, which stands for PREgnant MAREs' urINe, is composed principally of estrone, the very estrogen that postmenopausal women who get cancer have too much of naturally. The work of Siiteri and MacDonald, which dates back to 1966, gives the lie to comforting theories, espoused by ERT promoters, that high levels of estrogen protect against cancer in older women. Siiteri and MacDonald provided the framework that helped all the 1975 studies to fall into place.

Harry Ziel and William Finkle of Kaiser-Permanente Medical Center in Los Angeles:
In a study that cost only $1,900, Ziel and Finkle gathered the hospital records of 94 Kaiser-Permanente patients who had endometrial cancer. These were matched with 188 carefully selected control women—2 for each cancer patient—who were much like the cancer victims in age, area of residence, and general health.

The records were evaluated by "blind" analysts who did not know which patients had developed cancer. Women who had used conjugated estrogens for seven years or longer, it was demonstrated, developed endometrial cancer at a rate *14 times as high* as comparable women who had never used it at all. Women who had used such products for one to five years developed this cancer at a rate that was about *5½ times as high as non-users.*

The overall risk, including longer and shorter term ERT patients, was computed to be almost 8 times as great as normal.

ERT, according to Ziel and Finkle's research, may be far more dangerous than heavy smoking. If you smoke for twenty years or longer, your risk of lung cancer increases seventeen- or eighteenfold. Your risk of endometrial cancer increases fourteenfold *after only seven years of ERT use.*

Donald Smith, Ross Prentice, Donovan Thompson, Walter Herman, of The Mason Clinic, University of Washington, Seattle:

Donald Smith and his colleagues compared 317 endometrial cancer patients with an equal number of women who had *other female cancers,* usually of the cervix or ovaries. All were matched for age at diagnosis.

Smith and his colleagues made an observation that should interest and concern the prevention minded. While ERT may trigger endometrial cancer in any woman, the risk factor is greatest in those who have no other predisposing conditions. In a sense, ERT is more dangerous to a slim woman than a heavy one, for example. The heavy woman has a greater risk to start with, but the ERT partially cancels out the difference.

Thomas Mack, director of Cancer Surveillance at the University of Southern California Medical School, with M.C. Pike, B.E. Henderson, R.I. Pfeffer, V.R. Gerkins, M. Arthur, S.E. Brown:

Thomas Mack and his colleagues studied the residents of a southern California retirement community. Here again the odds of developing endometrial cancer increased eightfold among ERT users, the same average figure arrived at by Ziel and Finkle. And, like the Smith group in Seattle, the Mack group also noted that the dangers of estrogen therapy appear most striking in healthy women with no other risk factors.

While Ziel and Finkle brought in evidence concerning *length* of ERT use, the Mack group was interested in *dosage.* They report that higher doses of estrogen also enhance the risk. Thus, dose and duration of ERT are implicated in different studies.

We know now that length of ERT use increases the risk of cancer, and that size of dosage adds to this effect. What about differences in specific products?

Most of the women recently studied were taking conjugated estrogens of the Premarin type. Some doctors are switching their patients to alternative products, in the hope that these may prove less virulent. Unfortunately, the Mack group—which looked at product variations— concluded that other estrogens are similarly carcinogenic.

Donald Austin, chief of the California Tumor Registry:
Early investigators such as Saul Gusberg, who maintained that estrogens stimulate cancer of the endometrium, did not appear, at first, to be supported by national health statistics. Our Third National Cancer Survey, covering the period from 1947 to 1971, revealed no increase in this diagnosis.

But that was before the Youth Pill mystique led to a tripling or quadrupling of the ERT prescriptions. On December 16, 1975, Dr. Donald Austin informed the FDA that among white women 50 and over, living in California, there was more than an 80 percent increase in uterine cancer just in the years from 1969 to 1974.

The increase was noted in seventy-five hospitals, and was most pronounced in areas of greatest affluence where ERT use is high. In Alameda County, Austin reported, the annual incidence of endometrial cancer has *tripled*.

This unfortunate trend in now confirmed in other states that keep good registries, including Washington and Connecticut. Since 1969, endometrial cancer has steadily and rapidly increased.

FDA spokesman Crout has commented: "The chronic users tend to be middle- and upper-income women, the kind of people who go to doctors and the kind of people who would most value the longed-for youthful appearance. It's an interesting example of the poor being spared, if you will, some of the adverse effects of estrogens that are now coming to the fore."

Bruce Stadel of the National Institutes of Health, Bethesda, and Noel Weiss of the School of Public Health and Community Medicine, University of Washington, Seattle:
What are the women who take ERT getting for all their risks? Is it helping them in other ways?

Possibly yes, in some cases, but no in a great many others, according to the most reliable data we have on who uses it and why.

In an elaborate study of Seattle area residents, Bruce Stadel and Noel Weiss estimated that 51 percent of all women over 50 had, by 1973 to 1974, used ERT for over three months' duration. Most amazingly, of those who first responded that they had *not* used it, more than a quarter were found to be ERT patients after all. This was established during personal interviews at which estrogens were identified by a pill display, and by further discussion with the women's doctors.

The estrogen users were—again—more educated and affluent than non-users. One in every 20 was under 39, 1 in 5 was 40 to 49, almost half were 50 to 59, and 1 in 3 was 60 or older. The median use was slightly over ten years, while the longest was over thirty.

More than half of the ERT patients had tried at least two preparations, and some as many as four. One in 3 took straight Premarin; 1 in 5 used Premarin combination products; the remainder used other oral brands or received injections.

The women on ERT were more apt to have suffered troublesome hot flashes before taking it—about 2 out of 5 reported this complaint—while the frequency in non-users was less than 1 in 7. Clearly then, the flashes drove some women to ERT, but not the majority who took it. Weiss and Stadel conclude that "the frequency of menopausal estrogen use . . . is much higher than the estimated frequency of severe menopausal symptoms. . . . It appears that physicians in King and Pierce counties do not follow a conservative approach to hormonal treatment of menopausal problems."

Cancer of the Uterus

Cancers of the reproductive system—the uterus, ovaries, and cervix—constitute 1 out of every 5 malignancies diagnosed in women. As cancers go, they have a relatively high cure rate, for only 2 in 15 of these cause death.

The probability that endometrial cancer will occur in a postmenopausal woman with an intact uterus who *does not use estrogen* is *1* in 1,000 a year. The risk among estrogen users is *4 to 8* in 1,000 a year, or higher, depending on length of use. According to Noel Weiss, no other cancer—not even breast cancer, which is much on the increase—occurs with even as high an annual frequency as 3 per 1,000.

Thomas Mack explains it like this: *A woman who has a uterus and uses estrogens has a risk of developing endometrial cancer that is greater than her usual combined risk from cervical, breast, and endometrial cancer.*

It would be reassuring if endometrial cancer, now presumed to be the number one cancer, by far, in ERT users, was readily detectable by Pap test. The simple Pap test is highly reliable in diagnosing cancer of the cervix, and death rates due to cervical cancer have therefore dropped significantly.

Unfortunately the Pap catches endometrial cancer only about half the time. For a sure diagnosis, the tests are quite elaborate, expensive—and painful. Doctors are still uncertain which procedures are most accurate. Some advise dilatation and curettage, often requiring hospitalization, but others maintain that an endometrial smear and biopsy, in the hands of a specialized expert, is as good or better.

A procedure called the Gravlee jet wash is favored by Dr. George L. Weid, editor of the *Journal of Reproductive Medicine*. Jet-wash screening requires an involved laboratory work-up, making it costly, but Weid advises it be done routinely for all "high-risk patients" including long-term ERT users.

Women whose menopause menstrual irregularities persist unduly long, whose bleeding ceases only to recur many months later, or whose menstruation is unusually painful are also considered potentially at risk.

Should cancer occur, a hysterectomy is usually performed. Radiation treatment is added when the patient has more cancer than simple surgery can handle. Some women, who either have advanced disease or other conditions, such as heart trouble, which preclude surgery, are treated with massive radiation alone.

On the theory that they have an "opposing" effect to estrogen, progestins are added by some doctors to their therapy program, most frequently a product called Depo-Provera. Even if these hormones help, their effect is temporary.

When endometrial cancer is fatal, progestins may produce "subjective improvement" just prior to death. Unless the family is warned, "the illusion can be devastating," according to *Emergency Medicine*.

Breast Cancer

For many years, most breast specialists opposed the use of estrogen in women who have a family history of breast cancer (in mother, sister, or daughter), or who have had prior breast surgery for mastitis or dysplasia, or who react with severe breast congestion to hormone pills. There was much suggestive evidence linking estrogen and breast cancer, but, until very recently, no large-scale study that could be called conclusive.

Robert Wilson claimed that ERT kept the breasts lovely and youthful. But among the women *we* interviewed —and there were some who are very fond of ERT—not one suggested seriously that it had benefited her breasts.

Quite the opposite. We heard story after story of breast discomfort, and worse, among former ERT users. In many instances, a woman's general doctor urged her to stay with the medication, while the breast specialist she finally consulted took her off. Here are excerpts from three of our tape-recorded interviews which illustrate the medical confusion, and sometimes poor judgment, that characterizes the prescribing of ERT:

Aviva S., a 45-year-old writer: "Fifteen years ago, when I was 30, I read an article about estrogens. I had great faith in my gynecologist. When I mentioned the article, he put me on Premarin, which I continued taking until recently. My periods became irregular, and I repeatedly called my doctor, but he was unconcerned. Whenever I asked him about the advisability of the drug, he hit the ceiling and voiced strong disapproval of lay opinions. He was adamant about the strong points of Premarin, its beneficial effects on bones, dowager's hump, and vaginal secretions. I developed lumpy breasts, but my doctor said not to do self-examination, as I would be unable to distinguish between a 'normal' lump and a tumor.

"Recently I had a complete checkup at HIP [a prepaid medical plan in New York City, similar to Kaiser-Permanente]. A breast lump was disclosed, and I was referred to a surgeon. He discovered an even larger lump in the second breast. The gynecologist at HIP told me: 'If the lump turns out to be benign, continue the Premarin.' The surgeon said to stop. A second surgeon said that if fluid could be drawn from the lump there was no indication for biopsy. Such fluid *was* drawn, and I was told that I was lucky. I asked the second surgeon if there was any connection between the condition of my breasts and Premarin. He said: 'Absolutely.' He went on to tell me never to touch another hormone in my life, and that if I get hot flashes I should ask for a nonhormonal drug. 'Don't ever use Premarin again,' he warned me.

"Now I have to go to the doctor for a breast exam every three months. I worry a lot."

Aviva's case illustrates the standoff that so frequently occurs between gynecologists and breast surgeons. Two gynecologists urged her to take Premarin—which one later denied, by the way—and two breast specialists advised against it.

June W., a 54-year-old physiotherapist: "When I turned 47, my gynecologist put me on Norlestrin, which I took for two years with no problems. Then I fell and had to have surgery, so I was told to stop. I started having flashes, and after a time the doctor put me on Premarin—6.25 mg.

"For a while I was fine, but a year later I noticed my breasts enlarging. A clear fluid started oozing out of my left breast, just like after I had a baby. After about six months, the doctor decided to operate and found a benign tumor. I stopped the Premarin, but when the flashes came back, the doctor said to resume it. The one breast became much larger and heavier than the other, with a lump as big as my thumb, and the surgeon grew very concerned. He took me off Premarin for the last time.

"I'm okay now. I went through menopause with no medication. I had a mammogram two weeks ago and everything was fine. When I was on the Premarin, it helped my arthritis. In some ways I never felt so good. But if I had one thing in my whole life to do over differently, I would not take Premarin again!"

(One wonders why June's doctor prescribed it again, after her first experience. The breast surgeon wondered, too.)

Gloria B., a 37-year-old administrative assistant: "In 1971, in the course of a checkup, my GP took a Pap smear and said: 'You're not producing enough estrogen in your body. I want you to take Premarin.'

" 'But why?' I said. 'I'm only 32 and I have a breast lump that we're watching. And there's nothing else wrong with me. I've read enough to know that you shouldn't take hormones if you have a lump.'

" 'Well, ruff-ruff-ruff—' he said, 'that hasn't been decided yet—it's still controversial—and I think you need a little bit more estrogen.'

"So I took Premarin. But the lump kept worrying me. My doctor and his partner never once mentioned anything about a biopsy or a mammogram or breast cancer. 'What we're looking for,' they said, 'is a pea-sized three-dimensional lump, and this isn't it, so good-bye.'

"The only reason my cancer was discovered was that my husband changed health plans. Under the new plan I had to have an examination. Within four days I was in the hospital, and my breast lump turned out to be cancer. It was three years between the time I had discovered the lump and the time I was operated on—and meanwhile, I had been taking Premarin for no reason at all. My surgeon said: 'I think you have a malpractice case, but I can't put my name on it in court. I have to live with those doctors at the same hospital.'

"Here I had done everything a layman can do, had never neglected myself, and I ended up with cancer."

Gloria B.'s case illustrates why some gynecologists and GPs never see the harm their drugs may do. Serious conditions are treated by *other* specialists, and the patient is often too angry to tell the original doctor what happened. The specialists sometimes don't either, for they fear offending referral sources.

These cases are typical of the era just before the bombshell of August 1976. Perhaps the stories women hear and tell will be different from now on.

On January 21, 1976, at Senate hearings, Dr. Robert Hoover, of the National Cancer Institute, hinted that bad news was coming on ERT and the breast. He referred to an "unpublished study" of several thousand women in Louisville, Kentucky. Hoover's prestige notwithstanding, most reporters and doctors ignored the hint. After all, we can only absorb so much bad news at once. The American public was still reeling from the newly proven association between ERT and uterine cancer. Uterine cancer is highly curable with early detection, but breast cancer is not.

Hoover could not then say much about the "unpublished study," but he did venture his opinion of earlier research which claimed to show that ERT is "a cancer preventive or even a general youth-maintaining tonic." This work, he said firmly, was incompetent, and invalid—"conducted by gynecologists who, while I am certain they were well intentioned, had little or no experience in how to do an epidemiologic study. The result is a group of studies so heavily flawed in design, conduct, and analysis as to make any conclusions reached from them meaningless." Hoover went on to point out that "breast cancer is a disease notorious for the long intervals between relevant events and the appearance of the effects of these events." In other words, any sound study assaying the risks of ERT and breast cancer would have to compare women who had taken it at least a decade earlier with women who never had.

For seven months longer, until August 1976, women who no longer had a uterus went on thinking they could safely take ERT without risking cancer. Their doctors often assured them of this. Hoover had tried to warn otherwise, but was unheeded for the time being.

Once again, the *New England Journal of Medicine* carried the actual report. The study was authored by Hoover himself, with coauthors at the University of Louisville School of Medicine and the Harvard School of Public Health.

Here is what the Louisville study showed: During the first five years of estrogen use, breast cancer does not increase. It may even occur less frequently than it does among women who are not taking hormones. But after five years the risks start rising.

Fifteen years after commencing therapy, ERT patients have *twice as much breast cancer* as women who never used it. The length of time a woman stays on ERT does not seem to matter. What counts is simply the number of years that have passed since her first exposure. Dosages do matter, though, and the usual daily dose prescribed in the United States—1.25 or 2.5 mg—*is* associated with breast cancer many years later.

Estrogen therapy also seemed to negate the relative protection against breast cancer enjoyed by women who had had children, or had had their ovaries removed before menopause. Women who have had benign breast diseases ordinarily face twice the usual risk of developing breast cancer later. If, however, the benign breast disease occurred after taking ERT, cancer risks increase sevenfold.

As 1976 drew to a close, it was patently clear that the estrogenizing of American women is a major factor in our rising rates of female cancers. Breast cancer alone kills 33,000 women annually, and 89,000 new cases are diagnosed each year.

There is one regrettable sidelight on Hoover's report. The Senate hearings at which he hinted that a link had been suggested between breast cancer and ERT took place in January; the report in the *New England Journal of Medicine* was published in August. Why did *seven months* elapse?

The reason has to do with a policy of the *New England Journal*, probably the most distinguished medical periodical in the United States. The *Journal* forbids contributors to give out any of the contents of their articles to the media before they appear in the *Journal*. The seven months time lag in this case seems regrettable, especially it one happens to be a woman on ERT who thought she was "safe" from breast cancer.

CHAPTER 30

Products and Dosages

Mary D., who is healthy and high-spirited at 70, has been using Premarin for thirty years and smoking cigarettes for more than fifty.

"Now they want to take away all my comfort," she sighs. "The Premarin I might give up. The cigarettes—never."

What does the Premarin do for her? Has it kept her young?

"I look no better nor worse for the wear than women my age who don't take it," says Mary. "Anyone with eyes or a head on her shoulders can see it makes no difference in that respect. It's just for my flashes. I had an early menopause—a natural one, no hysterectomy—but the flashes were very bad. None of my friends were using Premarin—they weren't the type. I wasn't either, but the flashes were not in my head. I could have survived the daytime, although I often wanted to jump out of all my clothes, but at night I just couldn't sleep.

"My GP said that there was something I could take, but he didn't want the responsibility—he said I might get cancer and sue him. He sent me to a gynecologist. The gynecologist gave me yellow Premarin [1.25 mg, an intermediate dose] and told me to take it two weeks out of the month. That was thirty years ago.

"I was fine. My son grew up, my husband died, and several years ago I retired. Every so often my GP has advised me to stop the Premarin, or else I have thought, is this expense still necessary? Besides, in the wintertime, at my age, you like being a little bit warm.

"So I have stopped at intervals, but in a month's time the flashes have come back, just at night, less severely than before, but enough to wake me every hour or two. So I call the gynecologist, and he mails me a new prescription."

Mails her a prescription? Doesn't he do a Pap smear, or, better yet, a biopsy, D&C, or jet washing—any one of the tests recommended for high-risk patients such as long-term ERT users like Mary?

"Oh, yes," Mary explained. "From time to time the GP says I should get a Pap smear, so I see this gynecologist in person. I've had exactly five Pap smears in thirty years; the last one was just a few months ago—at the gynecologist's request. I called him for my prescription, but he wouldn't send it. 'Haven't you been reading the papers?' he asked.

"I told him that I had, but I've always known Premarin can cause cancer—that was what my GP warned me in the first place. My cigarettes might give me cancer, too. I didn't know what the new fuss was about. So the gynecologist renewed my prescription. He said: 'I guess after thirty years you're able to handle it.' He didn't do any special checkup either, just the usual Pap."

We asked Mary if she'd ever had any Premarin side effects. She said no—no bleeding, no breast tenderness, no weight gain or skin rash.

Did Premarin do anything for her energy or mental outlook? No, none of that either. She felt exactly the same on it or off it, except that the flashes would return.

Mary was puzzled about dosages, however. She had met a woman who took it every other day, and others who used it three weeks a month or four, instead of two. She asked her gynecologist how dosages were arrived at.

"He just blinked at me, as if it were an extraordinary question," she said. "He told me to take it the same way I always had."

Monitoring of ERT Patients

Mary D. is not being adequately monitored for harmful side effects of ERT. She has had only five Pap tests in thirty years, and no further assays of her endometrial condition. She should, from time to time, have an endometrial biopsy or one of the alternative procedures described in the previous chapter.

ERT patients today are understandably confused about the expensive lab tests and evaluations that some doctors require. Sometimes hospitalization is involved, even when the patient feels perfectly well. Are these procedures necessary, or are they excessive?

Long-term ERT is so chancy to any woman with a uterus that careful monitoring is no frill—it is essential. Most doctors and patients who doubted this were convinced by the cancer statistics that emerged in 1975.

The standard tests for estrogen deficiency are a different matter. Vaginal smears are not reliable, and they are much overused. Levels jump all about, depending on where you are in your biological cycles, and what cells the doctor happens to catch on his swab. Vaginal smears may be of some help in adjusting estrogen dosage, but no woman should be placed on ERT solely on the basis of her smear. Laboratory tests of pituitary output are more precise. Measured in "mouse units," pituitary gonadotropins always rise—to about eight times the premenopause level—in women whose ovulation has ceased. In a few menopausal women, the levels are higher yet.

Later, pituitary output may diminish, but still remains much higher than it had been in the fertile years. The body adjusts, in time, to these higher levels, and flashes—if they occurred—usually stop, provided no ERT has been used to delay them.

The ERT Products

Women take ERT in any of the following forms (this list contains most of the common brand-name products. Generic versions are also available):

ORAL PRODUCTS WHICH ARE STRAIGHT ESTROGEN:
>   *Amnestrogen* by Squibb: red-coated tablets (.625 mg), yellow-coated tablets (1.25 mg), purple-coated tablets (2.5 mg).
>   *Premarin* by Ayerst: reddish-coated oval tablets (.625 mg), bright yellow-coated oval tablets (1.25 mg), purple-coated oval tablets (2.5 mg), green-coated oval tablets (.3 mg).

Estratab by Reid-Provident: yellow-coated tablets (.625 mg), red-coated tablets (1.25 mg), pink-coated tablets (2.5 mg).

Evex by Syntex: orange-coated tablets (.625 mg), pink-coated tablets (1.25 mg), yellow-coated tablets (2.5 mg).

Ogen by Abbott: yellow tablets (.625 mg), peach tablets (1.25 mg), blue tablets (3 mg), light green tablets (6 mg).

Estinyl by Schering: beige-coated tablets (.02 mg), pink-coated tablets (.05 mg), peach-coated tablets (.5 mg).

Diethylstilbestrol by Lilly: red-coated tablets or white tablets (.1 mg, .25 mg, 1 mg and 5 mg).

Hormonin by Carnrick: pink and white tablets (1.13 mg), green and white tablets (2.27 mg).

Estrace by Mead Johnson: lavender, scored tablets (1 mg), turquoise tablets (2 mg).

ORAL PRODUCTS WHICH COMBINE ESTROGEN AND
OTHER DRUGS:

This group includes preparations containing male hormones (testosterone), vitamins, tranquilizers, and other more unusual ingredients. They are his 'n' her compounds, frequently recommended for aging *men* with osteoporosis. In Australia, young men take them, too, as contraceptive pills!

These ERT products contain testosterone:

Gynetone 02 by Schering: salmon-pink-coated tablets (.02 mg estrogen and 5 mg methyl-testosterone).

Gynetone 04 by Schering: green tablets (.04 mg estrogen and 10 mg methyltestosterone).

Halodrin by Upjohn: small pink-scored tablets (.02 mg estrogen and 1 mg fluoxymesterone).

Estratest by Reid-Provident: long green-coated tablets (1.25 mg estrogen and 2.5 mg testosterone).

Test-Estrin by Marlyn: capsules, tablets or sublingual tablets (.25 mg estrogen and 1.25 mg testosterone) or (.5 mg estrogen and 2.5 mg testosterone).

Premarin with methyltestosterone by Ayerst: dark red-coated tablets (.625 mg estrogen and 5 mg methyltestosterone), yellow-coated tablets (1.25 mg estrogen and 10 mg methyltestosterone).

These ERT products also contain vitamins:

Formatrix by Ayerst: long red-coated tablets (1.25 mg estrogen, 10 mg methyltestosterone, and 400 mg vitamin C).

Mediatric by Ayerst: long black capsules or red-coated tables (.25 mg estrogen, 2.5 mg methyltestosterone, and a generous selection of of vitamins). (Just in case all those vitamins didn't get you going, Ayerst thoughtfully added 1 mg methamphetamine hydrochloride, commonly known as *speed*.) Mediatric is also available in a liquid formula which, in every 3 teaspoonsful, contains the same doses of estrogen, methyltestosterone, vitamins, and speed, plus 15 percent alcohol. Whee!

Gevrine by Lederle is also a "togetherness" hormone compound. Recommended for both males and females it contains an array of vitamins and minerals, in addition to .01 mg estrogen and 2.5 mg methyltestosterone in a purple capsule.

Another "togetherness" compound is manufactured by Geriatric Pharmaceutical. In addition to .005 mg ethinyl estradiol and 1.25 mg methyltestosterone, it contains a variety of vitamins and minerals plus amino acids.

These ERT products contain tranquilizers:

Menrium 5-2 by Roche: light green tablets (.2 mg estrogen and 5 mg chlordiazepoxide (Librium)). *Menrium 5-4:* dark green tablets (.4 mg estrogen and 5 mg Librium). *Menrium 10-4:* purple tablets (.4 mg estrogen and 10 mg Librium).

Milprem-400 by Wallace: dark pink-coated tablets (.45 mg estrogen and 400 mg meprobamate— better known as the tranquilizer Miltown). *Milprem-200:* light pink-coated tablets (.45 mg estrogen and 200 mg Miltown).

PMB 400 (red tablet) and *PMB 200* (green tablet) by Ayerst contain the same ingredients as Milprem-400 and Milprem-200 respectively.

ORAL PROGESTIN PRODUCTS:

Amen by Carnrick: beige tablets (10 mg medroxy-progesterone acetate, a derivative of progesterone).

Provera by Upjohn: orange, scored tablets (2.5 mg medroxyprogesterone acetate); white, scored tablets (10 mg medroxyprogesterone acetate).

Micronor by Ortho Pharmaceutical: small lime tablets (.35 mg norethindrone).

Gynorest by Mead Johnson: white, scored tablets (5 and 10 mg doses dydrogesterone).

Norlutate by Parke, Davis: scored tablets (5 mg norethindrone acetate).

Norlutin by Parke, Davis: white, scored tablets (5 mg norethindrone).

INJECTABLE ERT PRODUCTS:

Injections that are straight estrogen: *Delestrogen* (Squibb), *Depo-Estradiol Cypionate* (Upjohn) and *Estradurin* (Ayerst).

Injections that combine estrogen with other drugs: *Depo-Testadiol* (Upjohn), *Depotestogen* (Hyrex), *Deladumone* (Squibb), *Test-Estrin* (Marlyn).

Injectable progestin products: *Progynon* (Schering), available in 25 mg pellets for implantation under the skin, *Depo-Provera* (Upjohn).

TOPICAL ERT PRODUCTS:

Premarin cream (Ayerst), *Dienestrol cream* (Ortho) and *Diethylstilbestrol suppositories* (Lilly).

How These Products Are Used

THE PILLS

Most manufacturers suggest a regimen of three weeks on and one week off. Cautious doctors—and the FDA—now maintain that "the aim of proper hormonal therapy for acute symptoms is to *control these as rapidly as possible, with as little medication as possible, and to discontinue treatment as soon as possible.*" Some doctors advise their patients to take the pills only every other day, or only as needed when they feel "flushy."

It is argued that estrogen alone may be more carcinogenic—and also more productive of other great and small side effects—than preparations that combine additional hormones. Some doctors therefore prefer combination products, and may also prescribe 5 to 10 mg of progestin daily for five days or a week each month, to induce regular shedding of the endometrium. The "withdrawal flow" resembles menstruation, and, according to gynecologist Charles Debrovner, "never allows the lining of the uterus to build up dangerously, as it does with estrogen alone.

"Obviously," adds Debrovner, "it is very difficult to get all patients to be willing to menstruate, and those not willing are certainly more of a problem." Debrovner's present philosophy is shared by many of his colleagues. He states his rules succinctly:

> All patients who do not need ERT for menopausal symptomatic relief should be taken off.
> All patients should be evaluated as to whether they are on the lowest possible dose.
> Those who will not agree to menstruate should be subjected every six months or annually to diagnostic surveys of the endometrial cavity. These are not the most comfortable procedures in the world and probably, after one or two, the patient will either agree to menstruate or stop her estrogens altogether.

It is not established whether endometrial shedding, induced by progestins, really does protect the ERT patient against cancer. Dr. Herbert Kupperman, a long-standing Youth Pill enthusiast, admits, in a paper published by the Wilson Foundation, that shedding "prevents *the physician* from becoming unduly alarmed" by episodes of intermittent natural bleeding (from endometrial overstimulation) which might otherwise occur. Kupperman also maintains that the addition of progestin (he suggests 10 mg Provera twice a day for the first seven days of each calendar month) spares the breasts from overstimulation.

Kupperman used to recommend sequential birth control pills for some of his menopause patients. He believed that, like the combination of ERT and Provera, they might protect against cancer—at bargain rates. Kupperman was wrong about the sequentials, and in 1976, after they were shown tentatively to be more carcinogenic than other oral contraceptives, they were withdrawn by their manufacturers at the request of the FDA.

And so, in a recent editorial, the *British Medical Journal* warned that there is "no proof" that progestins "counteract the carcinogenic properties of estrogen." Further, the editorial stated, "we know for certain that the addition of progestins *does not* prevent blood clots or metabolic disturbances."

However, the main ingredient in Premarin is estrone, the very cause of endometrial cancer, according to some researchers. The *British Medical Journal* is hopeful that newer products such as Hormonin and Estrace, which have less estrone and more estriol and estradiol, may truly be less carcinogenic. This too is an "iffy" hypothesis, since it seems that almost any hormone may be converted to estrone within the body. The product literature concerning Estrace states that it produces "marked and rapid increase in circulating levels of 17B-estradiol *and estrone*."

Estrace only came on the market in 1976, having been made possible by a new process called micronization, which reduces particle size. Until then, 17B-estradiol had not been well absorbed orally. Estrace is selling well, according to Roland Eckels, director of public affairs for the Mead Johnson Laboratories. It may produce less nausea than other ERT products. Side effects in the women on whom it was tested included edema (31 percent), breast tenderness (24 percent), uterine bleeding (18 percent), and weight gain.

In sum, many doctors now hope that the use of either added progestin, or low-estrone products, or both, may protect their ERT patients from harm. Others say that such notions are just wishful thinking. For now it seems likely that low-estrone products will capture a growing share of the market, and increasing numbers of gynecologists will, like Debrovner, insist that their ERT patients take progestins too, so that they maintain "menstruation."

THE INJECTIONS

Estrogen injections may be quite long acting and are usually given at weekly or monthly intervals. Progestins, oral or injectable, are frequently added to the regimen.

Products combining estrogens and androgens are also available.

Injections are more expensive than pills, and have the further disadvantage that if side effects develop the patient must endure them until the medication wears off. In spite of this, says Youth Pill advocate Robert Greenblatt, "many patients prefer such a method since they do not need to remember to take tablets every day."

THE PELLETS

Estradiol pellets, implanted under the skin, are the most expensive method of all. The hormones are released to the body slowly, over a period of three to six months. Sometimes the dosages are one to three pellets of estrogen alone. Other patients may receive testosterone pellets also. A popular combination is two estrogen and one testosterone pellet, or vice versa.

Pellet implantation is considered minor surgery, whether it is done by incision or with a special instrument called a Kearns Pellet Injector. Aseptic precautions must be observed. Common sites for implantation are the armpit or region of the shoulder blades; some doctors implant pellets internally during surgery for removing a patient's ovaries.

THE TOPICAL PREPARATIONS

Estrogen creams, applied daily or as needed to the vulva and vagina, are used to control the vaginal discomforts experienced by some aging women. Applicators are available to aid insertion, but some women find suppositories more convenient. In cases of severe itching or chronic inflammation, cortisone preparations may be prescribed as well.

As we noted in chapter 26, estrogen from these vaginal preparations is absorbed systemically, It is not known how much, or which systems or organs may be most affected. The labeling for Premarin Vaginal Cream warns: *Overdosages may result in systematic hyperestrogenic effects such as abnormal or excessive uterine bleeding, edema, breast tenderness or reactivation of endometriosis.* The labeling for Lilly's Diethylstilbestrol Suppositories states: *Indiscriminate or injudicious administration may be dangerous; patients receiving the drug should be under continuous medical supervision. Although systematic absorption of Diethylstilbestrol in suppository form will be less than that ensuing from oral or parenteral [injections] administration, precautionary measures are urged. The breasts and pelvic organs should be examined before treatment is begun and at intervals during therapy.*

It is easy to be lulled into thinking that a cream cannot be too potent or dangerous, but these preparations, like any hormones, are nothing to take lightly. Consider the alternatives first.

Menopause: Wholesome Remedies

Just as some women think they must choose between the pill and pregnancy, other women fear that without ERT they will lose their well-being and their good looks.

There are far better ways to achieve good health at menopause and after than by taking a dangerous hormone. We discuss these ways in the following chapters, and at the end suggest a basis for your personal regimen.

There are time-honored *herb remedies* and we will name them. We advise our readers to use them judiciously, however. Although many herbs have been prescribed for thousands of years, their pharmacology (in most cases) is not fully understood.

Vitamins, a 20th-century discovery, are of great help at menopause. As we point out, they should also be chosen and used carefully. In a recent *Medical Tribune* interview, Dr. Theodore Cooper at HEW, then our nation's highest government physician, acknowledged that he personally, and his family, use substantial supplements of C and the B's. Yet government policy is still uncommitted, or even negative, on vitamins as a preventive measure.

Why should this be so?

First, Myron Winick, M.D., director of the Institute of Human Nutrition at Columbia University, has observed: "The state of nutrition education as it relates to health is in complete chaos. One cause of that chaos is the medical profession's failure to take responsibility for this area.

"This lack of interest and of adequate training in

nutrition, which is common to all medical specialties, has resulted . . . in poor care for many patients who are under direct management of a physician. Some pregnant women are still told to gain no more than 15 lbs. . . . Solid foods are given to babies too early and on no rational basis. . . . The nutritional needs of . . . the elderly are not generally being considered. . . . Special needs of certain segments of our population are not being addressed. The physician who prescribes a contraceptive pill often does not know that this imposes special nutritional requirements, let alone what they are. . . . Physicians believe a subject that isn't taught in medical school cannot be important. Most medical schools still do not teach a single required course in nutrition."

Second, let us hear from Linus Pauling, Nobel Laureate: ". . . of all the sciences, nutrition is in the worst state with the poorest people in the field . . . [it was] explored to some extent in the '30s, especially in regard to vitamins . . . It was definitive in respect to the deficiency diseases, but provocative with respect to the general question of nutrition in relation to optimum health. There were indications all along that you can improve your health by taking proper amounts of important nutrients but these weren't followed up. . . . We still don't know what proper amounts, are, the optimum amounts haven't been determined even now, forty years later."

Pauling and other esteemed scientists are working hard to clarify these issues, and hope that upon clarification, our life expectancies may increase dramatically. A high official at the National Cancer Institute confided to us recently that he is sure nutritional remedies to prevent and cure cancer will soon be identified.

Exposure to cancer-causing agents, of which there are enormous numbers in our environment, may cause changes in the genetic material of cells. Evidence is mounting that certain vitamins and minerals—A, C, E and selenium are currently under study—may help such cells to purify or repair themselves. While we recognize this to be an extremely promising field of research, it is still experimental, and whopping doses of some nutrients, without adding others, could upset the body's normal metabolic balance. Thus we advise proceeding with caution on megavitamins, until more is known. Therapeutic dosages, by contrast, appear to correct borderline deficiencies, and help the user *feel* much better.

Dosing oneself with megavitamins—unless one possesses a sound understanding of nutrition—can be quite chancy. This is especially true of vitamins A and D which are toxic for some persons at fairly low doses. But under some circumstances, they may cure or prevent serious illness. The vitamin supplements we advocate are in what is considered the safe "therapeutic" dose range. They are higher than the recommended allowance, in many cases, but lower than the megaranges in which toxicity is sometimes reported. To function normally, and comfortably, many menopausal and postmenopausal women quite clearly need somewhat more than the recommended allowances of E, B-complex, C, and the bioflavonoids and certain minerals, especially calcium. We base this statement, confidently, on the work of the few sound researchers who are concerned with the special needs of mature women, and the positive results so widely reported by nutrition-conscious women themselves.

Recommended allowances are derived from compromises arrived at by government committees. These are frequently revised, most often upward. Also, as Dr. Winick has noted, the needs of special groups and individuals seem not to be taken into much account. And as scientists have recently discovered, pollution may alter our dietary requirements, especially for E and C.

The food industry has far too much influence on our government committees, as is well documented in the reporting of Beatrice Trum Hunter, and Dr. Michael Jacobson, co-director of the Center for Science in the Public Interest and publisher of *Nutrition Action*. We refer the skeptical reader (who still thinks the government is protecting *us*) to their authoritative publications.

Murky relations between the food industry and our government agencies were recently highlighted by the ban on saccharin. The Delaney Amendment, the absolute ban, has *not* been invoked against DES, a proven *human* carcinogen even at low dosages, but *was* used against saccharin, which is proved to be tumor-causing in only one species of animal.

Such priorities make no sense to cancer researchers, some of whom attribute the move to the power of the sugar industry, while others suspect it may be a Machiavellian maneuver to get the Delaney Amendment overturned.

It isn't only packaged foods that don't deliver what they ought. The poor condition of our mineral-depleted soil and the problems with chemical fertilizers are so serious and widespread that even establishment sources, like the Rockefeller Brothers Fund have sounded alarms in their recent publications such as *The Unfinished Agenda*. At the University of Colorado, a center for zinc research, "think zinc" is the motto scientists have adopted when an infant or young child fails to thrive.

Contrary to the innocent beliefs of many parents, repeated epidemiological studies have now shown that these deficiencies exist in middle and upper income homes, as well as among the poor.

Exercise is essential for the welfare of aging bones, for the cardiovascular system, and to help along our program of therapeutic nutrition. Moderation is the word, at least to begin with. A sedentary woman may start out too strenuously and injure herself.

Two important new studies have established that even moderate exercise for thirty minutes three times a week provides some protection against coronary disease. It is never advisable to start a more strenuous program until one has worked up to it and gotten in condition.

Just as the weekend male athlete may seem to invite coronaries, the weekend female athlete invites back injuries, torn ligaments, and broken bones.

We hold a high opinion of the *gentle* get-in-shape exercise program devised by Marjorie Craig of Elizabeth Arden. Miss Craig was formerly a physical therapist at the Neurological Institute of the Columbia Presbyterian Medical Center. A program such as hers, available in her books and on tape, is the sort that mature women who are out of condition should start with.

Even our *dietary recommendations* must be approached with care. Since body chemistry *is* so personal, a change in eating habits could bring unexpected allergies.

Thus, we make no claims that any one health program is suitable for every woman. We include this section so the reader will know that there are many ERT alternatives to *try*.

CHAPTER 31

Ginseng: A Natural Remedy from the Orient

Traditional Chinese medicine (T'iao Ch'i or Li Ch'i) rests on theories of "normalizing" the body, or "balancing energies." These concepts are difficult at first for the Western mind to grasp. A leading interpreter has been Washington-based Dr. C. P. Li, former Chief of the Virus Biology Section at the National Institutes of Health.

Dr. Li is especially interested in ginseng and acupuncture, and has tried to explain their benefits to his Western colleagues: "[The] regulatory capability of the body can be made much more efficient by acupuncture or by ginseng, 'the root of life.'"

At menopause the body is in a state of temporary stress, or endocrine imbalance. Its "regulatory capability," as Dr. Li would put it, has gone awry. Yet, strictly speaking, the patient is not sick. To use powerful drugs, carcinogens, to treat a healthy woman with hot flashes seems excessive. To gently normalize the body oriental-style is a sounder approach—if it works.

Ginseng is the common name for several species of Panax herbs (its scientific name means panacea) belonging to the family Araliacaeae. Ginseng has been prized in the Orient for four thousand years. Its price has been so high that an ancient Chinese proverb warns, "Eat ginseng and ruin yourself financially." The finest ginseng of all, grown on Changpai Mountain in Manchuria, and known as Tung-Pei Wild Imperial Ginseng, sells today for 2,000 an ounce. In New York City, a bottle of 100 good-quality capsules sells for $10 or $11, while roots command prices as high as $170. More than two thousand years ago, the ancient Chinese pharmacopoeia, *Shen Nung Pen Ts'ao*, mentions ginseng for complaints of middle and old age. The Chinese native doctors still prescribe ginseng as a tonic for general weakness, and, specifically, for any kind of sweating, temperature or heat stress. It is combined with other medical herbs to speed recovery from a host of illnesses also. Modern research has confirmed that it dramatically reduces sweating and helps the body adapt to heat stress, and yet seems not to be toxic (poisonous) even at high doses. Ginseng would appear to be a safe, time-tested remedy to *try* for hot flashes.

Studies of Ginseng

Are we certain that ginseng will always cure hot flashes? No, we are not. Most of the modern experiments concerning heat stress have been performed on animals such as rats, rabbits and cats. The reason for this is that the Chinese consider it unethical to do double-blind studies on sick human subjects. As U.S. pharmacologist Louis Lasagna has explained, after a visit:

"The Chinese do not countenance double-blind techniques or placebo controls, considering them as inimical to the concept that patients must at all times be thoroughly informed about their diseases and the remedial measures planned."

Another pharmacologist who went to China as a member of an exchange delegation, Dr. Norman Farnsworth, told us:

"We kept asking them, 'How do you know this works?' The answer, every place we went—and we traveled 6,000 miles, to six cities and a dozen hospitals—was, 'We have used this for 3,000 years; we know it works.'" A frustrating answer for an American scientist, but insofar as animal work can confirm a human therapy, ginseng research has.

In 1958 two Peking investigators divided experimental rats into two groups; one was fed a regular diet and the other the same diet laced with 5 percent ginseng powder. When subjected to very high temperatures, the control rats were paralyzed or had convulsions. They did not regain normal activity for twenty to sixty minutes. The ginseng-fed rats "appeared normal" after the same stress, and none of them convulsed. The scientists who conducted the experiment believe that ginseng normalizes the pituitary, which is the gland involved in hot flashes.

Since the 1958 experiments, many others have confirmed that animals exposed to either heat or cold fare dramatically better when protected by ginseng. In other rat experiments, it was found that the animals not fed ginseng quickly drowned in *cold* water, but those who had had ginseng lasted for hours, even with lead weights on their tails.

The modern center of ginseng research is the Soviet Union, which has put its leading pharmacologists to work reviewing traditional folk remedies. Pharmacological and clinical investigations are now being carried out in Moscow, Leningrad, Vladivostok, Tomsk, and Khabarovsk, among other cities. Vladivostok is the coordinating center of all ginseng research, and the ginseng kingpin of Russia is Professor I. I. Brekhman, who heads a laboratory called the Institute of Biologically Active Substances. Many scientists consider Brekhman the world's leading authority on herbs. It was Brekhman who named ginseng an "adaptogen." He claimed:

• It is "innocuous" and does not disturb physiological functions, as most drugs do.

• It is "nonspecific" in that it increases resistance to a wide spectrum of adverse influences such as overheating, cooling, high barometric pressure, radiation, some tumors, and many poisons.

• It has a general "normalizing" action on the entire body.

The Soviets have made numerous human studies concerned with ginseng and its effect on work capacity and mental alertness. Here, in Brekhman's words, is how ginseng affects work performance; his findings should interest menopausal women (and anyone else) troubled by lassitude and fatigue:

"Numerous experiments on humans have shown that ginseng preparations increase physical and mental efficiency, improve accuracy . . . contribute to concentrating attention, and prevent overfatigue. As distinct from synthetic stimulants of the amphetamine type, ginseng neither provokes subjective excitation nor disturbs normal sleep.

Its administration can be prolonged and repeated, without any after-effects, . . . [unlike] amphetamines. . . . Increased work efficiency is retained from one to two months following a one-month administration of ginseng."

One experiment that bore out Brekhman's statements was a double-blind study performed by Soviet gerontologist M.A. Medvedev, in which 18 radio operators who transmit coded messages were given ginseng extract dissolved in cranberry juice, while 14 colleagues were given the cranberry drink alone. The number of mistakes made by the control group was *twice that of the ginseng group*.

There are some six hundred modern scientific papers, many by scientists of international reputation, which show that ginseng produces few side effects and yet "does something" remarkable for heat stress and endurance.

A doctor at a ghetto street clinic for teen-agers told us: "Sometimes you learn from your patients. Some of the kids coming down from drugs were talking about this ginseng. So I tried it one day for a hangover, and it worked. Then I tried it before a tennis game on a steamy hot day, and I beat an opponent I had never touched before. She was drenched with sweat [the doctor we cite here is also female], but I felt like it was twenty degrees cooler, spry as September. After that I read Brekhman's papers and I was convinced. It's certainly an adaptogen in some situations. The root is best if you can get it, but the powder and capsules are effective, too. Now I give ginseng to kids with drug problems all the time. I've also prescribed it for a couple of cigarette smokers, and it got them through cold turkey. . . . Combined with Midol, ginseng has gotten some of my teen-aged patients through very bad menstrual periods that used to knock them out.

"We don't know enough about it. It's criminal that we have no research on American patients. . . . I wouldn't take it every day, but I keep it handy in my medicine chest at home. I use it less often than vitamin C, but more often than aspirin.

"Yes, I am going to try it if I get hot flashes. It'll be the first thing I try."

We spoke to the medical director of a U.S. airline, who admitted, reluctantly, that he *had* recommended ginseng to his pilots and flight attendants. "The Russian spacemen use it for a balancing effect against weightlessness. I thought it might help jet lag—it does. Any unusual conditions that the body must adjust to—ginseng helps it adjust."

In the United States, ginseng has sometimes been promoted as an aphrodisiac or treatment for impotence. There is no scientific basis for this use. Some superstitious people believe that roots that are shaped like a man—with body, arms, and legs—do cure impotence, but the fact is that many roots have this same shape. In folk medicine, ginseng was a general tonic for the symptoms of aging, and for people who were debilitated, undernourished, and overworked; it was also often prescribed for change of life in women. In Korea and elsewhere, it has long been used against heat stress in summer, even by the young and healthy if they can afford it.

Ginseng and Hot Flashes

Advocates of ginseng for hot flashes have to rely on its reputation in folk medicine, on word of mouth, and on personal experimentation. There is no good study—by the standards of Western medicine—that proves that it cures hot flashes. Though some doctors do prescribe it, and claim excellent results, no one has produced a controlled study comparing ginseng with a placebo. (In point of fact, though, most of the claims for ERT have not been proven in placebo-comparison studies either.)

Robert Atkins, the diet doctor, told us that he has used ginseng to relieve 400 patients suffering from hot flashes. Eighty percent improved by taking ginseng alone, and most of the remainder improved on ginseng combined with high doses of vitamin E. Atkins has for many years been urging his patients to stay away from ERT, since he finds that it—and the pill—keeps his diet from working.

In our experience, women suffering from hot flashes take from ten days to six weeks to benefit from ginseng; two weeks is average time before some effects are felt. Some women with flashes do not benefit at all, but most say that (a) their flashes are gone or greatly diminished, or (b) they feel generally stronger and more resistant—they still get some flashes but do not feel "knocked out" by them.

If a woman asks her doctor about ginseng, he will

probably laugh. For years it has bounced in and out of the official U.S. pharmacopoeias, and has been out since the 1950s. The U.S. Agriculture Department made some studies of it, early in this century, but these were directed toward helping ginseng farmers increase their crops.

Farnsworth's Opinions

Norman Farnsworth, head of the Department of Pharmacognosy and Pharmacology at the University of Illinois Medical Center, is said by his colleagues to be open-minded and knowledgeable about Oriental herbs. He concludes that about half of the traditional remedies used by Chinese rural doctors (ginseng among them) have a "rational basis" that even Western minds could accept. Pharmacologist Louis Lasagna, of the University of Rochester School of Medicine, stated recently:

"Many Western physicians and scientists have a tendency to view skeptically the use of plant extracts as drugs, forgetting that many of our own drugs originated through an investigation of herbal medicines, and that even today perhaps 25 percent of U.S. prescriptions contain one or more ingredients consisting of a crude plant material, crude extracts obtained from plants, or a purified active principle obtained from plants."

We asked Farnsworth about Brekhman's studies in Russia, for Brekhman, as a Soviet scientist, is a kind of bridge between Eastern and Western belief about ginseng.

"Brekhman is first class," Farnsworth assured us. "But there's a funny semantic problem with Brekhman. A lot of scientists in this country say they can't accept his fundamental theory that adaptogens [or tonics] such as ginseng help you build up an immunity without an antigen-antibody response. I think what he's saying is just that adaptogens cause metabolic and hormonal changes. . . . In the last two years, the Japanese . . . have published studies on ginseng's metabolic effects that no one could quibble with. It changes cholesterol, and the liver, quite measurably."

"Could it be more like a food or vitamin than a drug?" we suggested. "It works mildly and slowly."

"The important chemists in this country aren't interested in that," Farnsworth continued impatiently. "They say that if something is good for everything, it's good for nothing. The reason ginseng is good for so many things is that it changes the metabolism of the body—increasing DNA, RNA synthesis, protein synthesis—over a long period of time. The picture is something that can't be discounted, but we won't do the expensive research."

Another interesting fact about ginseng, according to Farnsworth, is that it produces estrus [heat] in castrated animals. "This may be attributed to a . . . steroid in the roots," he says. "There is evidence of the presence of estradiol and estriol." This, in addition to ginseng's effect on the pituitary, could also explain its apparent ability to calm the symptoms of menopause.

Farnsworth does not advocate taking ginseng in the absence of symptoms or stress. A person who is feeling well and not subject to exceptional stress or fatigue should not fool around, even with an old herbal remedy like ginseng.

"The final reason that the American drug industry won't pick up ginseng," Farnsworth said, "is that they can't control the source of the material. It would be too expensive to extract the ingredients, and the active principles are so complex that they wouldn't be able to synthesize them. And they couldn't get a patent on them anyway, because the benefits have already been disclosed. They can't make any money, so they just sit back and say, well, that Russian pharmacology is no damn good. It's easier to do that than to prove that it isn't."

Farnsworth, a past president of the American Society of Pharmacognosy, is regarded by his colleagues as one of the top drug evaluators in the United States. On folk remedies, he has developed an influential theory of "convergent evolution." Farnsworth argues that if peoples who are geographically distinct use a given plant for the same purpose, this constitutes "prima facie evidence that the putative use is valid."

Ginseng was popular with frontier doctors in America, who learned about it from the Indians. All of the old American herbals contain extensive references to it, with the indications similar to those used in China. But it was always a folk medicine, popular in rough and rural communities, and viewed disdainfully by most "civilized" physicians.

Another of the world's leading pharmacognosists, E. J. Shellard of London University, puts it like this: "Ginseng is an old, much maligned drug that is being reexamined . . . It has anti-infective and anti-fatigue properties and there is accumulating evidence of anti-stress activity. . . . In many persons—but not all—it delays mental and physical fatigue." Shellard believes that glycosides, not found to date in any other plants, account for much of ginseng's effectiveness.

A few users, perhaps 1 in 10, are overstimulated by ginseng. Such reactions, Brekhman reports, are apt to occur in "hyperactive" types. For such persons, eleutherococcus— a plant related to ginseng—is preferable. Marketed in the United States as "Siberian ginseng," eleutherococcus capsules are carried by many health-food stores and some pharmacies. One distributor is the Solgar Company, Lynbrook, New York 11563.

Two additional ginseng "cousins" are goldenseal and Fo-ti-tieng. Goldenseal is a traditional cure for night sweats of any origin, while Fo-ti-tieng is considered, by some herbalists, to be more of a specific *for women* than ginseng and the other products. Some women who are knowledgeable about Eastern herbal medicine use ginseng and Fo-ti-tieng together for menopause complaints. Goldenseal is available at many health-food stores. Fo-ti-tieng is more scarce but can be ordered from Kiehl's Pharmacy, 109 Third Avenue, New York, N.Y. 10003. It is also available through Pacific Trends, Inc., Woodland Hills, CA. 91367. There seems little question that herbs of this general family prevent or relieve menopause symptoms in many women.

Dr. Sarah Roshan, a New Jersey gynecologist, cancer researcher, and estrogen authority, is appalled at the casual use of ERT and the pill. In the past she gave her patients Bellergal, a prescription drug combining phenobarbital and belladonna, to combat severe hot flashes. Recently, she has switched to dietary measures, along with ginseng and vitamin E.

Sarah Roshan says that hot flashes are almost unheard of in Iran, where she was born and raised. Her mother knows no one personally who has ever had one. Roshan now suggests that there may be factors in meat that aggravate menopause complaints (see chap. 33). She also believes that the spices most commonly used in Iranian food preparation—which include several in the ginseng botanical family—do much to help allay such conditions.

Dosages for Menopause

Ginseng is available in a confusing array of powders and instant teas, capsules, syrupy liquid "concentrates," and in the root itself.

To make matters worse, Norman Farnsworth cautions: "I would be willing to almost stake my reputation that half the preparations that are sold at these high prices don't even contain any ginseng. There's no way that the FDA can tell if there's real ginseng in these products, although we are working on tests."

As a general rule, then, it is essential to buy ginseng from a reliable health-food store, pharmacy, or other dealer whom you trust.

With one traditional exception—alcohol-based extracts—one should avoid combination products, those that contain ginseng along with other vitamins or herbs. Some such formulations are perfectly honest, but many are not. Be especially wary of products advertised as aphrodisiacs. These sometimes contain pepper or other irritants to the genital and urinary organs instead of ginseng.

Instant teas or "crystals," which are highly popular and quite delicious, contain 88 to 95 percent milk sugar and only a dash of ginseng proper. While some are made by reputable manufacturers and constitute a pleasant "pick-me-up," they are not sufficiently potent to control hot flashes, unless taken in large (and fattening) amounts.

The product for ginseng beginners is the capsule, as proper dosage is easiest to ascertain.

Correct ginseng dosage varies with body weight. A woman who weighs between 100 and 130 pounds should take one gram (or 1,000 mg) daily for menopause symptoms, half a gram (500 mg) before breakfast, and the same before dinner.

A woman weighing between 130 and 160 should take

a gram and one-quarter to a gram and one-half (three 500-mg tablets or capsules) per day. If her weight is higher, she should take two grams (or 2,000 mg) daily. A capsule is usually measured in grains—8 to 10 grains per capsule approximating 500 mg.

As a rule, ginseng is most effective when taken on an empty stomach, before or between meals, but not right after. It should not be taken simultaneously with vitamin C, which may weaken or neutralize its effects. Orientals also believe that the following foods should be avoided for three hours after taking ginseng: pineapple, tomato, grapefruit, lemon, orange, carrot, turnip. Vitamin E, however, and alcohol are believed to increase its effectiveness.

At low doses, ginseng has a body-building effect, and is often prescribed for athletes, or for weight gain in the elderly or debilitated. At high doses it appears to speed up metabolism in a way that contributes to weight loss.

Dr. Robert Atkins prescribes high doses for his diet patients, as much as three grams (six 500-mg capsules) daily in conjunction with their weight-loss regimen. *However, they are under his medical supervision* and on a controversial food program as well. More than the weight-indicated dosages are inadvisable to take on one's own.

A woman starting ginseng should track her weight. If she is gaining undesired pounds, she should slightly *increase* her dose. If she is losing, and doesn't want to, she should *decrease* it.

Buying Ginseng, Taking Ginseng

If you do not live near a health-food store or pharmacy that stocks herbals, you can order ginseng capsules by mail from several reliable sources:

Kiehl's Pharmacy (see address on p. 436) buys its own carefully selected roots and grinds them into powder themselves. It is available in loose or capsule form. They also sell the root, dried and chopped, and an alcohol-based elixir with the root included in the bottle. The root can be eaten when the elixir is gone.

Korean Ginseng Products Ltd., at 817 Lexington Avenue, New York, N.Y. 10021, maintained by one of the oldest and most respected ginseng exporters, stocks seventeen different preparations, including 5-, 8-, and 10-grain capsules, and has a showroom open to the public.

Most ginseng on the American market comes from Korea. Korean ginseng is strictly controlled and apt to be honestly graded. The top grade is Heaven, then Earth. Lowest are Good and Tails.

American ginseng is ranked below Chinese and Korean, but above Japanese. Canadian roots tend to be larger and sweeter-tasting than ours in the States, and some excellent ginseng is grown in Ontario.

Ginseng can even be grown as a house plant, though one must wait five or six years to harvest it. Precise gardening instructions are available in *The Ginseng Book* by Louise Veninga, P.O. Box 1072, Santa Cruz, California 95061. Instructions may also be available from the U.S. Government Printing Office.

The root itself is considered the most powerful form of ginseng, but it is the most trouble to buy and prepare. It may need to be steamed before eating, although the chopped variety, provided by Kiehl's and other suppliers, is easily munched on. To prepare tea from the root, place a ⅛- to ¼-ounce slice in three cups of water. Cook for about two hours on a low heat, until one cup remains. Folklore has it, and apparently some scientists agree, that ginseng and metal do not mix. The root is scraped with a wooden knife, and boiled in an earthenware vessel.

We have mentioned that alcohol potentiates or increases ginseng's effects, as do honey and vitamin E. A small root may be dropped into a bottle of light wine, vodka, gin, or brandy. Let it stand for two weeks to a month, shaking from time to time. Use as needed for a nightcap or for night hot flashes. After the liquor is gone, the root can be eaten.

Ginseng powder is often mixed with equal parts of honey and grated orange peel. It is then dissolved in hot water, as a tea, or may be taken dry. The combination of ginseng, honey, and orange peel is mentioned in the folklore as a cure for insomnia. Ginseng root tea or "broth" cooked with a bamboo leaf is also suggested for this purpose.

But ginseng alone is not apt to curb insomnia in most people. To the contrary: Twenty minutes to an hour after ingestion of real ginseng, one ordinarily feels a slight surge of energy and alertness, Brekhman's "stimulant" effect. If this is not discerned, the product may be ersatz.

The ancient Chinese were so confident of ginseng, they used to test the quality of imported roots by setting two runners, known to be equally matched, against each other in a race. One was given a root sample to chew, and the other not. If the chewer failed to win, the shipment was rejected.

In the words of Norman Farnswoth: "The use of ginseng as a general body tonic would seem to be well founded. . . . Some of the ginseng story is fantasy, but much of it is fact."

Stephen Fulder, a biologist studying aging at the British National Institute for Medical Research agrees. He predicts that the herb will be found to "delay the onset of degenerative conditions such as arthritis and arteriosclerosis." "But," he cautions, "no one yet knows how it works."

"An old story in Asia," as *Smithsonian Magazine* observes, "but elsewhere one that has scarcely begun." *Smithsonian* continues, "After at least 2,000 years, Western medicine is now starting to take acupuncture seriously. Next may be ginseng. . . . Britain, France, Italy, Finland, Bulgaria, Korea and Japan are among the countries that have been investigating the mysterious root . . . more research than anywhere else has been done in the Soviet Union. . . . In 1974, experts from seven countries attended the first International Ginseng Symposium, held in Seoul. Among the . . . findings announced were . . . ginseng can prevent change of body temperature in animals and help them withstand temperature stress."

CHAPTER 32

Vitamin E and Other Helps for
Menopause Symptoms

Skeptics say it's a "placebo" effect, but thousands of women claim they have cured their own menopause symptoms with vitamins and diet. Vitamin E and perhaps the B complex may be of especial value, according to *Novak's Textbook of Gynecology*, and many other medical sources confirm this.

Vitamin E as a relief for menopause symptoms recently surfaced almost by accident. In August 1974, *Prevention* magazine included a questionnaire on this controversial vitamin. Later, reporting the results, biochemist Richard Passwater, author of *Super-Nutrition*, explained:

"Actually, there was no mention of menopause on the questionnaire. *Yet, 2,000 women volunteered that they found vitamin E to largely or totally relieve the problems of menopause.* The most frequent comments written in were (1) more energy and a better sense of well-being, (2) relief of leg cramps, and (3) relief of hot flashes and other problems of menopause."

Passwater searched the medical literature and found a number of studies that confirmed what *Prevention* readers said. One, written in 1945 in the *American Journal of Obstetrics and Gynecology*, reported that 25 women, all with severe menopause symptoms, responded to the vitamin E treatment and showed either complete relief or very marked improvement. No untoward aftereffects were noted.

In 1949 another investigator, Dr. Rita Finkler, described vitamin E treatment of 66 menopausal patients in the *Journal of Clinical Endocrinology*. Good-to-excellent relief was obtained in 31 cases, fair in 16, and the remain-

441

ing 19 women evidenced no improvement. The dosages used by Dr. Finkler were relatively low—about 20 to 100 units daily, the average being 30. In 17 cases, when the real vitamin E was replaced with dummy pills, symptoms soon recurred.

Canada's controversial vitamin E advocate, Dr. Evan Shute, has long claimed a similar success ratio. He prescribes doses of 300 to 600 units and warns that "treatment must be persisted in, because no effect is observed for two to four weeks after commencing therapy."

Prevention readers also mentioned that vitamin E cured vaginal symptoms. "Corrected vaginal dryness. It's great," wrote one woman who was taking only 100 units daily. This effect had also been noted, back in 1949, by Dr. Hugh McLaren, writing in the *British Medical Journal*: "Vitamin E relieved severe menopausal flushing in 30 patients (64 percent) and failed in 17. The required dose varied, but averaged 500 units per day over 37 days. *Prolonged and heavy dosage seemed to cause healing in 50 percent of senile vulvar and vaginal lesions.*" McLaren, who was one of Britain's leading menopause researchers, predicted that E would soon become the treatment of choice for hot flashes since estrogen, he believed, would prove carcinogenic. McLaren was wrong on the first point (unfortunately) and right on the second.

Vitamin E is not as dramatic in curing hot flashes or vaginal symptoms as estrogen. The vitamin (alone) is said to bring marked relief in about half to two-thirds of cases, and it takes a while to work. Some women who seem to benefit from this treatment may just be naturally outgrowing menopause and the vitamin may be coincidental. In other cases, the cure could indeed be a placebo effect.

A few people are sensitive to E, and it should be taken only in low or moderate doses by persons with diabetes, rheumatic heart condition, or high blood pressure. Any user who develops blurred vision should give up E at once. Resumption of menstruation *is* an occasional outcome of E supplementation, sometimes desired and sometimes not. Some users complain that in higher dose ranges, E makes them feel queasy, or gives them gastric distress. Dr. Sarah Roshan notes that the dry or powdered form seems to be more digestible, and our own experience confirms her finding. So-called dry E is available from the Solgar Company in Lynbrook, New York, among other manufacturers.

Why Was E Abandoned by Most Gynecologists?

The earliest report on E therapy for menopause symptoms, authored by Dr. Evan Shute, appeared in the *Journal of the Canadian Medical Association* in 1937. Shute and his brother Wilfred continued their studies and published their work in many influential journals, including *Lancet* and the *American Journal of Obstetrics and Gynecology*. As we have seen, their research was confirmed by other less controversial investigators.

But in the 1940s, the vitamin was far more costly than most estrogen products. And estrogens do curb flashes in women who fail to respond to E, or even to the more potent E, B-complex, bioflavonoids, and ginseng combination.

We fear that another reason E was ignored by most doctors may lie partially in the way prescription and nonprescription remedies are regarded. Many women probably thought estrogen "better" than E because the hormone was available by prescription only. They may have been disappointed in doctors who told them to go out and buy a vitamin or eat wheat germ. In the wake of the Youth Pill craze, physicians forgot the research on vitamin E. Younger doctors may never have been introduced to it.

On the doctor's side, prescription drugs are sometimes more appealing because they give him or her *control*. Furthermore, vitamins, and especially E, fall under the same mantle of suspicion as remedies like ginseng because they are claimed to have such a wide range of benefits. In his book, *The Heart and Vitamin E*, Evan Shute remarks: "No substance known to medicine has such a variety of healing properties." This, he concedes, is a major drawback to acceptance.

Finally, we must again refer to the second- or third-class citizenship status of the older woman. Her complaints do not attract the attention of many qualified researchers or the interest of many journalists. Thus, E's proven effectiveness in curbing hot flashes had been obscured by other dramatic claims for the vitamin, such as its possible benefits to the heart.

Taking Vitamin E for Hot Flashes

The recommended allowance of 30 units daily for adults increases during periods of general stress, or during extra demands on the reproductive system. "Aging" also increases vitamin E requirements. The woman at menopause *fits into all three categories*, medically and biochemically. She is experiencing general stress, her reproductive system is going through a potentially difficult adjustment, *and* she is moving into a mature phrase of life where the E requirements of all humans, male or female, are raised.

When vitamin E is deficient, FSH and LH production increase. Too much FSH and LH production (see chap. 24) is now accepted as the central reason for hot flashes and related menopause complaints. Vitamin E also prevents the destruction of sex hormones. In a deficiency state, the hormone levels go down, pushing up the FSH and LH levels.

In addition, middle-aged women (and men) who are conscious of calories and cholesterol are especially apt to avoid many of the high-calorie foods that provide natural E.

The natural dietary sources of E are:

High: Cottonseed, corn, soybean, safflower, and wheat germ oils

Medium: Coconut, peanut, and olive oils; wheat germ, apple seeds, alfalfa, barley, dry soybeans, peanuts; chocolate, rose hips, yeast; cabbage, spinach, asparagus

Low: Brussels sprouts, carrots, parsnips, mustard, corn, brown rice, lettuce, cauliflower, peas, sweet potatoes, turnip greens, kale, kohlrabi, green peppers; bacon, beef, lamb, pork, veal, beef liver; eggs, butter, cheese; whole wheat flour, dried navy beans, corn meal, oatmeal, coconut, rye, oats, wheat; blackberries, pears, apples, olives

If the oils listed above are heated or stored for long periods, much of the vitamin E may be destroyed. For this reason it is essential to store vegetable oil in the refrigerator after it is opened.

Dosages of E

The recommended allowances of vitamin E and the other fat-soluble vitamins are usually stated and marketed in international units (IUs) rather than in the gram, milligram, and microgram allowances applied to many other vitamins.

An IU of vitamin E, in its various forms, is equivalent to about 1 to 1.5 mg in weight. In other words, the 30 IUs recommended daily E allowance would equal between 30 and 45 mg.

Like ginseng alone, E alone is well worth trying for hot flashes, and *the two together—according to our own interviews and those of clinicians who are prescribing them in combination—seem almost on a par with ERT in effectiveness*. E or ginseng, or the two together, take longer to work than ERT. Relief from hot flashes may take two to six weeks, while vaginal lesions heal yet more slowly.

Exact dosages for E cannot be given here. Women require different amounts of it, depending on whether they are already in a deficiency state (as might be the case for someone who has been on the pill or ERT or has been eating a lot of processed foods). Chemist Jeffrey Bland now recommends higher intake of E in the presence of environmental oxidants such as smog and cigarette smoking.

If a woman is in good health and not experiencing significant menopausal symptoms, she might want to try 30 to 100 units a day. If she is having marked hot flashes or other symptoms, she could start with 100 units, and build up the dose over a period of a few weeks, or months, until she begins to experience relief. Some women may have to go as high as 400 to 1200 units to alleviate flashes. *No one, as mentioned, who has high blood pressure, diabetes, or a rheumatic heart condition* should take over 100 to 150 units. And no one should take over 600 units a day without being under the supervision of a physician. There is a growing body of evidence that the trace mineral selenium works hand in hand with E and helps it do its job more efficiently. Women who have trouble tolerating higher dose ranges of E, though requiring them to curb hot flashes, should take one or two tablets daily of products that combine about 200 units of E and 25 mcg of selenium, such as Selene É.

Vitamin E is absorbed from the intestinal tract only in the presence of fats. It, in turn, aids in the absorption of unsaturated fats. Therefore, vitamin E should be taken at the end of a meal that contains fats, especially polyunsaturated vegetable oils. It should not be taken on an empty stomach. This is in contrast to ginseng, which may be better utilized by the body when taken before meals.

Sleep Remedies

Next to hot flashes, sleeplessness may be the major discomfort menopausal women suffer. Doctors are quick to prescribe ERT and possibly sleeping pills. ERT cures sleep disturbances caused by hot flashes (as so may ginseng and E) but not those caused by depression and other factors. Sleeping pills, taken by some 30 million Americans, are likely to be addictive and certainly—for long-term use—are ineffectual.

A relatively new Hoffman–LaRoche product, Dalmane, is currently regarded by sleep researchers as the least noxious of prescription sleeping aids. There is still a lot to learn about Dalmane, but, thus far, it *appears to be* less habituating than most such remedies, and to continue working over a somewhat longer period of days or weeks. (Dalmane is closely related to such antianxiety drugs as Valium and Librium, which are also relatively safe and effective for insomnia.)

Some other products not intended to be sleeping aids may work well nonetheless. These include two antihistamines, Benadryl and Phenergan, and common aspirin (without caffeine).

Sleep Remedies Found in Nature

Milk, especially warm milk, contains tryptophane, an amino acid that has sedative effects. Meats are also high in tryptophane, which is one reason that people often get drowsy after meals. Tryptophane tablets can be purchased in health-food stores. The sedative dose is about two to three grams. According to Dr. Nathan Kline of Rockland Psychiatric Institute and others, it also has antidepressant effects. In Britain, tryptophane is marketed as a natural antidepressant combined with vitamins C and B$_6$ because they all work together in brain metabolism. For unexplained reasons, wine, particularly red, may be more sedative than hard liquor (sweet wines may be extra effective).

Camomile tea and valerian root are two popular herbal sedatives. A pleasant brand of tea called Sleepytime, available at health-food outlets and some groceries, is camomile-based, and also includes spearmint, tilia flowers, lemon grass, blackberry leaves, passionflowers, orange blossoms, hawthorn berries, scullcap, rose petals, and hops.

Valerian has a strong odor that many people find offensive in tea form. It is available without the odor in various brands of tablets. One brand, called Nervenruh, imported from West Germany, combines valerian with passionflower, goosefinger herb, hops, and lecithin.

It's wise to be cautious and conservative in the use of herbal remedies. Even camomile, if taken nightly, may slow down the digestion.

Women who had severe menopause reported in our interviews that muscle cramps and backaches were often a cause of sleeplessness. Calcium, or calcium-magnesium products, such as dolomite, may alleviate these symptoms, as may the trace mineral manganese.

Attending a gym in the evenings, or taking a bike ride or just a brisk walk, can dramatically aid sleep induction. Swimming is especially recommended. So is sex.

Coffee, conventional tea, cocoa, and cola drinks contain caffeine and may affect you more than formerly; they should be avoided at the evening meal.

Depression

It used to be believed that depression was more common at menopause, but current research indicates that this is probably untrue. Nonetheless, it is a problem that can add significantly to menopausal complaints. *ERT is ineffective for treating depression.*

Significant depression that requires psychiatric care must be distinguished from a number of other reactions.

The everyday blues: Practically everyone has a bad morning, day, or even week now and then. Spirits are low, there is reduced drive, and a general feeling of pessimism. This is part of the human condition, and best taken in stride. Treatment is unnecessary.

Mourning (grief): Many women in their forties and fifties must endure traumatic events, including the loss of one or more older relatives and possibly their husbands, too. Mourning differs from depression. It is the world that seems impoverished rather than oneself. Suicidal thoughts, while they can occur, do not usually become a major preoccupation. Loss of appetite and weight loss are not commonly found in mourning, except perhaps in the first few days. In both mourning and depression, guilt is a common reaction, as are sleep disturbances and tears.

Mourning normally takes six weeks to six months for resolution. Someone to talk to, a friend or professional therapist, can be extremely helpful. Some mental health clinics offer group therapy for recently bereaved widows. If the symptoms persist beyond, say, six months, the mourning may have changed to a clinical depression, and more strenuous treatment should be sought.

Clinical depression is a serious condition. Among the symptoms: waking during the night or early morning, loss of appetite, weight loss, constipation, hopelessness, helplessness, low self-esteem, self-blame, suicidal thoughts and acts, forgetfulness, difficulty in concentration, indecisiveness, lack of drive, loss of pleasure, fatigue, stooped posture, sad facial expression, and either slowed or agitated thoughts and movements. In addition, there may be preoccupation with bodily ills, either real or imagined. Characteristically, the symptoms tend to be worse in the morning, and not quite so bad in the evening. One or a few such symptoms may not represent depression, but five or six of them may. No one (fortunately) will have all the symptoms listed.

There are a number of types of clinical depression:

Reactive depression occurs after a real-life loss, such as the death of a loved one, children leaving home, an unwelcome move, a loss of a job, illness in the family, a faithless husband, or financial reverses. A mild reactive depression may not require anything more than sympathetic understanding from friends and family. A change in life patterns and vocational counseling may be important. In a more severe reactive depression, psychiatric help and antidepressant medication are necessary.

Endogenous depression, which occurs in the absence of significant precipitating life events, is more apt to have a physical basis. Some people get recurrent endogenous depressions throughout their lives; others may experience only a single episode. Referral to a psychiatrist is advisable, as is a creative and thorough physical work-up that includes factors like metabolism and nutrition checkups. On her own, the woman should examine whether her diet and exercise are adequate. If she informs herself about physiology and nutrition, she may discover her own cure.

Although depressions are usually self-limiting (many terminate within weeks), they can go on for months or even years. The longer a depression lasts, the harder it is to shake off without pertinent medication.

There are two groups of antidepressant drugs. The tricyclics work in up to four cases out of five. They often produce minor side effects, such as dryness of the mouth and constipation, and occasionally increased sweating, which may be confused with that found in hot flashes. Brand names include Tofranil, Elavil, Sinequan, and Vivactil. These drugs should be used very carefully in the presence of heart disease. The tricyclics usually begin to bring relief within a few weeks. After full recovery they should then be tapered off gradually over a period of about six months to a year to ensure that symptoms do not recur. The patient may experience severe nightmares and other untoward effects if the drug is withdrawn suddenly.

A second group of antidepressants, called monoamine-oxidase (MAO) inhibitors, sometimes work where the tricyclics fail. They occasionally have dangerous side effects, including hypertension, and must be used with caution, including the avoidance of certain foods.

Bi-polar depression (manic-depressive illness) often responds to lithium treatment. Shock therapy is still employed by many psychiatrists, but we feel it should be used only in special cases and as a last resort. It may impair memory and intellectual functions, temporarily.

A curiosity of depression is that skipping a full night's sleep—staying up for a continuous thirty-six hours or more (from Tuesday morning, say, until Wednesday evening)— seems to lift it temporarily through unexplained changes in brain chemistry.

An unfortunate feature of depression, in our society, is that many doctors still prescribe ineffectual medication— Valium or Librium as well as ERT—instead of the anti-depressants that usually work. There is quite an amazing range in how people utilize these drugs biochemically, so it's important to seek a doctor who is thoroughly familiar with them. Some patients may require ten times the dose of others to get well. One way to find such a doctor is to call the chief of the psychiatry department at the medical school closest to where you live. Ask him which of his colleagues he would go to if he were depressed. We use the male pronoun deliberately because we are aware of *no* women psychiatrists who chair their departments at any of the 114 U.S. medical schools.

CHAPTER 33

The Real Keys to Osteoporosis

Nutrition Therapy

Osteoporosis, or loss of bone due to aging, is a complex problem, and thus far no totally successful medication for it has been developed. Increased vitamin D, calcium, and sodium fluoride seem to help—but are toxic in excessive doses.

How can the woman who is suffering from osteoporosis ensure that she is getting an adequate but not excessive therapeutic diet? Only a few foods contain vitamin D—fish liver oil, butter, egg yolk, and liver have the largest amounts.

Calcium, on the other hand, is comparatively easy to get in a daily diet, through green leafy vegetables, cheeses such as Swiss and cheddar, and fruits. (It is better to use a steamer in preparing vegetables, by the way, because nutrients are lost in the cooking water.) Other foods, high in calcium, also contain a great deal of phosphorus, which seems to stimulate secretion of parathyroids and thus draws calcium away from the bones. Such foods include turkey, ham, pork, fried potatoes, bread, processed cheeses, nuts, crackers, and soft drinks.

Phosphorus in various forms is also added to many foods as a preservative. Certain "health foods" contain large amounts of calcium and very little phosphorus, but few of us eat them regularly—sesame seeds, molasses, and seaweed (kelp)! Kelp tablets and powder are available at most health-food stores.

Decreased phosphorus intake is a distinct advantage of a vegetarian diet, according to Dr. Jennifer Jowsey, director of orthopedic research at the Mayo Clinic, who has done extensive work on osteoporosis. "Vegetarians who eat eggs and milk, but avoid meat, have a higher bone density than people whose diets include meat," she points out.

If a map were designed showing worldwide osteoporosis patterns, it would illustrate vividly how much the excess phosphorus in meat contributes to this disorder. Vegetarian societies have little osteoporosis, semivegetarians have an intermediate amount, and meat-loving cultures like ours have the most.

Many people, but especially women, observe that as they get toward middle age they are less attracted to meat, while finding dairy products, fruits, and vegetables more appetizing. Perhaps they are heeding their own body signals, specifically those issuing from the kidneys.

In newly reported research from Israel, the age-related ability of the kidneys to throw off excess phosphorus was evaluated. During childhood and youth, the body eliminates excess phosphorus efficiently. One of the earliest signs of aging is that this capacity diminishes. Excess phosphorus is much more apt to be retained by the body, where it makes mischief by drawing calcium from the bones. Older people are also apt to get less D-producing sunshine essential to help them utilize calcium well.

Since many American women are deficient in D, and some in calcium also, we advocate moderate supplements of both D and calcium for all women starting at around age 40.

The woman who does not get much sun or drink much D-enriched milk might aim for 800 units of vitamin D, or twice the average daily allowance. The woman who *does* get sun and milk might settle for 400 units, unless her dental x-rays reveal early signs of bone loss.

Every woman should get at least one gram (1,000 mg) of calcium daily. Here are some typical food values:

1 cup lamb's quarters, steamed	460 mg
1 cup mustard greens, steamed	308 mg
1 cup collard leaves, steamed	282 mg
1 cup spinach, steamed	124 mg
3 oz. Swiss cheese	810 mg
1 cube cheddar cheese	133 mg

1 cup canned blackberries	100 mg
2 large dried figs	80 mg
1 cup cooked rhubarb	112 mg

Some of the vegetables mentioned, collard leaves being an exception, may contain sufficient oxalic acid to bind the calcium, making it less available. Persons who rely on vegetables as their main calcium source should follow the ongoing research on this controversy. After natural or surgical menopause, calcium requirements probably increase to about one and one-half grams.

To prevent osteoporosis, your calcium intake must be balanced against proper amounts of both magnesium (so that the calcium isn't excreted but stays in the bones instead) and phosphorus. Intake of calcium should be roughly double the intake of magnesium and at least equal to the intake of phosphorus. If the magnesium *gets too low*, the body can become calcium-deficient even when dietary intake of calcium is adequate. If the phosphorus *gets too high* (and it *is* in most American diets), the over-stimulated parathyroids draw calcium from the bones.

We regret that in the space of this book we cannot present extensive tables of the relative calcium, phosphorus, and magnesium properties in most foods, although chapter 35 contains guidelines. We recommend that the reader buy a book giving nutrition tables (many are available in both paperback and hard cover), write down everything she eats in a typical week, and then, checking against her book, determine the amounts of calcium, phosphorus, magnesium, and vitamin D she is consuming. Then she can start adjusting her diet accordingly.

Chances are that the average affluent (i.e., meat-eating, weight-conscious) American woman will be shocked to learn she is consuming four or five times the amount of daily phosphorus as calcium. (And that is without considering the unmeasured amounts of phosphorus used as preservatives in some of her packaged foods.)

Her vitamin D intake may be practically zero, and, all told, she is inviting osteoporosis. The essentials, then, are to bring calcium and phosphorus intake into balance, and add sufficient D. Magnesium plays a secondary but important role.

Calcium not only helps to preserve bone mass, but also may lessen the symptoms of an achey and irritable menopause.

Exercise and Bones

But osteoporosis can occur at any age, often as a result of immobilization. Calcium is deposited in proportion to the load that the bone must carry. The bones of athletes, for instance, become considerably heavier than those of sedentary persons. Also, if someone has one leg in a cast but continues to walk on the opposite leg, the bone of the immobilized limb becomes thin and decalcified, while the other may grow thicker because of the increased load it must bear. Space physicians who worked with astronauts quickly learned that weightlessness is osteoporosis' best ally.

Since *bone density depends on the extent to which the bone is used,* it is not surprising that the incidence of osteoporosis is lower in populations where individuals exercise regularly all their lives.

In a study of the relationship between physical activity and osteoporosis in women, researchers at the University of Hong Kong compared the incidence of hip fractures in Swedish, British, Hong Kong and Singapore Chinese, and South African Bantu populations. They found that fractures occurred most frequently in the Swedish and British populations. Among both Bantu and Chinese, a shortage of mechanical aids results in much more physical work being done by women than in more developed societies. These women, the researchers noted, "take a full and equal place with men in all forms of manual labor until old age."

And so we know that bone thinning is part of the reason older people who fall tend to break their hips, and sometimes their backs. But bone thinning is only one factor in this process. Two additional factors that seem to influence the probability that a minor fall will result in a fracture are the condition of the discs between the vertebrae of the spine, and the strength of the ligaments supporting the skeleton. Convincing evidence exists that ligaments can be strengthened by regular excercise of almost any reasonable sort.

In 1966, work done at the San Fernando Valley State College in California revealed that rats whose opportunity for movement was restricted showed weakening of the ligaments. Rats exercised on an uneven surface showed even *greater* ligament strength after the experiment. The strengthened ligaments were heavier and also less tightly stretched between their bony attachments, thereby increasing the range of movement and reducing the probability of fracture.

These and other animal studies confirm that the strength of ligaments supporting the skeleton seems to increase with exercise, which in turn reduces the probability that a fracture will occur after minimal trauma, and also seems to speed up the healing of fractures that do occur.

Exercise, Health, and Longevity

The United States has about 3 centenarians per 100,000 people. The Russian republic of Georgia has about 39 centenarians per 100,000, and in Azerbaijan, close by, there are 84 per 100,000. The most impressive statistic comes from Vilcacamba, a little town in the Ecuadorean Andes, where 9 of its 819 citizens were over 100 years of age, roughly 366 times the ratio in the United States.

The one constant in these populations is that all these people do hard physical work throughout their lives and do not retire at 65.

Exercise seems also to be related to general well-being. In Durham, North Carolina, a ten-year study of 268 persons aged 60 to 94 revealed that of three health practices examined (inactivity, obesity, and cigarette smoking), the amount of exercise was most closely correlated to illness indicators such as physicians' visits, days spent in bed. The proportion of persons who rated their health as poor was more than four times as high among sedentary persons as among those who pursued an active schedule.

Oh, My Aching Back

The back pain associated with osteoporosis is of two types: an acute, sometimes severe pain near the small of the back that disappears over a period of weeks and is related to fractures of the vertebrae or to previous injuries, and a more chronic, diffuse, aching pain. Uusually the pain follows physical exertion such as bending forward or lifting heavy objects, but it sometimes can result from a seemingly trivial action such as simply turning over in bed. The more chronic pain is found in only a minority of individuals, and may not be related to osteoporosis at all, but possibly to arthritis or to muscle pain. (We wonder how many of the physicians who prescribed estrogen replacement therapy for the "back pain of osteoporosis" first investigated the possibility that the pain might be the result of muscle weakness due to inactivity.)

When our ancestors abandoned the trees to become terrestrial dwellers, whose weight was *supported* rather than *suspended,* as is that of tree-dwelling primates, our structure was radically altered mechanically and neurologically. Human feet and legs became enlarged and strengthened to bear the body weight, but the pelvis adapted itself to the upright stance in a way that is apparently unsatisfactory and probably incomplete. Our hindquarters remained similar to those of animals who walk on all fours, but the torso was set off at an angle, imposing an extreme mechanical disadvantage.

If back muscles are tense and underused, low back pain can result. Muscle weakness is also related to the familiar tension syndrome of stiff neck and headache. Exercise helps guard against painful, disabling episodes of "throwing the back out."

It is essential to work into condition *gradually.* Brisk walking and swimming are usually safe and satisfactory for beginners. Swimming exercises every muscle in the body. Calisthenics within the range of one's age and physical condition are also good. If a woman already has been diagnosed as having osteoporosis, she should see a rehabilitation or "physical medicine" specialist. A personal program must be prescribed; unsupervised exercise could only make matters worse.

Osteoarthritis and Diet

Can nutrition help the painful condition called osteoarthritis, occurring in the joints, from which an estimated

12 million Americans suffer? The Arthritis Foundation thinks not. It states that no food has been implicated as a cause of arthritis, and that none provides "effective protection" against it. However, the Foundation does acknowledge that a "normal well-balanced and nourishing" diet is essential for arthritis victims.

But Roger Williams, esteemed by his colleagues as the "grand old man" of American nutrition, is much more hopeful. "There is a good possibility," he states, "that individual arthritics will be able—if they are lucky and make intelligent trials—to hit upon particular nutrients or nutrient combinations which will bring benefit. . . . On the basis of reports presently available, that items that certainly need to be considered are niacin (niacinamide), pantothenic acid, riboflavin, vitamin A, B_6, magnesium, calcium, phosphate and other minerals. The objective is to feed adequately the cells that are involved in keeping the bones, joints, and muscles in healthy condition."

In Bridgeport, Connecticut, internist William Kaufman treats arthritis patients with massive doses of niacinamide—400 up to 2,500 mg daily. In London, researchers at the Rheumatic Clinic of St. Alfege's Hospital discovered that arthritics have only one-quarter to one-half the pantothenic acid levels of healthy people. Either injections of calcium pantothenate or oral doses may relieve symptoms in as little as one week. Symptoms return when the supplements are discontinued. Dosages as low as 50 mg daily can suffice.

In Mt. Pleasant, Texas, Dr. John Ellis reports that B_6 —again, 50 mg of it—may relieve such symptoms as finger pain, stiffness and numbness, pains in the shoulders, hips and knees and nighttime muscle cramps. Joints in the hands and wrists or bursitis following injury seem not to benefit.

Vitamins A and B_2 also occur in lower-than-normal concentrations in the blood of many arthritis victims. Vitamin C benefits some patients, perhaps through its effect on collagen and cartilage. An array of minerals, including calcium, magnesium and manganese are sometimes helpful.

When Dr. Williams, a past president of the American Chemical Society, urges giving a *trial* to such regimens, he means that precisely. Each individual responds uniquely.

CHAPTER 34

Healthy Skin at Menopause

Women have been led to believe that estrogen is essential to keep their skin youthful and moist. This is at best a half truth.

Just as we need vitamins, we do need a normal and balanced supply of hormones to maintain our skins in optimum condition. However, unlike vitamins, hormones are normally manufactured by our own bodies.

Two hormones contribute to skin health more than any others and are considered the real "basics" in this regard, comparable to vitamins A, B_{12}, and biotin. These two hormones are *aldosterone* and *vasopressin*.

An imbalance in vasopressin is seen quickly in the skin. Too little produces excessive dryness—the skin loses water and aging lines stand out. Too much produces a marked facial pallor.

There are thirteen additional hormones—and estrogen is only one among them—which lend further support functions to the skin. These are, in alphabetical order: ACTH (adrenocorticotropic hormone), cortisone, epinephrine, estrogen, growth hormone, insulin, norepinephrine, oxytocin, progesterone, relaxin, testosterone, thyroxine, and TSH (thyroid-stimulating hormone).

Estrogen does, however, have a specific target influence on the *lining of the vagina*. (See chap. 26.) In some severe cases of dryness and deterioration, locally applied estrogen creams work where other remedies fail. Concerning the face, the "youthifying" benefits of estrogen are both unproven and unlikely. In their official labeling for doctors, *estrogen manufacturers have never been allowed to claim that internal use of this hormone has unique benefits for facial skin.*

So blatantly has this myth been pushed on women that in September 1976 the FDA specifically ordered manufacturers to state:

"ESTROGENS ARE NOT INDICATED FOR CERTAIN CONDITIONS, I.E., NERVOUSNESS, PRESERVATION OF SUPPLE SKIN, OR MAINTENANCE OF A YOUTHFUL FEELING."

Estrogen and Facial Skin

Estrogen's adverse effects on facial skin are little publicized to women, but they can be found in the official labeling on estrogen products. Many women have a bad cosmetic reaction to hormones, including allergic rashes, extreme bloating, the loss of hair or growth of it in undesired places, skin discolorations resembling the mask of pregnancy, excessive dryness or oiliness, increased susceptibility to bruising and vein formation, herpes infections that scar the skin, and liver disorders that also discolor the skin or leave scars.

Some acne cases respond well to estrogen but others are intensified.

One reason surplus estrogen may harm the skin is that it interacts negatively or "antagonizes" two of the central skin vitamins, A and B_2. It also (see chap. 28) depletes a wide range of vitamins and minerals that influence liver health, resistance to infection, the state of collagen fibers and blood vessels, and so on.

Estrogen, like vasopressin, has an effect on water balance—although that is not its main function. The more water the skin retains, the more it puffs out, making fine lines less visible.

Water retention or loss at different points in the menstrual cycle is an estrogen-associated phenomenon. Thus, indirectly, estrogen can encourage the skin to hold water.

Hormone face creams also have a "plumping" effect on the skin. All creams help the skin to hold water to some extent. Recently, water-attracting compounds called NMFs (natural moisturizing factors) were isolated from epidermal tissue and reproduced in laboratories. They are now available in some cosmetics. Such creams probably encourage surface water retention as well as or better than estrogen products, and are not carcinogenic.

A woman who wishes to achieve this "plumping" effect can look for the ingredient NMF on the label of a moisturizer. But most women discover safe and natural moisturizing products that work well for them.

Another group of cosmetics that help conceal lines are those that form an invisible smooth surface, causing light to be reflected more evenly. Thus, there are two distinct groups of beauty products that help conceal lines temporarily—the "plumpers," such as estrogen, NMF creams, or other moisturizers, and the "light reflectors."

Vitamins and Skin

Dr. Jean Mayer considers A, "the moisturizing vitamin," to be central in maintaining a normal skin. B_{12} and biotin are next in importance, while B_2, D, and pantothenic acid have "indirect" but crucial effects.

Should any of these six be deficient, the skin will probably show it. *Any woman with any skin problem must make certain she is getting at least her daily requirement of all of them.*

But that's just the start of it, for a host of other vitamins and minerals—almost any of them—may influence the skin under certain circumstances. "Skin lesions" are an early sign of B_6 deficiency, and certain herpes infections that do not respond well to any drug *do* respond to massive doses of B_6. Niacin, C, and folic acid affect pigmentation, and also, it is thought, the collagen fibers beneath the skin which influence wrinkles and sagging.

When giving up a hormone product, the body may go through a major readjustment that can take a drastic toll on the skin. The best ways to speed one's return to normal are through nutrition, topical measures, and exercise.

Nutritionally, a high-protein diet is advisable, as is avoiding starches and junk foods. The woman at menopause should be sure that she is getting all of the skin vitamins at twice their recommended allowance, or more. *But she should not go further than tripling the recom-*

mended allowances of A, which means not more than 15,000 daily units. Also, she might try such "boosters" as lecithin, kelp, and especially yeast and organic desiccated liver, which sometimes seem to improve the skin quite noticeably. Zinc is probably the most central mineral in skin maintenance.

It is wise to remember also that rapid weight loss can cause the skin to sag, as can heavy consumption of alcohol and cigarettes and lack of sleep.

When the skin is going through a readjustment after giving up hormones (or through the milder readjustments of natural menopause), a program of twice-weekly steaming and home facials, *combined with a proper nutrition regimen and circulation-boosting exercise*, usually brings improvement within weeks. Many women return to hormone products out of desperation when it isn't necessary at all. The normalizing benefits of old-fashioned steaming have got to be tried to be believed. Steaming can do more for a dry skin than the most elaborate hormone products, more for an oily skin than the most abrasive medications.

To give herself a facial steaming, a woman can bring a large pot of water to a boil, drop in a tablespoon or so of appropriate herbs, and let them simmer for a minute. She then places the pot of water on a table and drapes towels over her head and the pot to create a "tent" that holds in the steam. She keeps her face a foot or more away from the steaming pot and lifts the towel when she needs to get air. The idea is to persist for five or ten minutes until she has worked up a thorough sweat.

The most commonly used herb in a facial steaming is camomile, which is cleansing, neutral, and soothing.

Another effective product, sold at many pharmacies and health-food stores, is Swiss Kriss, which is actually an herbal laxative. However, the ingredients in Swiss Kriss seem highly effective for removing excess oil and impurities.

After her steam tent, the woman (or man) should use an appropriate facial mask, depending on whether her skin is dry or oily. Masks blended from rich ingredients such as honey or avocado are excellent for dry skins, while clay or earth based masks help to draw out oil and control acne. More neutral masks, such as simple egg white, are excellent for general tightening and toning. For what are called "mixed skins" different preparations can be applied to appropriate portions of the face.

While many good commercial products are available, homemade masks are better yet as they do not contain preservatives or other irritating chemicals.

Georgette Klinger, the European-born cosmetologist who maintains skin care emporiums in New York, Los Angeles, and other cities, offers the following tip for women who have dry-skin-adjustment problems after giving up Premarin. "While bathing," she advises, "slather on lots of moisturizer which the steamy bath will help to work in."

In Europe, cosmetology—the optimum maintenance of normal skin through the life cycle—is a respected paramedical specialty, requiring years of training. Women who can afford a professional cleaning and consultation from time to time are often very pleased with the results.

Some dermatologists are very helpful also, but, as physicians, they tend to be more interested in disease than prevention.

CHAPTER 35

Vitamins and Minerals That All Women Need

The greatest nutritionist of our time, Roger Williams, who was born in 1893, and served as president of the American Chemical Society in 1957, has always maintained that our individual nutritional requirements differ genetically, and also because of the stresses that occur throughout our lifetimes. Pregnancy, menopause, aging, infections, our polluted air and water, the quality of our soil, the food additives and drugs we use all alter our needs.

Increasingly, Dr. Williams's theory of biochemical individuality appears borne out. Many or most of us feel better when we take certain supplements.

Supplements

The genetics of malabsorption is a fascinating issue, and many provocative research clues are starting to fall into place. In one family of our acquaintance the grandfather had diabetes, while the grandmother had arthritis and Parkinson's disease. A daughter has exceptionally severe dysmenhorrea, while a second daughter suffers from hypoglycemia. The son of a third daughter is a celiac.

All of these conditions are now tentatively linked to B_6 malabsorption, among other predisposing conditions. The surviving family members who take B supplements are responding very well. Originally, the family immigrated from an area in Europe where the normal diet was much higher in B_6 than it is in the United States, and these conditions did not appear until the move occurred. There is a mounting body of evidence that many serious illnesses, including some cancers, do not occur much in certain population groups until they change their place of residence and dietary patterns. In short, we may be bred for certain diets, and may succumb to illness when we alter them.

The general nutritional supplement guidelines that follow are particularly directed toward women in the reproductive and menopausal years. They are conservative, not faddish, and are geared toward long-range health and well-being, as well as the correction of what our grandmothers called "women's troubles."

Our tables are based on the current government allowances, and go up through what is considered the therapeutic dose range. Many individuals now take megavitamins, dosages much higher than those we are about to present. For example, a recent Menopause Roundtable in *Prevention* magazine quoted Dr. Jonathan Wright of Seattle: "Now some women are very successful with very high doses of vitamin E throughout the menopause— 2,000 to 3,000 units daily." Dr. Wright may be correct, but the dose range we suggest is only 30 to 600 units, which frequently suffices.

Similarly, mega-C is very popular, and many physicians and scientists are so impressed with Linus Pauling's important theories that they personally take several grams of C daily, or more. Many feel that they are greatly benefited.

But Pauling is the first to acknowledge that his work is experimental, not definitive. For the time being, it's important to know that minor ailments associated with C deficiency often respond quickly to dosages of only 200 to 750 mg, the much lower therapeutic range we advocate in this book.

In megaranges vitamins start to work like drugs. For better or worse they can alter the body's chemistry quite markedly. In time we may find that, as Pauling hopes, mega-nutrition could expand our average life expectancy to 100 years. On the other hand, megavitamins sometimes cause unexpected side effects, or withdrawal symptoms. On page 507 we describe a study of identical twins, in which the males around age 5 or 6 who received what were megadoses for their body-weight, showed greater height increase during only five months of vitamin C treatment. (This difference did not occur in the female twins; clearly, megavitamins have many secrets yet to yield.)

Our own position, as reflected in our tables and recommendations, can be summarized like this:

—Our overprocessed diets are much more deficient than the government acknowledges. Pollution, drugs, and other conditions of modern living potentiate our deficiencies. Many of us are not getting what we need, even when we do our utmost to eat sensibly. A simple apple, at the average supermarket, is *not* like an apple plucked fresh from the Garden of Eden.

—As a nation of immigrants, many of us were bred genetically for different diets, and many have higher specific needs for some nutrients than the American diet provides at its best. A very good clue to diet changes or vitamin supplements often lies in the success stories of one's nearest relatives.

A woman who was infertile after stopping the pill wrote to us for nutritional advice. From her description of her diet it sounded as if she might be quite deficient in the vitamins and minerals delivered by fresh vegetables, that are also depleted by the contraceptive. We suggested that she eat more raw fruits and vegetables, and save all her cooking water to return to the meal. Our correspondent was utterly dumbfounded. "That's what my grandmother told me! She had trouble conceiving also, and she claims that she cured it by saving her cooking water."

—Nutritional needs associated with aging, stress, and women's problems have been especially neglected. Dr. Thomas Brewer, who proved that severe weight restrictions in pregnancy can be lethal to mothers and babies both, continues to be ignored by many of his obstetrical colleagues. When a tragic pregnancy-malnutrition death occurred in his own community he wrote to us: "Now every woman has to safeguard her own health as best she can. . . . The medical and drug establishment are determined to deny the facts."

—While megavitamins are not yet understood, therapeutic ranges *are*. The latter have been prescribed for many years, and do not cause serious side effects or deaths, although some persons may experience minor discomforts, as in food allergies. Therapeutic dosages work most effectively when combined with other preventive measures. For example, a woman who takes B_6 for premenstrual acne should also deep-clean her skin. A woman who takes E for menopause distress should also find a regular exercise program that she enjoys.

Therapeutic vitamins don't cure every female disorder, but since they work frequently, and are safe, they seem a logical place to start. It's similar to our advocacy of the diaphragm and condom, or other benign contraceptives. We think that the dangerous contraceptives (like dangerous drugs for menopause) should be reserved as a backup, not pushed on women as a first choice.

General Advice

To decrease:
- Calories: eat less sweets, starches, fried, fatty foods.
- Cholesterol: eat less egg yolks, organ meats, shellfish.
- Saturated fats: eat less butter, coconut, fats, hard cheese, ice cream, lard, luncheon and breakfast meats, salt pork, whole milk.

To increase:
- Fiber (2 g daily): eat more bran, raw fruits and vegetables (with skin), whole grain breads and cereals.
- Iron (18 mg daily is the normal requirement; IUD users may need up to 20–100 mg): eat more beans, bran, dried fruits, green vegetables, liver or organic desiccated liver tablets, nuts, peanut butter, whole wheat breads and cereals.

NOTE: There is a growing concern that many middle-aged Americans may be avoiding eggs, dairy products and organ meats too assiduously. These foods have some essential nutrients that cannot be readily obtained from any other natural source. Like Aristotle, we would suggest moderation, not total avoidance and, as we have elsewhere commented, organic desiccated liver, about three tablets a day, provides the equivalent of a weekly liver serving without chemicals like DES and antibiotics, or much cholesterol.

Some consumers may succeed in finding organically

raised meat, free of dangerous chemicals, which constitutes about 15 percent of the American market, and usually issues from small producers.

Concerning cholesterol, we produce it in our bodies. Some studies have shown that a person's emotional state can have a greater effect on blood cholesterol levels than the amount of cholesterol in the diet.

Concerning saturated vs. unsaturated fats, there is still much controversy. Saturated fats may increase the risk of heart disease, while unsaturated fats may increase the risk of cancer. Increased dietary fiber may be valuable for many conditions, yet in children, at least, it may lead to some deficiency states.

Many important nutritional questions simply cannot be answered at this time; we just do not have the information. It seems to us that some medically-faddish regimens, including among others extreme versions of low cholesterol, high unsaturated fats, and high fiber diets, are probably unwise. There is far less evidence for them than there is for the safety and efficacy of moderate vitamin and mineral supplementation, combined with a balanced diet that has a minimum of processed foods.

Thus, we believe that some physicians who dismiss vitamin-taking as "faddish" while prescribing extreme diets for their patients are unwitting faddists themselves.

Key to Reading Tables

Some of the information concerning vitamins and minerals in the tables that follow is especially pertinent for women in certain categories. We have isolated the supplements of particular value to each group in the following manner:

* Pill or estrogen users, or those recovering from hormones, look for this symbol.
** Those suffering from hot flashes or other menopause complaints, look for this symbol.
*** Those 40 or over or experiencing symptoms of osteoporosis, look for this symbol.
**** Those suffering from fibrocystic breast disease, look for this symbol.
***** Those suffering from menstrual distress or loss of menstruation, look for this symbol.

† Those with skin problems associated with hormones or menopause, look for this symbol.

†† Those with gum and tooth problems, look for this symbol.

††† IUD users, look for this symbol.

†††† Those suffering from arthritis pain, look for this symbol.

Vitamin Selection

There is much confusion concerning "natural" vs. synthetic formulations, and also discount vitamins as compared to more expensive name brands. The organic producers claim that their products, based chiefly on plant sources, may contain still unidentified "associated factors." Sometimes this proves correct. The B-complex provided by the organic companies in the 1940s *did* contain a B vitamin that was not isolated, or added to synthetic brands, until later.

On the other hand, the dosages in synthetic vitamins are easier to control—rose hips, for example, growing on the *same* mountain vary in their C content from season to season depending on the weather—and with many nutrients the synthetic and organic forms are chemically identical.

A case can be made for either type of product and we suggest that the user herself determine which she prefers.

Some discount houses—Bronson Pharmaceuticals (4526 Rinetti Lane, La Canada, CA 91011) is one example—claim that they purchase their ingredients from leading brand-name manufacturers, including Hoffman-LaRoche, Merck, and Pfizer, but sell them at about one-half the price. Other discount companies are less forthright about sources. Then too, in some cases, while the raw materials may be the same, the coating on the name-brands may be more palatable.

The Fat-Soluble Vitamins: A, D, E, K

Do not exceed two to four times the recommended allowance of A and D except under medical supervision.

But don't take it for granted that you're getting

enough in your diet. Skin and vision problems *may* be due to A deficiency; osteoporosis to deficiency of D; hot flashes to E deficiency. Vitamin K supplements should not be taken at all except under medical supervision. If you think you may be deficient in K (see "Deficiency Symptoms" in vitamin K table), discuss it with your doctor.

VITAMIN A

Approximate Daily Requirement. Most Adults Under Normal Conditions

5,000 units. Some nutritionists recommend up to 20,000 units as a normal supplement. The need for A increases with greater body weight.

Conditions That Increase Need

Low bile and malabsorption problems, liver disease and damage, high intake of prepared and processed foods, low-fat diet, working in bright light, pregnancy, lactation; estrogen products either increase or decrease need in unsettled fashion, but estrogen is considered an antagonist to A. Overcooking destroys A.

Foods That Provide Daily Requirement

Calf and beef liver provide enormous amounts of A, as much as 6 times the daily allowance in an average portion. Chicken liver supplies twice the daily allowance, as does a serving of chard, spinach, or turnip greens.

Other foods that contain the daily allowance, or somewhat more, are an average serving of string beans, broccoli, carrots, yellow squash, apricots, sweet potatoes, and yams. A tip for calorie counters and fiber watchers: One raw carrot or one-half cup (4 oz) of kale provides the approximate daily A requirement. The carrot has only about 20 calories, and the kale about 35.

Many researchers now consider it desirable to attain about 2 g of fiber in the daily diet. The carrot provides one-quarter of the fiber requirement, and the kale provides half.

Deficiency Symptoms

Night blindness; abnormal dryness of the eyeballs; softness of the cornea; dry, rough itchy skin; mucous membrane abnormalities. Vitamin A sometimes helps dry skin conditions of menopause, but some women benefit more from adding E, which helps them use their A better.

Excess Symptoms

Loss of hair, cracked lips, dry skin, severe headaches, general weakness, blurred vision, bruising, nose bleeds, painful joints, tenderness and swelling of the long bones, emotional disturbance, fatigue, insomnia.

Therapeutic Dose Range

Toxic level 50,000 units. 10,000 to 20,000 daily units should be the maximum without medical supervision. Skip supplements when high dietary intake of liver, carrots, carrot juice, spinach is eaten. Consider that you may not require A supplements at all if you are a regular consumer of extremely A-rich foods.
* May be useful when recovering from the pill if skin symptoms occur. Do not take when recovering from the pill if planning to have a baby.
† May be useful for skin problems in menopause.
†††† 5,000–10,000 daily units may help ease arthritis pain, if blood levels of A are abnormally low.

VITAMIN A (continued)
Hormone Interactions

Too much estrogen keeps A from performing normally in the body.

Interactions with Other Vitamins and Minerals

Presence of E is necessary to prevent the destruction of A in the body; A cannot be stored if choline is undersupplied. Synergistic with B_{12}, B_2, C, and E. Dietary protein is required to mobilize liver reserves of A.

Other Comments

Vitamin A is stored largely in the liver. A descreases basal metabolism. The halflife of A is weeks or months, meaning that it can be stored (and then mobilized from the liver by protein), so it need not be taken daily.

VITAMIN D

Approximate Daily Requirement. Most Adults Under Normal Conditions

400 units. A few nutritionists advocate up to 4,000 or 5,000 daily units for all adults, but this occasionally produces serious side effects.

Conditions That Increase Need

D is essential for normal absorption of calcium. To prevent osteoporosis, persons over 40 require supplementation if dietary intake is low or exposure to sunlight reduced. Many adults who live in northern states, work indoors, and drink less than a quart of daily D-enriched milk are deficient in D.

Foods That Provide Daily Requirement

1 qt of D-enriched milk, fish liver oils, 3½ oz of sardines, herring, salmon, tuna, shrimp. Also in egg yolk and margarine. Low amounts in other dairy products and meats. 3 oz of salmon (120 calories) or tuna (170 calories) or 4 oz of shrimp (103 calories) are good sources of D for dieters.

Deficiency Symptoms

Softening of the bones, rickets, demineralization, decreased blood calcium and phosphorus, brittle bones, osteoporosis.

Excess Symptoms

Loss of appetite, nausea, headache, urinary problems, diarrhea, excessive thirst, weight loss, depression, irritability, psychoses, leg weakness, death from associated calcium deposits in the kidney and lung.

Therapeutic Dose Range

Serious toxicity has been found at 1,800 units in susceptible individuals. 800–1,200 daily units should be the maximum therapeutic dosage without medical supervision. (Some doctors give osteoporosis patients very high doses, but they monitor the effects.) Less is needed when exposure to sunlight is increased.
*** 400–1,600 daily units. Women are apt to get less D from sunlight than men because of sunscreens (to prevent wrinkles) and make-up. D is needed to utilize calcium and help preserve bone mass.
**** 400–800 daily units, in conjunction with dolomite or calcium pills to ease premenstrual tension and menstrual pain.

VITAMIN D (continued)
Hormone Interactions

D deficiency (like phosphorus excess) overstimulates the parathyroid, drawing calcium from the bones and contributing to osteoporosis.

Interactions with Other Vitamins and Minerals

Vitamins A and B₁ reduce D's potential toxicity or increase the body's tolerance for it. When taking more than double the recommended allowance of D, some A and B complex should be also added.

Other Comments

D is formed by the action of sunlight on the skin.

VITAMIN E

Approximate Daily Requirement. Most Adults Under Normal Conditions

30 units. Dosages of up to 1,600 daily units are advocated by a few nutritionists. Many more advocate 50–100 daily or up to 400 or 600, but not beyond. Vitamin E consists of at least seven related chemicals named alpha, beta, gamma, delta, epsilon, zeta, and eta tocopherols. The alpha form has been most studied and is deemed most potent, but other forms may have as-yet-undiscovered functions. Some nutritionists feel it is only necessary to take the alpha form; others recommend taking mixed tocopherols which contain alpha plus some or all of the other variants of E.

Conditions That Increase Need

Taking hormones; pregnancy; lactation and other stress on reproductive system; pollution or presence of other chemical and environmental toxins; ingestion of unsaturated fats, mineral oil; menopause (hot flashes), aging, post-pill syndrome.

Foods That Provide Daily Requirement

2 generous tbsp of wheat germ sprinkled on cereals or salads or used in baking, or 4 slices whole grain bread or a salad including the wilted leaves (higher in E) with oils such as safflower or wheat germ in the dressing. 1 oz of wheat germ (2 tbsp) provides one-third of the daily 2 g fiber need, as well as about 100 calories and most of the normal E requirement.

Deficiency Symptoms

Destruction of red blood cells, muscle degeneration, paralysis, hot flashes, possibly insufficient blood flow to extremities, some anemias, some reproductive disorders such as absence of menstruation; insufficient E may have adverse effects on skin health. This may be an indirect result of E's protective effect on A and other vitamins, on fat storage, or role in protecting against toxins in the environment that damage skin.

Excess Symptoms

Weight gain from increased fat storage, indigestion, possibly high blood pressure, skin rashes, sleepiness; if dose is too high, foods may start to seem unappetizing. At dosages of 4,000 daily units taken for 3 months diarrhea and soreness of the mouth, tongue, and lips have been reported.

Therapeutic Dose Range

Never more than 30–100 units daily for persons with high blood pressure, diabetes, or rheumatic heart. Those taking digitalis should not use E without medical supervision. Normal therapeutic range that most people can handle varies from 30 to 600 daily units.

VITAMIN E (continued)

More should be medically supervised. Users of E supplements should experiment to see if they prefer the dry or oily capsules. Products which include about 25 mcg of selenium for each 200 units of E increase E's efficiency. For people who cannot take E following a meal with fat, it may be desirable to swallow with their E, 1 or 2 lecithin capsules (or the equivalent in granules), which are a soybean extract containing choline and inositol as well as large amounts of unsaturated fatty acids, which work hand in hand with E. A warning about lecithin: 6 capsules also supply one-quarter of the daily requirement of 800 mg to 1 g of phosphorus, which may be undesirable for persons prone to osteoporosis, such as women whose ovaries were surgically removed or who are heavy eaters of meat. Amenorrhea has been effectively treated with wheat germ oil—20 drops three times a day for 10 days.

* 15–30 daily units for women taking the pill; up to 300 for women taking estrogens alone. 30–600 daily units for women with post-pill or post-ERT syndromes.

** 30–600 daily units for hot flashes. More (under medical supervision) for postmenopause vaginal problems.

*** 600 daily units for fibrocystic breasts.

**** 30–600 daily units for absent menstruation. 30–200 daily units for better health during premenstrual week and menstruation.

† 30–600 daily units for dry or prematurely aging skin.

Hormone Interactions

Deficiency increases production of pituitary hormones FSH and LH, which may be the key to E's effectiveness in subduing hot flashes.

E is highly concentrated in reproductive tissues, and also interacts closely with cortisone and adrenal and growth hormones.

Interactions with Other Vitamins and Minerals

E interacts with, preserves, or helps utilize C, A, B_{12} and folic acid, K and pantothenic acid. For vegetarians, who have few dietary sources of B_{12}, E may actually substitute for it, as well as potentiating the B_{12} they do get.

Other Comments

E is stored in muscle, fat tissue, and liver; 60–70 percent of daily dose is excreted in feces; the rest is absorbed, but has a halflife of under one week, closer to the water-soluble vitamins (B's and C's) than the other fat-soluble vitamins such as A, which has a halflife of months, or D, which has a halflife of weeks. This is why it's safer for most people to take relatively higher doses of E than A or D.

VITAMIN K
[K, the fourth fat-soluble vitamin, is also known as the antihemorrhagic or coagulation factor.]

Approximate Daily Requirement. Most Adults Under Normal Conditions

30 mcg, but it is normally manufactured by intestinal bacteria.

Conditions That Increase Need

Healthy people do not need to worry about K, or take any supplements. Supplements may be required when antibiotics, sulfa drugs, or mineral oil are used, or in the presence of gallstones, liver disease, severe diarrhea or colitis.

Foods That Provide Daily Requirement

The vitamin is stable to cooking and oxidation, but is lost when foods are irradiated. K occurs in cabbage, cauliflower, soybeans, spinach, other vegetables, organ meats, strawberries, and whole grains.

VITAMIN K (continued)
Deficiency Symptoms

Natural blood clotting does not occur. Increased bleeding and hemorrhage. Literally, vitamin K protects you from bleeding to death if you are injured.

Excess Symptoms

Possible blood clots, vomiting.

Therapeutic Dose Range

This is medically determined. Dosages of 5 mg or more are sometimes administered by doctors, but should never be self-prescribed.
††† Some doctors prescribe it temporarily when they insert an IUD.

Hormone Interactions

K works synergistically with growth hormones.

Interactions with Other Vitamins and Minerals

K works synergistically with E. The fragility of red blood cells correlates with vitamins A, C, and K.

Other Comments

Vitamin K is used to treat mothers in labor, newborn infants with neonatal hemorrhage, and persons who have been overdosed with anticoagulants as after a pill-caused blood clot, or in the presence of heart disease.
K is used experimentally as a painkiller.

The Water-Soluble Vitamins: B_1, B_2, Niacin, B_6, B_{12}, Folic Acid, Pantothenic Acid, Biotin, Choline and Inositol, and PABA; Vitamin C

Essential to energy and emotional health, they are often depleted by the pill or estrogen supplements. Among the B vitamins thiamine and B_6 are especially apt to be used "inefficiently" with advancing age, and dietary need increases.

Many women feel that they get the most mileage out of B complex when they take it in a stress supplement formula—that is, combined with C, and in two or three daily doses. However, it may be best for pill or estrogen users to take tablets containing folic acid and B_{12} separately from C (three hours or more later), as high doses of C may wash out some of their already deficient folic acid and B_{12}.

VITAMIN B₁ (Thiamine)

Approximate Daily Requirement. Most Adults Under Normal Conditions

1.5 mg. 10 mg daily is advocated by many nutritionists for older people, the very active, and those under stress.

Conditions That Increase Need

Pregnancy, lactation, eating sugar, smoking, drinking alcohol, surgery, taking pep pills, crash diets, taking the pill, eating processed meats.

Foods That Provide Daily Requirement

Essential to have every day, as it is not stored. Wheat germ, rice, bran, soybean flour, yeast, and ham are the highest sources. Other sources include vegetables, grains, beans, nuts, and other meats. Many B_1-rich foods are also excellent sources of fiber.

4 oz of sunflower seed (in the hull) provide 2.3 g of fiber, 343 calories and 1.8 mg of B_1. A 1 oz or ½ cup serving of commercial bran breakfast cereal provides the daily fiber requirement, half the daily B_1 requirement, and 70 calories, without milk, or 150 with it. For dieters, 1 tbsp of brewer's yeast provides most of the B_1 requirement, and only 25 calories.

Deficiency Symptoms

Loss of appetite, constipation, digestive disturbance, depression, irritability, inability to concentrate, numbness and prickliness in toes and feet, stiff ankles, loss of reflexes. In later stages of deficiency, nerves, muscle, and heart function are affected.

Beri-beri, the disease resulting from severe B_1 deficiency, occurs in two forms. In the wet form, edema is paramount, and in the dry form, emaciation. Death results from cardiac failure.

Beri-beri is most apt to occur where white polished rice is the mainstay of the diet.

Excess Symptoms

Edema, nervousness, sweating, rapid heart beat, tremors, herpes, fatty liver, and allergies.

Therapeutic Dose Range

4–15 mg daily. Should be kept in balance with other B's if possible, that is, proportional to other B's in terms of multiples of the recommended allowance unless special needs for a certain B are suspected.

* The daily allowance, or twice that, may be enough to replace lost B_1 in pill users.
** As part of B complex, is generally helpful for post-pill and menopause complaints.
***** As part of B-complex is generally helpful during premenstrual week and menstruation.

Hormone Interactions

Affects the thyroid and insulin production.

Interactions with Other Vitamins and Minerals

Increases activity of B_{12}, works with pantothenic acid, niacin, and riboflavin to release energy from carbohydrates. Overdose of B_1 may cause B_6 deficiency. B_1, riboflavin, and B_6 work together to produce niacin.

Vitamin C decreases requirement for B_1. Tolerance to D is increased by B_1.

Other Comments

B vitamin most vulnerable to heat. Not stored to any great length and is readily excreted in the urine. Has diuretic effect. Injections may produce allergies.

VITAMIN B₂ (Riboflavin)

Approximate Daily Requirement. Most Adults Under Normal Conditions

1.7 mg, but many nutritionists consider this too low and feel the requirement should be 5 mg for all adolescents and adults.

Conditions That Increase Need

Taking the pill and possibly other hormones, pregnancy, lactation, and stress.

Foods That Provide Daily Requirement

Deficiency occurs on a starchy or junk food diet, or a low-calorie, low-cholesterol, or zen macrobiotic diet. It is difficult to assure the 1.7 mg daily intake, much less the 5 mg some authorities favor—even without the further depletion that occurs during hormone use.

The richest sources are brewer's yeast and milk. 1 qt of whole milk contains only 1.64 mg, as well as 640 calories. Six tablespoons of brewer's yeast also supplies the daily requirement at 150 calories. 3 oz of beef liver provides about 4 mg at 195 calories. Those who fear the DES and cholesterol in liver might wish to substitute desiccated liver tablets; 3 or 4 tablets a day will equal about one weekly serving of liver, providing riboflavin, B₁₂, and other members of the B complex. 4 oz of beef heart, at about 160 calories, provides almost the daily requirement.

Persons who consume large amounts of asparagus, beans, and greens such as watercress may meet their daily allowance with relatively few calories.

An average serving of these items has about one-sixth to one-third the B₂ requirement. For fiber watchers who are unconcerned about weight, a cup of shelled almonds provides the daily riboflavin allowance, 3.7 g of fiber, and 849 calories.

Deficiency Symptoms

Riboflavin is needed for the metabolism of proteins, maintenance of the nervous system, skin and cornea, and resistance to disease. Deficiencies include lesions affecting the mouth, lips, eyes, skin, and genitalia. These sometimes appear as extended cracks on the upper or lower lip and may extend into the mucous membranes inside the mouth. Burning and itching sensations in the eyes, and scaliness of the skin—especially around the joints—may also occur; so may dandruff. Cataracts occur in severe deficiencies, and a discolored tongue or anemia are further symptoms.

Excess Symptoms

Riboflavin is considered essentially nontoxic in man. But occasionally, as with certain other vitamins, there are minor symptoms of excess which resemble deficiency symptoms. These include itching, or spontaneous sensations of burning, prickling, or numbness.

Therapeutic Dose Range

5–15 mg.
* 10–15 mg.
** Not specifically associated with hot flashes but, like other B's, may help energy and well-being at menopause.
***** As part of B-complex is generally helpful during premenstrual week and menstruation.
†††† 5–10 mg daily may help reduce arthritis pain.
  Estrogen users also see Hormone Interactions (below).

Hormone Interactions

Riboflavin contributes to the normal release and activity of many hormones, including estrogen, the pituitary growth and adrenal hormones, thyroxine and insulin.
  An unusual feature of riboflavin is that it inhibits the formation of liver tumors in animals.

VITAMIN B₂ (Riboflavin) (continued)

Thus, theoretically, its depletion by the pill could be a factor in the liver tumors associated with this contraceptive.

Interactions with Other Vitamins and Minerals

Works with A and niacin in maintaining the health of the eyes; interacts closely with thiamine in monitoring thyroxine and insulin; and also has synergistic relations with most of the other B complex.

Other Comments

Normally, one-third of dietary amounts are excreted daily. There are diurnal variations, that is, riboflavin may be better utilized at some times of day than at others.

NIACIN

Approximate Daily Requirement. Most Adults Under Normal Conditions

20 mg, but some nutritionists recommend 40 to 100 mg a day for adolescents as well as adults.
    See next paragraph for special dietary factors

Conditions That Increase Need

Pregnancy and lactation. The need is not increased during pill use, perhaps because the body can manufacture its own niacin from protein, specifically tryptophane, an amino acid. It is probably not advisable for women with hot flashes to take large supplements, for flushing, a side effect of niacin, is increased when antibiotics are taken, or when caloric intake is high. (Niacin releases energy from carbohydrates and protein as well as stimulating gastric and bile secretions.) The need for supplemental niacin is probably highest for persons whose diet is low in protein, and/or B_1, B_2, and B_6, but substantial in calories. (In the absence of B_1, B_2, and B_6, the body cannot perform its usual job of manufacturing niacin from trytophane.)

Foods That Provide Daily Requirement

Roasted peanuts; organ meats; the white meat of poultry; fish, including tuna, halibut, and swordfish; yeast. Fruits such as avocado, dates, figs, and prunes; whole grains; legumes; and dairy products are further sources.
    A serving of swordfish or chicken breast provides half your daily niacin requirement for only 150 calories. A half cup of shelled peanuts provides most of your daily fiber and niacin requirement and about 420 calories.

Deficiency Symptoms

Pellagra, the famous niacin-deficiency disease, is characterized by skin eruptions, mental disturbances, digestive disorders, and deterioration of intellect. It is still sometimes found in populations that depend too much on corn as a staple item in the diet. Early symptoms of niacin deficiency are said to resemble pellagra, and may involve personality changes such as suspiciousness and hostility, skin that is sensitive to sunlight, and indigestion.

Excess Symptoms

Niacin is considered to have "limited toxicity" in man. Some individuals are quite sensitive to it and may develop burning and itching skin; fatty liver, overstimulation of the central nervous system; increased pulse rate, respiration, and cerebral flow; and decreased blood pressure. Unlike most of the water-soluble vitamins, it can also produce paralysis and death in animals such as dogs.

NIACIN (continued)
Therapeutic Dose Range

For most adults 40 to 100 mg, but some psychiatrists use much larger amounts, experimentally, in the treatment of schizophrenia. Pill users and women with menopause symptoms are advised not to exceed 100 mg, and to find B-complex products with smaller amounts if they can. In the form of niacinamide, this vitamin is less apt to produce flushing, and niacinamide should therefore be selected by women with menopause complaints.

***** As part of B-complex is generally helpful during premenstrual week and menstruation.

† Sunlight sensitivity symptoms, such as skin discoloration or dryness, may be reduced by moderate supplements.

†††† 400 mg or sometimes (under supervision) much more may help reduce arthritis pain.

Hormone Interactions

Niacin is involved in the synthesis and distribution of many hormones, including estrogen, progesterone, testosterone, cortisone, thyroxine, and insulin.

Interactions with Other Vitamins and Minerals

Niacin works closely with almost all of the B's in food utilization, and the alleviation of deficiencies and deficiency symptoms. Many of the side effects associated with niacin deficiency cannot be corrected unless other B's are added, too. Niacin—and other B's—also cooperate with vitamins such as A, D, and C in maintaining the skin; D and E in maintaining digestion and food absorption, and A and C in helping to maintain the nerves and psyche.

Other Comments

Niacin is so essential in monitoring cholesterol metabolism that high doses of it can lower serum cholesterol. It also has a major effect on the metabolic rate and temperature.

VITAMIN B₆ (Pyridoxine)

Approximate Daily Requirement. Most Adults Under Normal Conditions

2.0 mg. Many nutritionists recommend 5–10 mg routinely. Some individuals need 30–50 or more mg routinely.

Conditions That Increase Need

Inborn deficiencies in utilizing pyridoxine are fairly common and are most apt to occur in the presence of a family history of diabetes, hypoglycemia, or malabsorption syndroms such as celiac disease. The pill makes most users marginally depleted in pyridoxine, and many others severely depleted. Gastrointestinal disease, irradiation, and various other drugs also deplete pyridoxine. The need may be increased when the diet is high in protein, for pyridoxine is instrumental in protein metabolism. The need is also increased in pregnancy and lactation.

Foods That Provide Daily Requirement

The typical modern diet is not abundant in pyridoxine. It is difficult for pill users or those with inborn malabsorption problems to get enough from diet alone. Such sources include brewer's yeast, wheat bran, wheat germ, organ meats and blackstrap molasses, walnuts, peanuts, brown rice; herring, salmon, and some fruits (bananas, avocados, grapes, pears) and vegetables (cabbage, carrots, potatoes) are further sources. Cheeses and milk contain still smaller amounts. A good source of B₆ for fiber watchers is commercial all-bran breakfast cereals, which provide about half the official pyridoxine daily requirements, along with the fiber daily allowance and 70 calories if eaten dry, or 150 calories if taken with a

VITAMIN B₆ (Pyridoxine) (continued)

half cup of whole milk. For calorie counters, generous servings of raw salmon or tuna (as prepared "sashimi" style at Japanese markets and restaurants) are among the best lean sources of the daily pyridoxine requirement. Of course, in our overprocessed and polluted food environment, there are reasons to hesitate about consuming breakfast cereals or raw fish. Among all the vitamins, pyridoxine seems especially hard to get from healthful dietary sources.

Deficiency Symptoms

Slowly coming to be recognized as one of the most crucial vitamins, pyridoxine is of central importance in the normal maintenance of emotional health and energy, skin, resistance to stress, and the metabolism of proteins and fats. Deficiency symptoms include severe depression and diabetic syndromes in pill users, skin lesions, certain anemias, convulsions, extreme nervousness, weakness and lethargy. Deficiency may play a special role in the development of certain herpes infections. B₆ has been used to ameliorate symptoms of epilepsy and cerebral palsy, and to counteract such pregnancy side effects as nausea and headache. Lack of dream recall is a sign of pyridoxine deficiency; and many post-pill disturbances, including skin eruptions and absence of menstruation, respond to supplementation.

Excess Symptoms

Except for too-vivid dream recall and night restlessness, toxicity has not been reported at dosages below 300 mg, which is 150 times the recommended allowance. Pregnant women should be wary of doses over 50 mg, for their infants may then demonstrate withdrawal symptoms. The long-range effects of very high B₆ supplementation are not yet clarified. (See chap. 10.)

Therapeutic Dose Range

For persons not taking the pill or evidencing B₆ malabsorption symptoms, 5 to 25 mg is the usual therapeutic dose. Pill users often require 30 to 100 mg to correct deficiency symptoms, such as depression or disturbed carbohydrate metabolism. Do not exceed 100, or at the most 300 mg without medical supervision. Many people require twice their normal requirement of B₆ when they are stressed. A good clue to this need is dream recall. Some people need 50 mg, others as little as 5, to correct malabsorption difficulties, but a few others benefit from extremely high dosages, as much as 800 or 1,000 mg daily. Many vitamin products are short on B₆ because it is expensive and difficult to extract from natural foods or synthetics. Users of many B-complex products may benefit from a separate pyridoxine tablet along with their general B supplement. All in all, B₆ is very tricky and individualized, especially since the need varies so much with environmental stress, as well as hormone and other drug use, inborn malabsorption problems, and dietary protein intake.
*
**
***
***** 50–100 mg is used as a specific treatment for premenstrual water retention, breast swelling and acne. In Europe 200 daily mg for 5 days is used as a lactation suppressant, and reported to be more effective than hormones.
†† All women in these categories should try supplements of at least 5–10 mg daily. Those who think they have deficiency symptoms, which can include generally poor metabolism, water retention, dental cavities, and overweight as well as the other conditions mentioned, might wish to start with 25 or 50 daily mg and cut back if sleep disturbances occur. While it appears safe to go up to 300 mg without medical supervision, it is inadvisable to stay on such high supplements for more than three months without cutting back experimentally (for a week or a month) in order to determine the effects and give any incipient toxicity a chance to wash out.
†††† 50 mg daily may help reduce arthritis pain.

Hormone Interactions

Pyridoxine helps sustain normal maintenance of both gonadal hormones (estrogen and testosterone) and pituitary hormones (FSH and LH) in such a way that its performance is

VITAMIN B₆ (Pyridoxine) (continued)

dramatically handicapped by the ingestion of estrogen preparations. The reasons remain unclear, but the evidence for this effect is overwhelming. Long-term hormone users are likely to develop measurable problems in their pyridoxine levels. This vitamin also affects thyroxine, insulin, norepinephrine, and epinephrine (adrenal hormones affecting nerve condition, balance, energy, work efficiency, resistance to temperature, stress, and the general state of the emotions) as well as growth hormone and ACTH.

Interactions with Other Vitamins and Minerals

It is suspected that B₆ and the mineral magnesium may have a special connection, as E does with selenium. Neither vitamin can perform its job as efficiently without some boost from the pertinent mineral. The requirement of magnesium is 400 daily mg. Pyridoxine interacts closely with almost all of the other B vitamins, C, and E. It helps K to maintain normal circulation and blood cells, helps the body adjust to stress, and is instrumental in food metabolism.

Other Comments

B₆ should never be used by patients who are under L-dopa treatment for Parkinson's disease. In obscure ways, it seems to be involved in dental cavities, water and electrolyte balance, and a great diversity of other symptoms. Some people feel like "new personalities" when B₆ supplements are added. They lose weight, have increased energy, recover from depressions and neurological symptoms, their skins clear, their menstruation is normalized. But they are in danger of becoming addicted to too high doses, for some of today's vitamin manufacturers (perhaps to compensate for the too low dosages in traditional supplements) may be pouring B₆ on too thick.

Always take a general B and C with it, as well as magnesium.

VITAMIN B₁₂ (Cyanocobalamin)

Approximate Daily Requirement. Most Adults Under Normal Conditions

6 mcg

Conditions That Increase Need

Genetic factors that block secretion in the stomach. Under these circumstances, shots instead of oral supplements may be necessary. This is called "lack of intrinsic factor." Pregnancy, lactation, intestinal malabsorption or disease, alcoholism; may be destroyed by cooking or food processing; cobalt deficiency; parasites, gastectomy; strict vegetarian diet without eggs or dairy products; aging. Hormone users often become quite deficient in B₁₂, but, mysteriously, anemia and other life-threatening symptoms do not seem to ensue. This is in marked contrast to the situation with pyridoxine and folic acid. B₁₂ is so closely related to protein metabolism that need may increase when protein consumption is high.

Foods That Provide Daily Requirement

Plants contain only traces, but soybeans are the best source for strict vegetarians. B₁₂ occurs in all meats, especially organs such as liver, kidney, brain, and heart; in egg yolk and in clams, sardines, salmon, crabs, oysters, herring, other fish, cheeses, and milk.

Deficiency Symptoms

Anemia, including skin pallor, heart palpitations, sore tongue, general weakness, disturbances of the spinal cord, nervous system, poor growth, disturbed metabolism, prickly sensations in extremities, weight loss.

VITAMIN B₁₂ (Cyanocobalamin) (continued)
Excess Symptoms

(Rare) An abnormal increase in the number of red blood cells.

Therapeutic Dose Range

Highly controversial. Some doctors give weekly or twice-weekly shots of 1,000 mcg. Persons lacking the "intrinsic factor" require enormous supplements to get the vitamin into the bloodstream, but ordinary deficiencies, associated with the other factors mentioned under "Conditions That Increase Need" above, often respond to dosages of only a few daily micrograms. Some people say that they have much more energy, and/or healthier-looking skin if they take supplements ranging from about 25 to 100 daily mcg. The lower figure can be obtained in many stress or B-complex vitamin formulas such as the Plus Company's Formula 72. The higher figure can be obtained by swallowing 3 daily 11-grain desiccated liver tablets of the type that includes cobalamin concentrate. Liver is such a rich source of B₁₂ that 6 or 8 daily tablets without cobalamin concentrate still provide the recommended allowance of around 6 mcg. To keep folic acid and B₁₂ normally balanced, it's advisable to eat a leafy vegetable every day, and liver at least once a week, preferably desiccated liver supplements or some other organic form without DES.

* 3 to 6 daily mcg is sufficient for most people. Those who think they may have become severely depleted with hormone use may benefit from 25 to 100 daily mcg.
*** Pallor may improve. There are some reports of shingles being cured by B₁₂ therapy. The beneficial effects of B₁₂ on skin may be due to its helping vitamin A work better.

Too much B₁₂ might, by stimulating the parathyroids, increase the probability of osteoporosis. Its low amount in vegetarian diets could be an additional feature in the low osteoporosis rate. Never exceed more than 100 daily mcg unless special need such as lack of intrinsic factor is established.
***** As part of B-complex is generally helpful during premenstrual week and menstruation.

Hormone Interactions

Abnormalities of the thyroid and parathyroid hormones are associated with B₁₂ deficiencies and vice versa.

Interactions with Other Vitamins and Minerals

Synergistic with A, E, C, B₁, folic acid, pantothenic acid.
B₁₂ given with folic acid aids in relief of fatigue. B₁₂ has further synergistic relations with almost all of the other B vitamins.

Other Comments

Cobalt, a trace element found in soil, is interconnected with vitamin B₁₂.
B₁₂ may increase the size of tumors (sarcoma), another good theoretical reason to stay away from megadoses unless they are proven necessary.

FOLIC ACID (Folicin)

Approximate Daily Requirement. Most Adults Under Normal Conditions

0.4 mg or 400 mcg. (A microgram is one-thousandth of a milligram, as a milligram is one-thousandth of a gram. The B vitamins—often measured in micrograms, meaning we need smaller amounts of these proportionally—are the blood vitamins, folic acid and B₁₂, and biotin. Among other essential nutrients, iodine is also measured in micrograms.) Some nutritionists advocate much higher doses of folic acid, as much as 2–5 mg daily. The latter figure is more than twelve times the recommended allowance.

FOLIC ACID (Folicin) (continued)
Conditions That Increase Need

Pregnancy, illness, alcoholism, and the use of drugs including estrogens, sulfonamides, phenobarbital, Dilantin. Taking vitamin C increases the urinary excretion of folic acid. Certain intestinal bacteria destroy folic acid. Some people evidence poor natural absorption.

Foods That Provide Daily Requirement

The richest sources are liver or organic desiccated liver, asparagus, spinach, wheat, bran, dry beans, and yeast. Small amounts are present in all fruits, many vegetables, meat muscle, cheese, milk, and nuts. Storage and cooking (if the water is thrown out) cause substantial folic acid losses. Estrogen users are advised to save all their vegetable cooking water for soup. Asparagus is the best source of folic acid for both fiber and calorie watchers. Depending on the method of preparation or packaged brand, a generous serving provides one-quarter of the daily folic acid requirement, one-third to two-thirds of the fiber requirement, and only about 20–40 calories.

Deficiency Symptoms

Deficiency symptoms are extremely serious, including a form of anemia. Less severe deficiencies cause shortness of breath, dizziness, fatigue, intestinal disorders, and diarrhea. Deficiencies during pregnancy produce hemorrhaging, miscarriage, premature birth, and a high infant mortality rate. Skin discolorations, called the "mask of pregnancy," are a frequent deficiency symptom in both expectant mothers and pill users. Pill users, who often evidence folic acid deficiency, get anemia, bizarre changes in their cervixes, and skin discolorations as a result. The higher rate of birth defects and miscarriages in women who conceive while taking or shortly after stopping the pill is believed by some researchers to be associated with folic acid deficiency (and possibly vitamin A excess). The more severe hot flashes that some menopausal and postmenopausal women experience when giving up estrogen may be a consequence of lowered folic acid, as well as E and C-complex levels. The post-pill syndrome, including amenorrhea, may be influenced by folic acid deficiency, as well as deficiencies of E, other B vitamins, and zinc.

Excess Symptoms

Scientists usually say "no toxicity reported" or "there is no known human toxicity." A few people do have allergic skin reactions, and there has been at least one death reported from the injection of an extremely large experimental dose to an epileptic, in the hope it might help control his seizures. There have also been reports of increased convulsions when large doses are given to persons with seizure disorders. Furthermore, because folic acid deficiency blocks the normal effects of estrogen, some cancer researchers are using folic acid antagonists to treat cancer experimentally. In other words, if a patient is growing a hormone-dependent cancer, high doses of folic acid might, through its effect on estrogen uptake, indirectly encourage the cancer along. Persons with a family history or personal history of either convulsive disorders or hormone associated cancers, such as tumors of the breast or reproductive organs, should avoid taking high folic acid supplements for long periods of time.

Therapeutic Dose Range

For reasons just mentioned, we cannot agree with those nutritionists who say that 5 daily mg is safe. On the other hand, there is ample evidence that pill users, women recovering from the pill, women taking other estrogen products and, indeed many drugs, and women with menopause symptoms or other "endocrine deficiencies" benefit from the pregnancy dosage of folic acid, which is twice the recommended allowance, or 800 mcg. Temporary dosages of 1–5 mcg daily, for only a few weeks, can reverse abnormal Pap smears and skin discolorations, as well as curing folic acid deficiency anemia. However, we would not advise going over 1 mg daily, or certainly 2, except under medical supervision. We would not advise staying on a dosage of more than 1 mg daily after symptoms improve.

FOLIC ACID (Folicin) (continued)

•
••
•••
••••• As part of B-complex is generally helpful during premenstrual week and menstruation.

†† Most nonprescription B-complex and multiple vitamin products do not contain nearly enough folic acid to correct the deficiencies we have discussed. The typical B-complex product has only about 100 mcg or sometimes none. A pill user, for example, could not hope to correct her folic acid deficiency symptoms without taking 4–8 tablets containing 100 mcg. Some multiple vitamins contain the recommended allowance of 400 mcg, but comparatively too much A for pill users. Pregnancy vitamins may provide 800 mcg of folic acid, but again, too much A for pill users.

The reader who suspects she is deficient in folic acid can either (1) be extremely careful about her diet; (2) ask her doctor to recommend a prescription vitamin; (3) buy separate folic acid tablets at a health-food store or drugstore. These are usually sold in 4 mcg dosages, and she would need to take one or two a day, along with a conventional B-complex product.

Hormone Interactions

Folic acid deficiency flatly eliminates the normal response of female reproductive organs to estrogen. It also has profound effects on the distribution of testosterone in men. Folic acid works synergistically with growth hormone, called STH.

Interactions with Other Vitamins and Minerals

C and folic acid maintain a delicate balance. On the one hand C is needed to metabolize it properly, and works closely with it forming red blood cells. But too much C in proportion to folic acid causes the latter to wash out. B_{12} and folic acid are also in delicate balance, working closely together in formation of marrow and blood. For some purposes, but not others, they are interchangeable. Niacin requires folic acid to be properly utilized. Biotin, pantothenic acid, and folic acid perform crucial interacting functions on the liver and other organs.

Folic acid, B_6, riboflavin, and B_{12} are jointly required for normal protein metabolism.

Other Comments

Antibody formation decreases when folic acid is deficient. Folic acid has analgesic properties increasing the pain threshold. As sulfonamides block intestinal synthesis of folic acid, the vitamin, in turn, may hamper the drug.

PANTOTHENIC ACID

Approximate Daily Requirement. Most Adults Under Normal Conditions

10 mg.

Conditions That Increase Need

Stress increases need—cooking losses are high.

Foods That Provide Daily Requirement

Meat, chicken, milk, eggs, peanuts, peas, broccoli, kale, sweet potatoes, yellow corn, whole grain cereals, and breads.

PANTOTHENIC ACID (continued)
Deficiency Symptoms

Neuromotor disturbance, tingling hands and feet, numbness, hypoglycemia, cardiovascular disorder, digestive disorders, susceptibility to infections and colds, physical weakness, depression.

Excess Symptoms

Essentially nontoxic in man, but respiratory failure has been reported in mice.

Therapeutic Dose Range

50–100 mg daily, especially during stress.
*
** Due to close interactions with progesterone it may be helpful for post-pill infertility, menopause complaints, or even cancer prevention in victims of hormone medication. Might also help reduce likelihood of sugar disturbance, stroke, and heart attacks in hormone users.
***** As part of B-complex is generally helpful during premenstrual week and menstruation.
†††† 50–100 daily mg may help reduce arthritis pain. Some doctors prescribe much higher amounts.

Hormone Interactions

Pantothenic acid required for synthesis of several hormones including progesterones.

Interactions with Other Vitamins and Minerals

Synergistic with biotin, folic acid, C, niacin, A, and E. Pantothenic acid, a B vitamin, releases energy from sugar, and the body cannot utilize PABA or choline without it.

Other Comments

May have anticarcinogenic factors. Used to treat vertigo, postoperative shock, curare poisoning. Aids wound healing. Helps cure Addison's disease, liver cirrhosis, and diabetes.

BIOTIN (a B-complex Vitamin Sometimes called Vitamin H)

Approximate Daily Requirement. Most Adults Under Normal Conditions

0.3 mg (300 mcg). Synthesized in the intestinal tract. Eating many raw eggs or egg nogs causes deficiencies as the avidin in egg white ties up biotin in the intestines.

Conditions That Increase Need

Taking antibiotics and sulfa drugs, cooking losses, excess intake of avidin.

Foods That Provide Daily Requirement

Yeast, organ meats are the highest sources. Available in grains, egg yolk, fish, nuts, and fruits.

Deficiency Symptoms

Eczema of face and body, hair loss, muscle pain, paralysis.

BIOTIN (a B-complex Vitamin Sometimes called Vitamin H) (continued)

Excess Symptoms

None are known.

Therapeutic Dose Range

About 0.25 mg or 25 mcg.
† Supplements may be useful for skin problems, especially when these occur in connection with use of antibiotics or sulfa drugs, or an imbalanced diet.

Hormone Interactions

May influence cortisone, growth hormone, and testosterone.

Interactions with Other Vitamins and Minerals

Ascorbic acid synthesis requires biotin. Niacin cannot be metabolized if biotin is deficient. Hair may lose color when biotin and pantothenic acid are deficient. Biotin is synergistic with B_2, B_6, niacin, A, and D in maintenance of normal skin.

Other Comments

The severity and duration of some diseases—especially protozoan infections—is increased when biotin is deficient.
Biotin is essential for normal metabolism of fat and protein.

CHOLINE and INOSITOL

[Choline, inositol, and PABA, partially accepted B vitamins, are usually included in health-food store brands, but are not yet included in most pharmacy brands of B-complex supplements.]

Approximate Daily Requirement. Most Adults Under Normal Conditions

Recommended allowances not clarified for choline and inositol, though FDA very recently accepted the need in human nutrition for choline. They appear to work jointly in fat metabolism, perhaps keeping cholesterol in an emulsified state so that it cannot settle on artery walls or collect in the gall bladder. While FDA is 5 to 15 years behind cancer researchers in acknowledging the hazards of drugs such as estrogens, it is equally far behind many biochemists in acknowledging the inadequacy of American junk food diets, and the need in human nutrition for nutrients we do not get.

Conditions That Increase Need

Some individuals feel that choline and inositol have a soothing effect on the nerves, and there is some evidence that nerve fibers are influenced by choline. There are also reports that choline may control high blood pressure and help the liver eliminate poisons and drugs.

Foods That Provide Daily Requirement

Six daily lecithin capsules, made from soybeans, contain 244 mg each of inositol and choline and help potentiate vitamin E and (unfortunately) 180 mg of phosphorus, or almost one-fourth the daily requirements.
(Lecithin users are advised to take calcium supplements such as dolomite with their lecithin tablets, so that phosphorus and calcium will not become unbalanced.)

CHOLINE and INOSITOL (continued)
Therapeutic Dose Range

The average therapeutic dose in B-complex formulas that contain these vitamins is about 100 mg of each.
* May help to control cholesterol and liver problems in users of estrogen products.
** May enhance vitamin E's effects in controlling hot flashes.
*** May help the fat soluble vitamins in moisturizing the skin.

PABA (Para-aminobenzoic Acid)

Approximate Daily Requirement. Most Adults Under Normal Conditions

Though not accepted by all investigators as essential to human nutrition, some claim it's useful against the complaints of aging. Procaine injections, advocated to preserve youthfulness by Dr. Anna Aslan of Roumania, are a form of PABA.

Conditions That Increase Need

Under medical supervision, the potassium salt of para-aminobenzoic acid is sometimes used to treat arthritis and rheumatic disorders. Exposure to sunlight in some sensitive individuals.

Foods That Provide Daily Requirement

It occurs with the other B's in natural foods such as whole grains, brewer's yeast, and organ meats, and is also applied externally as a sun screen lotion.

Therapeutic Dose Range

20 to 30 mg daily. Like choline and inositol it is more readily found in health store B-complex products than those sold in pharmacies.
*
** Since it is linked to estrogen uptake by female organs, women with signs of estrogen excess, such as premenstrual breast cysts and tenderness, or hormone-associated cancers, should probably avoid it. Perhaps DES daughters should avoid it, too.
† The hormone or pill user who is exposed to sunlight and starting to develop blotchy spots (the mask of pregnancy) on her face may find it useful to include PABA in her supplements. By serving as a sun screen PABA may also help delay formation of wrinkles by collagen breakdown.

Hormone Interactions

PABA probably plays a role in the maintenance of female reproductive organs, and the normal utilization of estrogen.

Interactions with Other Vitamins and Minerals

It is linked to folic acid and occurs as part of the folic acid molecule.

VITAMIN C and Its Mysterious Relative, Called P, or C COMPLEX

[Women taking ginseng for menopause complaints should take it three hours before or after C supplements, or juices and other foods high in C.]

Approximate Daily Requirement. Most Adults Under Normal Conditions

40–60 mg. 200–500 mg daily is advocated by many nutritionists.

Conditions That Increase Need

During infections, illness, allergies, exposure to pollution, during stress, smoking, late pregnancy, when taking the pill, when taking aspirin, to help other vitamins work better.

Foods That Provide Daily Requirement

4 oz of fresh orange juice, or one medium orange.

Fiber and calorie watchers may wish to get some of their C from the following: Broccoli, one cup has almost 3 g of fiber, 140 mg of C, and only 40 calories. Brussels sprouts, one cup has 2.5 g of fiber, 135 mg of C, and 55 calories.

Strawberries, one cup has almost 2 g of fiber, 88 mg of C, and 55 calories.

Cabbage, raw or cooked, is a fair source of both C and fiber, at the cost of very few calories. One cup of cooked cabbage, for example, provides .5 g of fiber, 48 mg of C, and 30 calories.

Deficiency Symptoms

Bruising easily, tiny hemorrhages in blood vessels under the skin, bleeding gums and dental problems, failure of wounds to heal promptly, weakness, listlessness, fatigue, aching joints, rough skin, edema or water retention, weakness in connective tissues that hold skin, muscles, tendons, and bones together.

Scurvy, severe C deficiency, is characterized by extreme muscular weakness, bleeding under the skin, and spongy and bleeding gums.

Excess Symptoms

Excess C is excreted in the urine. Occasional diarrhea, excess urination, kidney stones, abdominal pain may develop. Allergic rashes. If taking more than 750 mg of daily C, use magnesium supplements to help prevent kidney stones. Be sure to take at least the daily requirement of folic acid and B_{12}, as mega C can wash these out.

Therapeutic Dose Range

Highly controversial. Linus Pauling and his followers feel that several grams daily can be beneficial, but 500 to 750 mg (½–¾ g) is the usual therapeutic dose for deficiency symptoms. C should be taken in 2 or 3 divided doses. For some conditions it seems more effective when taken with the associated factors discussed under "Vitamin P."

* 750 mg.

*** 200–500 mg.

***** Enhance the effectiveness of B-complex in curbing premenstrual and menstrual problems.

Women who have the special problems that benefit from C complex should not take an ordinary stress (B complex with C) formula. Instead a therapeutic B complex and a therapeutic C complex should be taken twice daily after breakfast and dinner.

The P factors are clearly most helpful for people with gum disease, excessively heavy menstrual periods, and, in some cases, hot flashes. Those who use C supplements not containing the P factors should take some citrus fruit or juice simultaneously to assure ingestion of the Ps.

VITAMIN C and Its Mysterious Relative, Called P, or C COMPLEX (continued)

Women taking ginseng for menopause complaints should separate it from any C supplements or C-rich foods by 3 hours. Ginseng is best metabolized before meals, and C afterward.

††† Many doctors prescribe 200–500 mg at insertion, and to help control spotting and heavy menstruation.

Hormone Interactions

Required for the normal functioning of adrenal, pituitary, and other glands.

Interactions with Other Vitamins and Minerals

Needed for the metabolizing of proteins and amino acids, as well as absorption and storage of iron. Helps conserve A and E, potentiates B_{12}, folic acid, B_6, and pantothenic acid.

Other Comments

Stored in the adrenal cortex. Other target tissues are pituitary, ovary, connective tissue, bone, liver, teeth, and gums. C maintains oxygen turnover, and is needed for normal respiration.

P or C COMPLEX (Citrus Bioflavonoids, Rutin, Hesperidin)

Approximate Daily Requirement. Most Adults Under Normal Conditions

The need in human nutrition has not been established.

Conditions That Increase Need

Reported to be useful in conjunction with C for skin hemorrhages, gum problems, and probably hot flashes.

Foods That Provide Daily Requirement

Found in the white skin and segment part of fruit and some vegetables.

Deficiency Symptoms

Capillary fragillity that is resistant to C treatment alone.

Excess Symptoms

Possibly citrus allergies. Some people who can handle C alone get rashes from bioflavonoids, in natural foods or supplements.

Therapeutic Dose Range

Is usually taken in proportion to C. For each 500 mg of C:
bioflavonoids—100 mg
rutin — 50 mg
hesperidin — 25 mg
* Take above type formula for pill users and convalescents with gum problems or easy bruising.
** Take above type formula in divided doses for hot flashes.
† Above type formula in divided doses for capillary problems.

P or C COMPLEX (Citrus Bioflavonoids, Rutin, Hesperidin) (continued)

†† Above type formula in divided doses for gum and tooth problems.
††† Above type formula for IUD users and others with excessive menstruation.

Users who are already taking sufficient C, in stress supplements or multiple vitamins, may be able to purchase separate bioflavonoid tablets. Nature's Plus is one such brand. Some nutritionists advocate taking equal proportions of C and these associated factors.

Hormone Interactions

May intensify some of C's normalizing effects on adrenal pituitary and other target tissues. This may help explain its reported usefulness in hot flashes, so may its effect in strengthening capillaries.

Interactions with Other Vitamins and Minerals

May help prevent the destruction of C in the body.

Other Comments

P is also called the "capillary permeability factor."

Essential Minerals and Trace Elements

Dust thou art and unto dust shalt thou return, literally. Our bodies contain the same minerals as the earth; they pass to us through our food. We need a small but constant supply for our bones, especially in childhood and after middle age, to prevent osteoporosis, and in lesser quantities for the maintenance of our soft tissues.

The major minerals comprise four or five pounds of our body weight. These are calcium (a couple of pounds), phosphorus (one pound), and a few ounces down to a fraction of an ounce of: potassium, sodium, chlorine, magnesium, and sulfur. Some dozen and a half other minerals or metals are present in only trace quantities, among them iron, iodine, zinc, fluorine, selenium, copper, and cobalt. Further trace elements include chromium, manganese, molybdenum, aluminum, boron, silicon, cadmium, vanadium, tin and nickel.

We obtain minerals and trace elements from unrefined foods, such as whole grain breads and cereals, raw vegetables and fruits, nuts, organ meats, and shellfish. The recommended allowance of most trace elements has not yet been settled.

CALCIUM, PHOSPHORUS AND MAGNESIUM

Intake should be in good balance. The recommended allowance for each has been set at about 1 g (1,000 mg). Phosphorus is in almost every natural food including meat, fish, poultry, eggs, cheese, milk, nuts, legumes, bread, and whole grain cereals. Furthermore, phosphates are widely used as preservatives in processed foods, greatly adding to our load. In most North American diets, phosphorus intake greatly exceeds the desirable level, possibly averaging 5 g a day. This in turn increases our body's need for calcium, setting the stage for osteoporosis and other complaints of aging if calcium intake is not raised. Since calcium is apparently used less efficiently after menopause, many researchers argue that the normal calcium requirement (even without excess phosphorus) is probably raised to about one and one half grams daily.

Small amounts of calcium are required almost everywhere in the body. It works with vitamin E to help ensure normal blood clotting, as well as contributing to muscle tone and nerve function. When calcium is needed by the blood or other tissues, it is drawn from the bones and distributed. Normal heart function requires a proportionate balance of calcium, potassium, magnesium, *and* sodium.

If this all seems too complex, nobody ever said that the human body is a simple organism! However, under natural conditions most people select diets that are balanced in these factors.

In addition to phosphorus, and magnesium (of which intake should be about half that of calcium) and sodium, at least two other dietary factors—protein and vitamin D—affect our utilization of calcium. Excessive protein raises calcium need. Vitamin D is essential to calcium absorption in the intestines. Fluoride also plays a role in calcium utilization.

The evidence mounts that the U.S. diet, with its emphasis on meat, which is high in phosphorus and protein, is a major factor in our soaring rate of osteoporosis. Vegetarian societies have little osteoporosis.

One of the first internal signs of aging is that, after 35 or 40, the kidney's ability to throw off excess phosphorus declines. Thus, changes in kidney function (in meat consumers) stimulate excess parathyroid activity, which draws calcium away from the bones.

At 40, at the latest, it's good prevention to cut down on meat (servings should not exceed four ounces) and foods preserved with phosphates (read the label), while increasing dietary intake of calcium, magnesium, and vitamin D. Leafy vegetables are good calcium sources that do not have a lot of calories. A daily quart of D-enriched skim milk, providing generous calcium and D, contains 360 calories, while whole milk contains 640 calories.

The recommended allowance of magnesium is 400 mg. Cooking washes away magnesium and processed bread fails to deliver it. To obtain magnesium one must consume whole grains such as bran or wheat germ breakfast cereals, and leafy salad greens. The water from boiled vegetables should be added to soups and stews.

Magnesium deficiency symptoms include irritability and belligerence, foot and leg cramps, irregular pulse, muscle weakness and twitching or tremors, calcium loss through excess urinary excretion and degenerative changes in the bones, teeth, and possibly kidneys.

Severe magnesium deficiency may produce brain deterioration. Persons on magnesium-rich diets appear to have fewer heart attacks and less arteriosclerosis.

One of the greatest favors a person approaching middle age can do for her or his bones is to cultivate a taste for certain greens—beet, chard, endive, kale, mustard, and collards—which offer an exceptionally favorable balance of calcium to phosphorus. We recommend at least one daily serving. The fact that collards are a dietary staple of many black persons in the United States may help account for their much lower rate of osteoporosis. All of these products are low in calories. A cup of collards, for example, has only 55. Many of these greens provide generous magnesium, too.

FLUORIDE

We know of fluoride's importance to healthy teeth, and now scientists have found consistently that osteoporosis is much rarer in areas that have fluoridated water. Fluoride-containing bone crystals are more durable than those without fluorides. This is significant in old age.

Dietary sources include tea and sardine bones.

Too much fluoride is dangerous, however, and high doses should never be used without medical supervision. Those living in areas where the water is fluoridated can assume they are already receiving 1 mg of fluoride daily. Two cups of tea a day will add another milligram. In the absence of fluoridated water, a daily supplement of 2 mg may be advisable, taken with water. Ten mg is too much and we suggest consulting a bone or nutrition specialist to determine the most sensible amount in any particular area. Dentists tend to be more up-to-date on fluoride research than physicians.

Tea lovers should be advised that the beverage (especially with lemon) aids weight loss, but supplements containing thiamine, the B vitamin, should be taken with it as tea depletes this nutrient, causing fatigue.

IRON

When iron is deficient the body cannot manufacture normal amounts of hemoglobin. The blood transports too little oxygen. Fatigue ensues and resistance to infection is lowered.

††† **IUD users often require five times the normal requirement of iron, or about 100 mg a day as compared to 18 or 20.**

Vitamin C helps the absorption of iron, which explains why it's desirable to take orange juice with eggs. The richest sources of iron are liver, egg yolk, wheat germ, brewer's yeast, apricots, beans, and peas.

SODIUM AND POTASSIUM

Sodium and potassium work jointly to maintain the balance of body fluids. In general the body regulates sodium without too much difficulty, but habitual heavy use of salt may promote high blood pressure.

Nerve and muscle functions are impaired when the sodium-potassium balance is upset and, as we have mentioned, the mineralization of bones may also be affected. When a diet is too high in phosphorus (i.e., too "acidic") the sodium, potassium, and magnesium found in fruits and vegetables help neutralize its effect. Increased intake of fruits and vegetables can therefore alleviate premenstrual and menstrual disorders, as well as prevent osteoporosis.

Besides table salt, sodium is abundant in milk, as well as fruits and vegetables. High-potassium foods include bananas, oranges, tomatoes, and soybeans.

Echoing the problem with phosphorus and calcium, it is believed that most North Americans get too much sodium (about 5 g daily) and too little potassium. Our recommended allowance of potassium has been estimated at a gram or so a day, but this may well throw the two chemicals out of balance. Many nutrition experts contend that we should obtain slightly *more* potassium than sodium, perhaps in a ratio of about five to four. Edema is a common symptom of potassium deficiency as is low blood sugar (hypoglycemia), gas and indigestion, and possibly heart attack.

** , *** Increase intake of calcium, magnesium, potassium, and fluoride; reduce phosphorus and possibly sodium.

***** Increase intake of calcium, magnesium, potassium and iron; reduce sodium.

Reminder: Also add 400–800 units of vitamin D.

Other Minerals and Trace Elements

IODINE

Iodine is concentrated in the thyroid; minor deficiencies may produce lethargy, chilliness, dry skin, husky voice, fatigue, low blood pressure and weight gain. Major deficiencies cause goiter and cretinism.

Iodine requirement varies with body weight. The average person needs slightly under one microgram for each pound. Thus a woman weighing 125 pounds should obtain around 100 mcg daily of iodine. Growing children and pregnant or lactating women need more.

One tablet of kelp or pressed seaweed provides about the average allowance for most people. Some dieters feel they benefit from taking as many as 15 or 20 tablets a day. Skin rash is an occasional side effect.

It is essential to use iodized salt, since much of the

iodine once present in our land has been washed into the sea.

Seafood and seaweed are excellent sources of iodine.

While endemic goiter still exists in some areas of the United States, there are nutritionists who contend that many of us get too much iodine, which may have the paradoxical effect of *depressing* thyroid activity.

ZINC

The required allowance is 15 mg, and possibly much more when the body is physically stressed. Evidence mounts that many or most of us do not get more than 11 or 12 mg from our dietary sources (see chap. 10), and that excess copper from our water pipes further drives out zinc, as do the pill and other medications.

Because zinc is essential to hormone metabolism, zinc deficiency may produce diabetes, dwarfism, anemia, slow wound healing, poor resistance to infection, many skin abnormalities, white spots in the fingernails and infertility. The offspring of zinc deficient animals have shown abnormalities of the brain, kidneys, eyes, and bone. Seafood, meat, and eggs are rich sources of zinc. Green leafy vegetables, nuts, and whole grains, *would be* if the soil in which they grew were not depleted in zinc. Processed foods deliver little zinc.

*, **, † In recent years, startling improvements have been demonstrated in the health of many children and adults when zinc supplements averaging 10–30 mg daily were given. Under present conditions it is one of the hardest nutrients to get reliably in our diet, and one of the most crucial to supplement.

COPPER

Copper is essential for healthy blood and the production of RNA (ribonucleic acid), a part of the nucleus of every cell. The recommended allowance is only 2 mg daily and most of us average five.

Excess copper accumulates in the tissues and can become toxic.

Copper occurs in green leafy vegetables, seafood, organ meats, whole grain breads and cereal, and dried fruits.

When symptoms of copper excess exist, it may be advisable to test one's drinking water (copper can leach off pipes and get into drinking water) and switch to bottled products if necessary.

* **Supplements should be *avoided*.**

CHLORINE

Chlorine is supplied by table salt, and foods containing natural or added salt. In the form of chloride it assists potassium and sodium in the maintenance of water balance, stimulates the production of digestive juices, aids in waste removal, and helps to distribute hormones.

MANGANESE

Manganese assists in the utilization of proteins, carbohydrates, and fats, is essential to milk production in females, and appears to affect the glands of reproduction as well as the adrenals, liver, and pancreas.

Sources are green leafy vegetables, wheat germ, nuts, beans, whole grain breads and cereals, and organ meats.

* **1 mg daily, estimate.**

SELENIUM

Selenium assists vitamin E in its functions. It occurs in brewer's yeast, garlic, liver and organic desiccated liver, and eggs.

*, ** **Women with post-pill syndromes, or hot flashes and menopause complaints, are advised to take 25 mcg of selenium along with each 200 units of E. New products are available that combine the two.**

There is growing evidence that selenium provides protection against some cancers, but that too much zinc (a hormone booster) cancels out this effect. Until more is known, it's advisable to take only moderate supplements of either unless special indications exist. *Chromium* levels drop sharply in menopausal and older women, but this element is not sufficiently understood, and accurate requirements have not been established. There are certain new products such as Sel-E-Chrome, combining selenium, E and chromium, which some nutrition specialists now prescribe for older women.

SULFUR

A nonmetallic element, it occurs in amino acids and in the
B vitamins thiamine and biotin. Sources are high protein
foods as well as onions, lentils, and brussels sprouts.

Sulfur assists in the metabolism of other minerals and
is needed for the maintenance of skin, hair, and nails.

CHAPTER 36

A Personal Nutritional Profile

Today we have a pretty good idea of what optimum diets are for various strains of laboratory mice and rats; tomorrow perhaps we will have similar information for humans.

But until we do, each individual must personally find out what combination of supplements is best. Trial and error will reveal what makes one feel and look better. In general, one can detect a change after a three months' trial. The supplements recommended to ward off osteoporosis are an exception; with them the proof is in subsequent metabolic effects.

Arianne H., a disbeliever in all pills, was extremely skeptical about our program, and only tried it because she feared hormones even more. "I have to be almost terminal before I'll even take two aspirin," she said. She promised to stick to the vitamin regimen for three months. (Arianne was suffering from severe hot flashes, and we had also suggested ginseng, which she considered too much like a drug.)

At the end of the first month Arianne stated that she was "feeling a little stronger—perhaps. I still get hot flashes, but they don't bother me as much. I'm not sure if the flashes have actually diminished at all." We urged Arianne to raise her E dosage from 100 to 200 units, and to keep a daily record of her flashes.

At the end of the second month, Arianne announced that her flashes had diminished, from a dozen or more daily to four or five. She increased her dose to 400 units in the dry form of alpha and mixed tocopherols, and also started taking desiccated liver tablets (11-grain size, 6 tablets daily) to get a bit of folic acid, which was missing from both the multivitamin and the B complex she had selected.

At the end of the third month, Arianne was better, down to three or four mild flashes a week, which she found "eminently manageable." She also reported that she hadn't "had as much energy since high school."

Vera C., aged 46, had just completed her Ph.D. Despite her cum laude status, she was still having trouble finding a job. Her youngest daughter was leaving for college and her husband was in the throes of "male menopause," as Dr. Sheldon Cherry calls it. In the midst of this, Vera's father died, leaving her mother with less insurance than expected, and placing an added financial strain on Vera's family.

Vera felt terrible, and it showed. She wondered whether it was her life stresses, the start of menopause, or a reaction to giving up the pill, which she had done some months earlier on learning of the British heart attack studies.

She was also suffering badly from the air pollution in her city, which, she said, blinded her and made her "feel crazy" when she was caught in it outdoors.

Vera began supplements at an intermediate level. She selected a multivitamin formula with 200 mg of C; a B complex including PABA as well as another 100 mg of C; and E at 200 units daily.

She bought a jar of wheat germ to get associated factors, for her E and B complex, and also added 15 mg of zinc daily.

Vera felt more energy almost at once, and was also "calmer" and "much more able to face pollution." Her skin had been severely dry and itchy. Most of the itch was gone at "around two or three weeks" and by six weeks Vera's general skin condition was noticeably improved. "What I'm saving in moisturizers almost pays for the vitamins!" As extra bonuses, her hair regained some of its earlier gloss, and a chronic vaginal discharge cleared up. The throbbing she had frequently experienced in a "bad vein" disappeared.

Our friend Vera may have had fairly severe deficiencies, for at first she adapted "hungrily" to all of her supplements. At about six weeks, she began to "feel aversive toward all but the E and zinc." She was also having to urinate too frequently, and the fact that her urine turned a deeper yellow concerned her, although this is a normal consequence of B therapy in many persons.

On cutting out C and B complex entirely—for a week—her sensitivity to pollution started to return, as did her vein discomfort. She also thought that the "little pucker lines" around her mouth (associated with lack of thiamine) might be reappearing.

By trial and error, Vera adjusted her dosage. She now takes the multivitamin formula and stress formula on alternate days, lowering her daily C from 300 mg to 150, but has increased her E dosage to 400 units, taking her two daily tablets after breakfast and after dinner.

"I've discovered I'm an E person," she observes.

Other people, heavy drinkers among them, are more apt to describe themselves as B persons. Still others explain that they "do C."

In other words, many vitamin enthusiasts conclude that the body—as Pascal said of the heart—may have its own wisdom, which "wisdom knows not of."

Was it the extra E that finally brought Arianne around or the folic acid, or time? What makes Vera an E rather than a B or C person?

We don't know and we would like very much to hear from readers about successful—or unsuccessful—variations in their own regimens.

Meanwhile, here is a suggested regimen designed for both the menopausal woman who has never taken ERT, and the one who has but is no longer taking it.

1. Vitamin E. **What to take.** Vitamin E comes as alpha-tocopherol and as mixed tocopherols. Which form is more beneficial is still debated. **How much.** 200 units (on the average), though 30 units are enough for some and up to 600 or more are required for others. **When to take.** a) After meals or bedtime snack containing fats, or b) with two lecithin capsules at any time. (Lecithin contains fatty acids which help the E to be absorbed.) **Caution.** Those with heart problems, diabetes, or high blood pressure should take no more than 30 units without medical supervision. **Note.** Some women find the dry form more agreeable.

2. Vitamins B complex and C. **What to take.** Traditionally, such terms as "stress formula" or "stress supplement"

are used to describe therapeutic or "high potency" vitamins that combine B complex with C. Select one that includes some folic acid and a minimum of 5 mg of B_6 (pyridoxine). The niacin should be in the form of niacinamide. A good moderate-level preparation is Plus Products' Formula 72. Some newer stress formulations may also include vitamin E, iron, or other ingredients. One such example is Lederle's Stresstabs 600 with iron. **How much.** Usually one or two daily. Read directions on the label. **When to take.** After meals. **Note.** If symptoms of water retention, weight gain, depression, hypoglycemia, or lack of dream recall suggest a deficiency, take additional B_6, from 30 to 100 mg as needed. **Note.** Other special conditions, such as joint pains, sometimes respond to additional supplements of other Bs including niacinamide and pantothenic acid (see vitamin tables). **Note.** To strengthen capillaries, thereby helping to diminish hot flashes, correct gum problems and reduce excessive menstrual bleeding, or if living in a polluted city or smoking heavily, add separate C-complex (C, combined with bioflavonoids, rutin and hesperidin) or a separate bioflavonoids tablet. Another way to get the C complex factors is to eat a lot of fresh citrus fruit.

3. Vitamin D. **What to take.** D is available in separate capsules, in combined A and D capsules, and in multivitamin preparations. **How much.** 400 units daily is the recommended allowance. In winter those living in northern climates may wish to double this, unless they drink a quart of D-enriched milk every day. **When to take.** After meals or bedtime snack. Combined with calcium at bedtime may have mild sedative effects.

4. Calcium. **What to take.** Calcium is available alone as calcium lactate, calcium carbonate, and calcium gluconate (there being little difference among them), combined with magnesium as in dolomite, or combined with vitamin D, phosphorus, and other minerals as in bone meal. We prefer calcium alone or dolomite for the menopausal woman. **How much.** 600 to 800 mg daily, which can be obtained in one large calcium tablet or in several dolomite tablets (see label). **When to take.** Plain calcium is best to take after bedtime snack along with vitamin D to take advantage of sedative effect. Dolomite may be taken in divided doses after meals.

5. Further dietary supplements. **What to take.** Depending on their own normal diet, and symptoms, women may

want to consider some of the health-food products discussed in other chapters and in the vitamin tables. Either desiccated liver or liver itself (from an organic supplier) is often reported helpful for skin and energy. It probably provides associated or undiscovered B factors that cannot be derived from vitamin products alone. Yeast and wheat germ are often beneficial and may improve the efficiency of B and E supplements.

Various minerals and trace elements (besides the all-important calcium) are often deficient at menopause and after. Moderate supplements of zinc, selenium, chromium, magnesium, manganese, iron, iodine and fluoride are all reported to benefit some women. A good multi-mineral supplement several times a week provides extra insurance.

Women who have dry scaly skin, poor night vision, or joint pains may benefit from vitamin A, 5,000–10,000 units daily (see vitamin tables).

6. **Ginseng. What to take.** Ginseng (Korean) comes in many forms. We recommend the capsules for hot flashes. If Korean ginseng has too much stimulant effect, try "Siberian ginseng" instead. Buy only from a reliable dealer and avoid combination products and teas. A capsule usually contains 8 to 10 grains, approximately 500 mg. **How much.** For women weighing 100 to 130 pounds, 2 capsules daily; 130 to 160 pounds, 3 capsules; over 160 pounds, 4 capsules. **When to take.** Before meals, in divided doses. Try to allow a few hours separation from foods or vitamins that are rich in vitamin C. **Note.** If undesired weight gain occurs, increase dose; if undesired weight loss occurs, decrease it. **Note.** Ginseng can be stopped when flashes are under control. Effects may last a month or longer. If flashes resume, ginseng can be resumed. Since ginseng is an herb, rather than a vitamin, greater caution needs to be exercised.

Finally, for women who want to keep their regimen as simple as possible, here is what we suggest:

1. **No Hot Flashes** (or gum problems or excess menstrual bleeding)
   —Take a good stress supplement (B complex with C) once or twice daily after meals.
   —After dinner or a bedtime snack, take a good therapeutic strength multiple vitamin, containing at least 30 units of E and 400 units of D.
   —Also add a calcium supplement.

2. Hot Flashes
   —Instead of a stress supplement take separate B complex and C complex twice daily after meals.
   —In addition to your daily multivitamin formula, and calcium, add 100–600 units of E or E with selenium.
   —Also take ginseng before meals.

NOTE: Please see remarks on page 160 about vacationing from vitamins.

Sources by Mail

Vitamins, Minerals, Ginseng:

Willner Chemists, 300 Lexington Avenue
New York, N.Y. 10016

Tiger-Mite Health Foods, 2071 Broadway
New York, N.Y. 10023

Freeda Pharmacy, 100 East 41st Street
New York, N.Y. 10017

Bronson Pharmaceuticals, 4526 Rinetti Lane
La Canada, Calif. 91011

Ginseng:

Kiehl's Pharmacy, 109 Third Avenue
New York, N.Y. 10003

Korean Ginseng Products, 817 Lexington Avenue
New York, N.Y. 10021

Siberian Ginseng and Dry Vitamin E:

The Solgar Company
Lynbrook, N.Y. 11563

The Grotesque Limits of
Sex Hormones

The breakfast of champions ain't Wheaties.
Dick Schaap, reporting on the
1976 Olympics

At first it was only women (and animals) to whom hormones were given promiscuously, but now the abuse has extended to grown men and children.

The use of hormones to resculpture the human body grows out of the fantastic notion, fostered by technologists, that our bodies are machines. We raise our children on fairy tales where locomotives speak and have feelings, then expect our sports heroes to *perform* like locomotives. The living and the inanimate are all mixed up. In an unending circle, metabolism, nutrition, and hormones interact with one another. But artificial hormones upset the delicate balance among all three. They alter the way we utilize food, the flow of our blood, our mental state and sex drive, susceptibility to infections, heart disease and cancer, and possibly our genes.

Athletes, Nutrition, and Hormones

In Europe there are still many sports physicians who believe in dietary supplements. "They do a lot of work with trace minerals—magnesium, manganese, phosphates . . . on the premise they help prevent muscle cramps and fatigue," explains Dr. John Anderson, head physician for the 1976 U.S. Olympic team.

In addition, in Europe, and in the United States, other physicians give *hormones* to athletes. The most popular products, called anabolic steroids, are synthetic testosterone derivatives, which have body-building properties and increase muscle mass. Approved by FDA as a medical treatment for pituitary dwarfism, some anemias, and breast cancers and conditions of old age, anabolic hormones are, in fact, used routinely by athletes in many disciplines, especially throwing, weight lifting, judo, and wrestling.

The *Manchester Guardian* estimates that, worldwide, about half of the serious competitors in these sports take massive doses of anabolic steroids. Many football players use them also, and several years ago *all* the members of a professional U.S. football team were placed on these and other hormones by the team doctor. The experiment was discontinued because of side effects. These could include phallic enlargement and increased frequency of erections; also sterility, occasional loss of sex drive, and growth of male breasts, including the secretion of milk; nausea; loss of appetite, vomiting, burning of the tongue; acne; jaundice; abnormal thyroid and liver function, electrolyte imbalance; abnormal retention of sodium, chloride, water, potassium, phosphates and calcium; possible clotting disorders; and diabetes. Like estrogen, excess testosterone has been increasingly linked to cardiovascular disease.

Women athletes who take anabolic steroids may develop facial hair, male pattern baldness, deepening of the voice, and clitoral enlargement. These changes are usually *irreversible*.

Other side effects in women include menstrual irregularities, and, should pregnancy occur, masculinization of a female fetus. The child, while genetically female, may have male external organs, or appear to be a hermaphrodite.

Brand names of anabolic steroids available in the United States include Dianabol, Winstrol, Durabolin, and Deca-Durabolin. The first two products are supplied in oral tablets, while the last two are given by intramuscular injection.

Anabolic steroids—as well as other drugs such as strychnine and amphetamines—have grown so popular with athletes that a team physician at the 1976 Olympics admitted: "It was obvious that doping was getting out of control. After every competition they were finding all sorts of syringes and needles in dressing rooms."

Another doctor observed sadly that there was little "camaraderie" left among athletes, as competition was so fierce.

And so, in recent years, methods were developed for discovering anabolic steroids in the urine. The reliability of these tests remains uncertain. Some authorities state that the hormones can be detected if the athlete has used them within *three days*. Others claim or hope that residues may remain, even if the competitor went off steroids *three weeks before*.

The Sign of the Yellow Cross

At the Montreal Olympics, in 1976, twenty-nine separate dope-control stations were established and manned by volunteer Canadian doctors. These were marked by a yellow cross to symbolize urine. Selected contestants were ordered to report for urinalysis after events. Among the competitors who flunked their hormone-detection tests were Peter Pavlasek of Czechoslovakia and Mark Cameron of the United States, both weight lifters, and a woman discus thrower, Danuta Rosani of Poland.

Some athletes tried to beat the system by smuggling in plastic baggies containing the dope-free urine of their coaches. Medical students from McGill and the University of Montreal were rounded up to supervise the athletes while they voided.

Will Frank Shorter Keep It Clean?

Frank Shorter is one of the finest long-distance runners in the world. He won the Olympic marathon in 1972 (the first American to do so in sixty-four years) and was hoping to garner a second gold medal in 1976. Instead he came in second.

Shorter has a wholesome reputation. He does not pop steroids, Dristan, Listerine lozenges, Vicks 44 Cough Mixture, Pertussin 8-hour Cough Formula, or any other medicines banned by Olympic committees. Neither does he utilize the "vampire" technique, which is practiced by many other champion runners, who drain their own blood, a pint or so, as if they were making a donation, then store it away. On the day of a big race, they reinject it into their veins, increasing their red blood cells, oxygen, and stamina.

Moments after his second-place finish in Montreal, Shorter was asked if he planned to compete again in 1980. "Yeah," he replied cynically, "if I find some good doctors."

And doctors aplenty are lining up to slip athletes special boosters. Quietly, the U.S. Olympic Committee has formed a new medical panel to "look into areas considered taboo" in sports. The panel is headed by Irving Dardik, an aggressive 40-year-old cardiovascular surgeon, and will also include orthopedists, exercise physiologists, and pharmacologists. Nutrition will be studied, but so will the use of drugs. There will be "extensive research" into anabolic steroids and the vampire technique.

The Search for the Double X Chromosome

Women contestants face a second ordeal, a chromosome test or skin scraping from the inside of their mouths. After the 1972 Olympics Kathy Schmidt, a javelin thrower, complained: "I had two friends, one on each arm, drag me in while I screamed, 'No, no I can't go through with it.'"

And yet, in this transsexual age, other women athletes welcome chromosome tests. Chris Evert, who heads the Women's Tennis Association, states testily that California ophthalmologist Renée Richards "is not a sister under the skin." Dr. Richards is a head taller, and 19 pounds heavier than Wendy Overton, one of several competitors who resigned from a recent tournament rather than face Renée Richards on the court. Olympic physician John Anderson agrees with Ms. Evert and Overton. Dr. Richards, he explains, "would flunk the genotype test performed on females in Olympic competition . . . the lack of androgens and the administration of estrogens postoperatively does not lead to a decrease in muscle mass."

A Tragic Case

In 1975, a 29-year-old person "of indeterminate sex" was admitted to the Mt. Zion Hospital and Medical Center in San Francisco. He, as it turned out, was a transsexual taking 5 mg of DES daily in preparation for a sex-reassignment operation. Like many other estrogen users, he'd had a pulmonary embolism, a blood clot in the lung, which he barely survived.

The doctor who saved his life predicts that with the increase in hormone prescriptions for healthy young males, we will soon be hearing many such stories. Men given estrogens, for any purpose, have an increase in clotting as well as cardiovascular deaths. Some develop breast cancer. Like women who take the pill, a yet undetermined number of transsexuals are bound to die for their "sexual freedom."

More Tragic Cases

Estrogens are so potent that men, and women, who merely work around them develop serious complications. On April 1, 1977 Dr. Malcolm Harrington, an epidemiologist at the Center for Disease Control in Atlanta announced the results of a year-long study of workers at a birth-control pill factory. Some of the men developed enlarged breasts, and a decline in sex drive. Harrington said there was no evidence that such conditions might cause cancer but, he added, "I am suspicious."

Women in the factory had abnormal vaginal bleeding. "I would not recommended that a pregnant woman work in such a plant," Harrington cautioned.

The plant Harrington studied is in Puerto Rico, and is owned by Ortho Pharmaceutical. Apparently, the mere presence of estrogen in the air caused these effects, although, according to Harrington, "The Company . . . was exemplary in its effort to control dust. . . ."

Tall Daughters and Short Sons

Countless children who are merely tall for their age, especially if female, or short, if male, are given artificial hormones to alter their growth patterns. Hormones can change ultimate height, but only by one and one-half inches, or less.

FDA has never approved the use of hormones for height alteration, but neither has it issued any warnings against them.

Increasingly, circumspect endocrinologists seem to agree with Dr. Claude Migeon of Johns Hopkins: "Tallness," he observed to Nadine Brozan of the *New York Times*, "is not a disease; the problem is really one of psychological adjustment to society. . . ."

After genes, nutrition, sleep and the emotions are probably the most important determinants of growth. Depression can so affect the hypothalamus and pituitary that release of natural growth hormone is suppressed. But psychotherapy, or a change of environment, such as going away to boarding school, can produce a six-inch-growth spurt in less than a year in extraordinarily short children of either sex.

Which Twin Has the High-C Vitamin?

Good nutrition obviously influences growth, but so, specifically, may extra-high-potency vitamins. Early in 1977, an unusual cover on the *Journal of the American Medical Association* depicted nothing but an appetizing platter of citrus fruit, arranged artistically. The big news *inside* the issue, the cover story, was a report from Judy Miller and her colleagues at the genetics department of the University of Indiana.

The Miller group had given high doses of C to identical twins, ranging in age from 6 to 16. Depending on body weight, the children took 500, 750 or 1,000 mg daily. In each case the second twin received a placebo, and codes were not broken until the study was finished. However, to ensure that the second twin was not C-deficient, he or she did receive the recommended allowance of the vitamin.

The object of the investigation was to test the Pauling theory that high dosages of C help prevent infections and colds. Here the results were ambiguous. In general, the younger girls and, to some extent the younger boys, had fewer or shorter infections if they took the high C. This was not so with older children. All of the subjects were carefully evaluated, and one unexpected and dramatic finding emerged. *Among the youngest boys, the treated twins grew notably taller than their brothers by an average of 1.3 cm in just five months.*

Biochemists speculate that high C might influence growth, either by altering the equilibrium between ascorbic acid levels in blood and bone, or by stimulating collagen synthesis.

Hot Flashes, Impotence, and Libido in Men

Despite all we hear of sex clinics and Masters-and-Johnson-type therapy, the use of testosterone as a cure for impotence is rapidly gaining favor. In the words of Dr. Jerome Feldman of Duke University Medical School: "A good many men do have testosterone deficiencies, and within the past couple of years radioimmunoassay techniques for determining testosterone levels have become widely available and relatively inexpensive. . . . *If the level is low, testosterone replacement* will probably help. . . . Loss of libido occurs in a lot of men as they get older, but it frequently has a psychological basis. Testosterone levels will often be completely normal in men who are 50, 60, or 70 years old."

Feldman urges, however, that all men with potency problems have their testosterone levels checked.

Sometimes men who have surgery on their testicles, for repeated hernias or, perhaps, cancer, develop hot flashes and sweats similar to those occurring in some menopausal women. One example, reported in the *Archives of Internal Medicine*, was a 48-year-old man who had fathered three children *after undergoing three separate hernia repairs.* But following his fourth and fifth operations, he noted a decrease in libido, and inability to maintain an erection. Simultaneously, he developed attacks of hot flashes, ten times daily, and frequently awakened at night, with drenching sweats that required a change of pajamas. Intramuscular testosterone cured his flashes, and enabled him to resume having intercourse every other day.

What happens apparently, is that after frequent surgery involving the testicles, the blood supply to these organs "may be compromised." The flashes—as in women

—are thought to result from *increased levels of pituitary hormones,* which are urging on the testicles to continue sperm production.

Some men have an opposite problem from the one just discussed—they have too much libido. In Britain a product called Androcur is already on the market as a treatment for sex offenders. Rapists and exhibitionists are placated with large doses, while in smaller quantities the chemical is undergoing clinical trials as a male birth control pill. One way or another the drug companies will find a use for it.

The Place of Hormones in Medicine

Synthetic hormones have a place in medicine, a limited place for people with true deficiencies or rare diseases. In most cases they have taken from life much more than they have given. To use hormones is to tamper with the unknown, at the profoundest levels of biochemistry.

But secretly, many of us believe ourselves to be freaks. We all desire the wisdom of 70, combined with the glamor of 18. We'd like to practice carefree birth control with no responsibilities or interruptions. We'd like to be perfect—lovelier, swifter, saner, more vigorous, or orgasmic. Some of us wish to change our height or our sex, and most of us wouldn't mind gaining or losing a bit or a lot of weight. Most women say that their breasts are either too large or too small, and their hair is either too limp or too curly. The average male describes his penis as "below average" in size.

We aren't going to get all our wishes—and certainly not out of any bottle or syringe. In most cases the healthy patient who takes hormones is courting illness only to fulfill the dream of perfection and eternal youth created by the salesmen to a gullible society.

Even now, it may be too late to avert widespread genetic disasters, resulting from second- and third-generation effects of the pill, DES, pregnancy tests, or the hormones in our food.

We have passed a point of diminishing returns with many wonder drugs and chemicals. The life expectancy of certain subgroups of Americans has already started to decline, and, for all of us, it is far less than in some other advanced countries, where prevention and good sense are emphasized.

Dr. John Knowles of the Rockefeller Foundation is correct; we must take more responsibility for ourselves.

This means approaching health care as consumers, or in partnership with our doctors, not as passive patients. It means informing ourselves and asking pertinent—or impertinent—questions.

All prescription drugs should have complete consumer labeling, for, obviously, it is apt to be the user who notes a complication first. The doctor must explain which side effects are dangerous, and which are not. An inexcusable number of hospital admissions in the United States are due to reactions to prescription drugs.

Great care should also be taken in selecting a hospital (which means ascertaining the affiliation of one's primary physician), for mortality associated with *the same procedures* can vary greatly from one institution to another.

Except for emergencies, no surgery, especially on the female organs, should be agreed to without a second opinion. Remember that more than 40 percent of the uteri and ovaries removed in this country are normal, and the five-year survival rate for breast cancer, in selected patients, is as high or higher when radical mastectomy is *not* performed.

Traditional Attitudes of Doctors

In supporting consumer labeling for the birth control pill, Michelle Harrison, a family physician in Princeton, New Jersey, wrote to the FDA:

"My experiences with patients on oral contraceptives have included stroke in a 22-year-old, now crippled permanently, severe thrombophlebitis, post-pill amenorrhea, vaginal infections, and chronic cervicitis. I can usually tell by the appearance of a cervix that a woman has been on contraceptive pills.

"Physicians are often reluctant to discuss with patients the full range of side effects and dangers. That has not traditionally been a part of physicians' training. The doctor's role has often been one of reassurance. Without complete warnings to women receiving pills, the current tragedies will continue. The labeling will not only inform the patient, but will force the physician to deal with the dangers of the prescribed medications."

The doctor's traditional role is one of "reassurance," the patient's to "let doctor do the worrying." Even today, many doctors and some patients still prefer the old system. For those who don't, concrete information may be difficult to extract. Traditionally minded doctors won't change until their patients demand that they be treated like adults.

Some doctors fear that if patients "know too much," malpractice lawsuits will increase, but preliminary studies indicate that the opposite is true. *Where the patient is informed of the full risks and benefits of any treatment— and alternatives—as well as the probable outcome of getting no treatment at all,* he or she is much less apt to blame untoward effects on the doctor. Medicolegal experts concur that physician liability drops (and so does that of any drug company, hospital nurse, or technician concerned) when a treatment has been entered with *informed consent.*

Thus, we must listen to what our own bodies tell us as we test different regimens and drugs, or even vitamins. And we must respond to the news of medical miracles or fountains of youth with healthy skepticism.

Sound Mind, Sound Body

As women turn away from hormones—and men turn increasingly toward them—we muse on Frank Shorter, the runner, and hope that he and all his fellow athletes—and fans—consider the wise words of Lord Killanin, president of the Olympic Committee: "Our ideal is the complete and harmonious human being, which is the essence of the Olympic movement. We must therefore prevent the creation of artificial men and women."

Appendix

Selected Sources of Information and Help

Overall Issues and Referrals

General clearinghouse on federal policies and women's health issues. Publishes newsletter and information packets. Refers to local health groups.
National Women's Health Network
1302 18th Street, N.W.
Suite 203
Washington, D.C. 20036
202-223-6274

DES Mothers and Daughters

DES-Action
P.O. Box 1977
Plainview, New York 11803

Menopause

University of Washington YWCA
4224 University Way, N.E.
Seattle, Washington 98105

Pill and IUD Deaths and Disasters

Report them to:
Dr. Donald Kennedy
Commissioner, FDA
5600 Fishers Lane
Rockville, Md. 20852

Dr. Heinz Berendes
Chief, Contraceptive Evaluation Branch
Center for Population Research
NICHD

Landow Building Room A-716
7910 Woodmont Avenue
Bethesda, Maryland 20014

National Women's Health Network
(address given above)

Jim Luggen, a pill widower, has organized a support group for
the bereaved.
Jim Luggen
992 Manhattan Avenue
Dayton, Ohio 45406

Sterilization Abuse

Committee to End Sterilization Abuse
P.O. Box 839
Cooper Station
New York, N.Y. 10003

Obstetrics Care

Doris Haire
American Foundation for Maternal and Child Health
30 Beekman Place
New York, N.Y. 10022

International Childbirth Education Association
P.O. Box 20852
Milwaukee, Wisconsin 53220

Birth and the Family Journal
110 El Camino Real
Berkeley, California 94705

Nutrition During Pregnancy

SPUN
Gail and Tom Brewer
14 Truesdale Drive
Croton-on-Hudson, N.Y. 10520

Breast Cancer

Rose Kushner / Breast Cancer Advisory Center
9607 Kingston Road
Kensington, Maryland 20795

Rape

Center for Prevention and Control of Rape
National Institute of Mental Health
5600 Fishers Lane
Rockville, Maryland 20852

Information on Cervical Caps, Sponges, and other Barrier Methods

Send stamped self-addressed envelope
Boston Womens Health Book Collective
Box 192
W. Somerville, Mass. 02144

Abortion Rights

CARASA (Coalition for Abortion Rights and Against Sterilization Abuse)
P.O. Box 4103, Grand Central Station
New York, N.Y. 10017

Notes

These references are arranged by chapter, section, and paragraph. To find the reference(s) to a particular statement in the text, note the chapter and the section of the chapter (these appear set off in large italic type throughout each chapter), and then, starting from the section heading, count paragraphs until you reach the one in which you are interested. Locate that paragraph in boldface type in these Notes; the references to that paragraph follow. In some instances the references apply to an entire section and not to specific paragraphs. And, often, at the beginning of a chapter there is no section heading, so you will find here only paragraph numbers. Where a reference is abbreviated, with only a name and date or a name and book title, the full reference can be found earlier in the Notes.

Preface

What this book is about, what it can do for you—paragraph 2:
1. *Wall Street Journal*, Mar. 22, 1976.
What this book is about, what it can do for you—paragraph 3:
2. D. Janerich, testimony before the Subcommittee on Health of the Committee on Labor and Public Welfare, and the Subcommittee on Administrative Practice and Procedure of the Committee on the Judiciary, U.S. Senate, 94th Congress, 2nd Session (Kennedy hearings), Jan. 20, 1976.
What this book is about, what it can do for you—paragraph 5:
3. B. Seaman, "Bringing medicine to heal," *Washington Post*, Mar. 31, 1974, p. C2.
What this book is about, what it can do for you—paragraph 6:
4. "Metabolic effects of oral contraceptives," *Lancet* 2:783–784 (1969).
What this book is about, what it can do for you—paragraph 7:

5. D. Small, "Hormone use to challenge physiology: is the risk worth it?" *New England Journal of Medicine* 294:219–221 (1976).

What this book is about, what it can do for you—paragraph 8:

6. V. Wynn, "Vitamins and contraceptive use," *Lancet* 1:561 (1975).

7. A. S. Prasad et al., "Effects of contraceptive agents on nutrients: I. Minerals," *American Journal of Clinical Nutrition* 28:377–384 (1975).

8. Charles Dodds, interview, 1969.

9. U.S. Senate, hearings on the present status of competition in the pharmaceutical industry, held before the Subcommittee on Monopoly of the Select Committee on Small Business, U.S. Senate, 91st Congress, 2nd Session, Jan. 14, 15, 21, 22 and 23, 1970. (Nelson hearings), vol. I, pp. 6426–6445.

10. Nelson hearings, vol. I, pp. 6296–6333.

11. H. A. Salhanick, D. M. Kipnis and R. L. Vande Wiele, eds., *Metabolic effects of gonadal hormones and contraceptive steroids* (N.Y.: Plenum, 1969).

12. Chris Chilvers, interview, Feb. 20, 1976. Chilvers now operates C.L.O.T. (Center for Lipid Observation and Testing) at 14 E. 95th Street, New York, N.Y. 10028. For $15 to $25 the patient can have more than 16 different risk factor tests, including blood pressure, cholesterol, triglycerides, glucose, uric acid, and an electrocardiogram. Special rates are offered for people on fixed incomes including students. Tests take 10 to 15 minutes and results are available within two days.

What this book is about, what it can do for you—paragraph 9:

13. Small, 1976, pp. 219–221.

What this book is about, what it can do for you—paragraph 10:

14. C. A. B. Clemetson, "Ceruloplasmin and green plasma," *Lancet* 2:1037 (1968).

What this book is about, what it can do for you—paragraph 11:

15. D. Janerich et al., "Oral contraceptives and congenital limb reduction defects," *New England Journal of Medicine* 291:697–700 (1974).

16. J. J. Nora and H. A. Nora, "Birth defects and oral contraceptives," *Lancet* 1:941–942 (1973).

THE AMAZING STORY OF DES

Paragraph 5:

1. Joint hearing before the Subcommittee on Health of the Committee on Labor and Public Welfare and the Subcommittee on Administrative Practice and Procedure of the Committee on the Judiciary, U.S. Senate, 94th Congress, 1st Session (Kennedy hearings), Feb. 27, 1975. Statement of Mrs. John Malloy, San Diego, California, p. 5.

Chapter 1: More Normal Than Normal

Paragraph 2:
1. Kennedy hearings, 1975, p. 32.
Paragraph 3:
2. E. C. Dodds, "Stilboestrol and after," in: British Postgraduate Medical Federation, *Annual Review of the Scientific Basis of Medicine* (London: University of London, 1965).
Paragraph 4:
3. Kennedy hearings, 1975, p. 32.
The Boston Disease: Its Origins—paragraph 1:
4. Interviews with Paul Rheingold, 1976.
The Boston Disease: Its Origins—paragraph 4:
5. Interview with George and Olive Smith, Mar. 20, 1976.
The Big Boston Success—paragraph 1:
6. O. W. Smith and G. V. S. Smith, "Diethylstilbestrol and treatment of complications of pregnancy," *American Journal of Obstetrics and Gynecology* 58:821–834 (1948).
The Big Boston Success—paragraph 3:
7. O. W. Smith and G. V. S. Smith, "The influence of diethyl-stilbestrol on the progress and outcome of pregnancy as based on a comparison of treated with untreated primigravidas," *American Journal of Obstetrics and Gynecology* 58:994–1009 (1949).
The Big Boston Success—paragraph 7:
8. Smith, 1949, p. 1003.
The Big Boston Success—paragraph 8:
9. Smith, 1949, p. 1008.
The Big Boston Success—paragraph 10:
10. Smith, 1949, p. 1007.
Troublesome News from New Orleans and
Chicago—paragraph 1:
11. J. H. Ferguson, "Effects of stilbestrol on pregnancy compared to the effect of a placebo," *American Journal of Obstetrics and Gynecology* 65:592–601 (1953).
Troublesome News from New Orleans and
Chicago—paragraph 3:
12. W. J. Dieckmann et al., "Does the administration of diethyl-stilbestrol during pregnancy have therapeutic value?" *American Journal of Obstetrics and Gynecology* 66:1062–1081 (1953).
Troublesome News from New Orleans and
Chicago—paragraph 6:
13. M. B. Shimkin and H. L. Grady, "Mammary carcinomas in mice following oral administration of stilbestrol," *Proceedings of the Society for Experimental Biology and Medicine* 45:246–248 (1940).
14. M. B. Shimkin, "Carcinogenic potency of stilbestrol and estrone in strain C_3H mice," *Journal of the National Cancer Institute* 1:119–127 (1940–41).

Chapter 2: The Time-Bomb Effect

The Herbst Report:
1. A. L. Herbst, J. Ulfelder and D. C. Poskanzer, "Adenocarcinoma of the vagina: association of maternal stilbestrol therapy with tumor appearance in young women," *New England Journal of Medicine* 284:878–881 (1971).
2. A. L. Herbst, S. J. Robboy, R. E. Scully et al., "Clear-cell adenocarcinoma of the vagina and cervix in girls: an analysis of 170 registry cases," *American Journal of Obstetrics* 119:713–724 (1974).
3. A. L. Herbst, R. J. Kurman and R. E. Scully, "Vaginal and cervical abnormalities after exposure to stilbestrol in utero," *Obstetrics and Gynecology* 40:287–298 (1972).
4. R. E. Scully, S. J. Robboy and A. L. Herbst, "Vaginal and cervical abnormalities including clear-cell adenocarcinoma, related to prenatal exposure to stilbestrol," *Annals of Clinical Laboratory Science* 4:222–223 (1974).
5. A. L. Herbst, S. J. Robboy, G. J. Macdonald and R. E. Scully, "The effects of local progesterone on stilbestrol-associated vaginal adenosis," *American Journal of Obstetrics and Gynecology* 118:607–615 (1974).
6. "Stalking a killer." *Wall Street Journal,* Dec. 23, 1975.
7. Hearing before the Intergovernmental Relations Subcommittee of the Committee on Government Operations, U.S. House of Representatives, Nov. 11, 1971 (Fountain hearings), Part IV, pp. 4–9.
8. A. L. Herbst and R. E. Scully, "Adenocarcinoma of the vagina in adolescence: a report of 7 cases including 6 clear-cell carcinomas (so-called mesonephromas)," *Cancer* 25:745 (1970).
9. K. Weiss, "Epidemiology of vaginal adenocarcinoma and adenosis: current status," *Journal of American Medical Women's Association* 30:59–63 (1975).
The Greenwald Report:
10. Fountain hearings, Part IV, 1971, p. 12.
11. Fountain hearings, Part IV, 1971, p. 16.
12. P. Greenwald, J. J. Barlow, P. C. Nascal et al., "Vaginal cancer after maternal treatment with synthetic estrogens," *New England Journal of Medicine* 285:390–392 (1971).
13. Fountain hearings, Part IV, 1971, p. 14.
14. Fountain hearings, Part IV, 1971, p. 15.
The Fountain Committee—paragraph 1:
15. Fountain hearings, Part IV, 1971, p. 48.
The Fountain Committee—paragraph 3:
16. Fountain hearings, Part IV, 1971, p. 81.
The Fountain Committee—paragraph 4:
17. Fountain hearings, Part IV, 1971, p. 50.
The Fountain Committee—paragraph 5:

18. M. F. Jacobson, *Food for people, not for profit* (Westminster, Maryland: Ballantine, 1975).

19. B. T. Hunter, *Consumer beware* (N.Y.: Simon and Schuster, 1971).

The Fountain Committee—paragraph 10:

20. Fountain hearings, Part I, 1971, p. 77.

The Fountain Committee—paragraph 12:

21. K. Weiss, "Vaginal cancer: a iatrogenic disease," *International Journal of Health Services* 5:235 (1975).

The Fountain Committee—paragraph 15:

22. Kennedy hearings, 1975, p. 13.

The Fountain Committee—paragraph 16:

23. Kennedy hearings, 1975, pp. 13–14.

Two DES Women Speak—paragraph 2:

24. Kennedy hearings, 1975, pp. 7–8.

Two DES Women Speak—paragraph 9:

25. Kennedy hearings, 1975, pp. 6–7.

Two DES Women Speak—paragraph 17:

26. D. H. Mills, "Prenatal diethylstilbestrol and vaginal cancer in offspring," *Journal of the American Medical Association* 229: 471–472 (1974).

Two DES Women Speak—paragraph 18:

27. Mills, 1974, p. 472.

Pantell and the Idaho Women—paragraph 1:

28. Kennedy hearings, 1975, pp. 89–93.

Chapter 3: Who Pays the Piper and for What?

Townsend and Those Office Fires—paragraph 4:

1. A. L. Herbst, R. E. Scully and S. J. Robboy, "Effects of maternal DES ingestion on the female genital tract," *Hospital Practice*, pp. 51–57 (1975).

Herbst's Cancer Registry—paragraph 1:

2. Herbst, 1975, p. 52.

Herbst's Cancer Registry—paragraph 3:

3. Herbst, 1975, p. 52.

Herbst's Cancer Registry—paragraph 4:

4. Herbst, 1975, p. 55.

DES Abnormalities—paragraph 2:

5. A. Stafl, R. F. Mattingly et al., "Clinical diagnosis of vaginal adenosis," *Obstetrics and Gynecology* 43:118–128 (1974).

6. Herbst, 1975, pp. 51–57.

DES Abnormalities—paragraph 7:

7. Stafl, 1974, p. 118.

DES Abnormalities—paragraph 8:

8. Stafl, 1974, p. 119.

DES Abnormalities—paragraph 9:

9. M. Bibbo, "Cytologic findings in female and male offspring

of DES-treated mothers," *Acta Cytologica* 19:568–572 (1975).

10. M. Bibbo, "Follow-up study of male and female offspring of DES-treated mothers: a preliminary report," *Journal of Reproductive Medicine* 15:15 (1975).

11. M. Bibbo et al., "Follow-up study of male and female offspring of DES-exposed mothers," *American Journal of Obstetrics and Gynecology* 49:1–7 (1977).

DES Abnormalities—paragraph 12:

12. John Lewis, personal interview, Feb. 16, 1976.

Treatment—paragraph 1:

13. Herbst, 1975, p. 53.

Treatment—paragraph 2:

14. B. O'Malley, "Hormones, genes, and cancer," *Hospital Practice* 65:73 (1975).

15. Herbst, 1975, p. 56.

New Light on Birth Control for the DES Daughter— paragraph 1:

16. L. Burke, "Management of vaginal adenosis at Beth Israel Hospital, Boston," *Journal of Reproductive Medicine* 16:291–292 (1976).

17. D. E. Townsend, "Management of adenosis," *Journal of Reproductive Medicine,* 16:290 (1976).

18. Adolf Stafl, personal communication, Aug. 1976.

Anger and Guilt—paragraph 1:

19. Burke, 1976, p. 291.

Anger and Guilt—paragraph 4:

20. Burke, 1976, p. 293.

Anger and Guilt—paragraph 5:

21. J. A. Celebre, "Management of vaginal adenosis at the hospital of the University of Pennsylvania," *Journal of Reproductive Medicine* 16:293 (1976).

Anger and Guilt—paragraph 7:

22. J. W. Scott, "The management of DES-exposed women: one physician's approach," *Journal of Reproductive Medicine* 16:285–288 (1976).

Anger and Guilt—paragraph 11:

23. Scott, 1976, p. 287.

Anger and Guilt—paragraph 14:

24. Scott, 1976, p. 286.

The Treatment of Adenocarcinoma:

25. J. T. Wharton et al., "Treatment of clear-cell adenocarcinoma in young females," *Obstetrics and Gynecology* 45:365–368 (1975).

26. Y. Tsukada et al., "Clear-cell adenocarcinoma (mesonephroma) of the vagina: 3 cases with maternal synthetic nonsteroid estrogen therapy," *Cancer* 29:1208 (1972).

27. "Experts discuss problems of DES-related cancer," *Journal of the American Medical Association* 234:585 (1975).

Advice to DES Daughters and Mothers—paragraph 11:

28. Progress report from Dr. Marluce Bibbo, Chicago Lying-In Hospital, to Dr. Heinz Berendes, Chief, Contraceptive Evaluation Branch, Center for Population Research, NICHD, Landow Building, Room A-716, 7910 Woodmont Avenue, Bethesda, Maryland 20014, August 31, 1977.

29. Letter from Dr. Sidney Wolfe, Director, Health Research Group, 2000 P Street, N.W., Washington, D.C. 20036 to the Honorable Joseph Califano, Secretary of the Department of Health, Education and Welfare, December 12, 1977.

30. Analysis of Chicago data by Dr. Robert Hoover, Head, Environmental Studies Section, Environmental Epidemiology Branch, Division of Cancer Cause and Prevention, National Cancer Institute, Landow Building, Room 3C07, 7910 Woodmont Avenue, Bethesda, Maryland 20014, at meeting of DES Task Force, March 3, 1978.

Advice to DES Daughters and Mothers—paragraph 15:
31. Interview with George and Olive Smith, March 20, 1976.

Advice to DES Daughters and Mothers—paragraph 18:
32. "Three in suit say drug produced cancer," *New York Times*, March 4, 1976.

Chapter 4: Of Mice and Men

The Mini Mop-up—paragraph 2:
1. D. Cistele, interview, Apr. 1976.

Bibbo's Study—paragraph 3:
2. "DES: Potential risk for men too," *Medical World News*, Jan. 1976, p. 99.

3. Marluce Bibbo, interview, Feb. 1976.

4. Bibbo, *Acta Cytologica* 19:568–572 (1975).

5. Bibbo, 1977.

DES Sons—paragraph 2:
6. T. B. Dunn and A. W. Green, "Cysts of the epididymis, cancer of the cervix, glandular cell myoblastoma and other lesions after estrogen injection in newborn mice," *Journal of National Cancer Institute* 31: 425 (1963).

DES Sons—paragraph 5:
7. J. A. McLachlan et al., "Reproductive tract lesions in male mice exposed prenatally to diethylstilbestrol," *Science* 190:991–992 (1975).

Chapter 5: After the Morning After

Paragraph 2:
1. Smith, 1949, p. 1007.

Paragraph 5:
2. J. M. Morris and G. Van Wagenen, "Compounds interfering with ovum implantation and development," *American Journal of Obstetrics and Gynecology* 96:804–815 (1966).

3. J. M. Morris, "Post-coital oral contraceptive," presented at the Eighth International Conference, International Planned Parenthood Federation, Santiago, Chile, April 1967.

4. J. M. Morris, "Interception: the use of post-ovulatory estrogens to prevent implantation," *American Journal of Obstetrics and Gynecology* 115:101 (1973).

Paragraph 7:

5. C. Tietze, "Probability of pregnancy resulting from a single unprotected coitus," *Fertility and Sterility* 1:485–488 (1960).

Paragraph 9:

6. V. Jones, "Effectiveness of diethystilbestrol as a contraceptive in rape victims," presented at the American Public Health Association, Oct. 17, 1976.

The Michigan Health Service—paragraph 1:

7. "Report on the morning-after pill," *Health Research Group*, Dec. 8, 1972, p. 1.

The Michigan Health Service—paragraph 3:

8. L. Kuchera, "Post-coital contraception with diethylstilbestrol," *Journal of the American Medical Association* 218:562–563 (1971).

The Michigan Health Service—paragraph 5:

9. Kennedy hearings, 1975, p. 170.

The Cowan Study—paragraph 7:

10. *Health Research Group*, 1972, p. 4.

The Cowan Study—paragraph 8:

11. Kennedy hearings, 1975, Belita Cowan testimony.

Second Thoughts About the Morning-After Pill—paragraph 1:

12. Mills, 1974, p. 471.

Second Thoughts About the Morning-After Pill—paragraph 2:

13. Kennedy hearings, 1975, p. 71.

Second Thoughts About the Morning-After Pill—paragraph 3:

14. Kennedy hearings, 1975, p. 33.

The Kennedy Committee Hearings—paragraph 6:

15. Kennedy hearings, 1975, p. 140.

The Kennedy Committee Hearings—paragraph 8:

16. "Diethylstilbestrol as a morning-after contraceptive," *Medical Letter* 15:19 (1973).

The Kennedy Committee Hearings—paragraph 10:

17. Kennedy hearings, 1975, p. 56.

The Kennedy Hearings—paragraph 15:

18. Kennedy hearings, 1975, p. 29.

The Kennedy Committee Hearings—paragraph 20:

19. Kennedy hearings, 1975, p. 27.

DES As a Milk Suppressant—paragraph 2:

20. Doris Haire, personal communication, 1976.

21. E. Gerstenberger, "DES . . . mothers who don't breastfeed," *Ann Arbor News*, Feb. 8, 1976, p. 17.

DES As a Milk Suppressant—paragraph 3:

22. *Physicians' Desk Reference* (P.D.R.), 30th edition (Oradell, N.J.: Medical Economics Co., 1976).

23. In its proposed patient package insert on estrogens, published in the Federal Register in 1976, FDA included the following warning: ESTROGENS TO PREVENT SWELLING OF THE BREASTS AFTER PREGNANCY

If you do not breast feed your bady after delivery, your breasts may fill up with milk and become painful and engorged. This usually begins 3 to 4 days after delivery and may last for a few days up to a week or more. Sometimes the discomfort is severe, but usually it is not and can be controlled by pain relieving drugs such as aspirin and by binding the breasts up tightly. Estrogens can be used to try to prevent the breasts from filling up. While this treatment is sometimes successful, in many cases the breasts fill up to some degree in spite of treatment. The dose of estrogens needed to prevent pain and swelling of the breasts is much larger than the dose needed to treat symptoms of the menopause, and this may increase your chances of developing blood clots in the legs or lungs. Therefore, it is important that you discuss the benefits and the risks of estrogen use with your doctor if you have decided not to breast feed your bady.

DES As a Milk Suppressant—paragraph 5:

24. T. N. A. Jeffcoate et al., "Management of normal pregnancy, labor and puerperium: Puerperal thromboembolism in relation to the inhibition of lactation by oestrogen therapy," *British Medical Journal* 4:222 (1968).

"The incidence of puerperal thromboembolism is three times higher in those women whose lactation is inhibited by administering [estrogen] than in those who breast fed their babies. [3.4 vs 1.0 per 1000] . . . [it is] . . . increased six times [7.6 compared with 1.3 per 1000] when delivery is complicated."

This means that women who had a complicated delivery should absolutely refuse to take post-partum hormones. Try 200 mg daily of B_6 instead, as it works better. In the Foukas double-blind study of B_6 compared to estrogens, 95% of the vitamin-treated women suppressed lactation within a week, but only 83% of the estrogen-treated. A placebo was effective for 17 percent.

25. S. Wessler et al., "Estrogen-containing oral contraceptive agents: a basis for their thrombogenicity," *Journal of the American Medical Association* 236:2179–2182 (1976).

DES As a Milk Suppressant—paragraph 7:

26. Doris Haire, personal communication, 1976.

27. Gerstenberger, 1976.

DES As a Milk Suppressant—paragraph 9:

28. M. D. Foukas, "An antilactogenic effect of pyridoxine,"

Journal of Obstetrics and Gynaecology of the British Common-wealth 80:718–720 (1973).
DES and Other Types of Cancer—paragraph 6:
29. B. S. Cutler, "Endometrial carcinoma after stilbestrol therapy in gonadal dysgenesis," *New England Journal of Medicine* 287:628 (1972).
DES and Other Types of Cancer—paragraph 9:
30. Telephone interview with American Cancer Society, 1976.

Chapter 6: Fed Up with DES

Paragraph 3:
1. Hunter, 1971, pp. 103–104.
Paragraph 5:
2. Fountain hearings, Part I, 1971, p. 91.
Paragraph 6:
3. The Animal Health Institute (AHI) press conference on Thursday, April 8, 1976 (Food Day), at the Overseas Press Club in New York City. The AHI, located at 1717 K Street, N.W., in Washington, D.C. is a lobby group that defends the use of these products to government officials, Congress and the press. Scheduled speakers at the "Food Day" celebration were R. M. Hendrickson, president of AHI and president of Pfizer Inc.'s agricultural division, Fred Holt, executive vice-president, and Dr. Jerry Brunton, director of scientific activities for AHI.
DES-Fed Animals and the Consumer—paragraph 1:
4. M. E. Royce, "DES and meat prices," *FDA Consumer*, May 1974.
DES-Fed Animals and the Consumer—paragraph 4:
5. Hunter, 1971, pp. 103–104.
FDA and the Pellets—paragraph 3:
6. Hunter, 1971, p. 141.
FDA and the Pellets—paragraph 4:
7. Hunter, 1971, p. 141.
FDA and the Pellets—paragraph 7:
8. Hunter, 1971, p. 103.
FDA and the Pellets—paragraph 8:
9. Interview with Joseph Conrey, USDA Analytic Chemist, Staff Officer, Residue Evaluation and Plant Health Inspection Service, Mar. 9, 1976.
FDA and the Pellets—paragraph 9:
10. In our household, we found this mysterious ingredient in Friskies Buffet Chicken and Kidney for cats.
11. Interview with William Leese, USDA Residue Planning and Evaluation Staff National Residue Coordinator.
FDA and the Pellets—paragraph 10:
12. Hunter, 1971, p. 142.
The Delaney Amendment—paragraph 1:
13. Hunter, 1971, p. 87.

14. Jacobson, 1975.

The Delaney Amendment—paragraph 3:

15. Fountain hearings, Part I, 1971, p. 33.

The Delaney Amendment—paragraph 8:

16. Fountain hearings, Part I, 1971, p. 33.

No Ultra-ban from FDA—paragraph 4:

17. J. Mayer, "FDA plans to halt use of DES," *New York Daily News*, Mar. 10, 1976.

No Ultra-ban from FDA—paragraph 9:

18. Hearing before the Subcommittee on Health and the Environment of the Committee on Interstate and Foreign Commerce, U.S. House of Representatives, 94th Congress, Dec. 17, 1975 (Rogers hearings).

No Ultra-ban from FDA—paragraph 12:

19. Rogers hearings, 1975, p. 50.

No Ultra-ban from FDA—paragraph 13:

20. U.S. Food and Drug Administration, press release, Jan. 9, 1976.

No Ultra-ban from FDA—paragraph 14:

21. FDA is *considering* paying consumer groups expenses to participate in hearings, according to *Consumer Reports*, Mar. 1977, p. 124. The National Highway Traffic Safety Administration, and the Consumer Product Safety Commission have already made such provisions.

"Safe Levels"—paragraph 3:

22. Interview with Richard P. Lehmann, Feb. 1976.

Piecemeal Legislation—paragraph 2:

23. Alexander Schmidt, prepared text for Kennedy hearings, 1975, p. 21.

For Appearance's Sake—paragraph 4:

24. Fountain hearings, Part IV, 1971, p. 50.

For Appearance's Sake—paragraph 5:

25. Fountain hearings, Part IV, 1971, pp. 52, 54, 55, 56, 57.

26. An additional class of drugs called 5-nitrofurans, which are "antimicrobial" or "antiinfective," are also added to our food supply. Residues are known to accumulate in edible tissue. FDA and USDA admit that they "lack practical testing methods" to establish how much.

In addition, there are organic products that go into animal food. Natural or "organic" products are not necessarily good. (Organic simply means that a chemical is composed of the building blocks of the living world.)

Let us take organic arsenical compounds, which are less immediately lethal than the inorganic arsenic of, say, rat poison, but which are somewhat lethal or toxic and have also been associated with human cancers of the respiratory tract. Four organic arsenicals are permitted in animal feed: (1) Arsanilic acid, (2) Sodium arsanilate, (3) 3-nitro-4-hydroxyphenlyarsenic acid, (4) Carbarsone.

Residues of organic arsenic have been found in as many as 27.5 percent of edible chicken livers sampled. Van Houweling, FDA's top veterinarian, has suggested correcting this problem *not* by banning arsenic but by doubling the "tolerance limitations" legally permitted.

The feed use of antibiotics, as contrasted to the much more limited therapeutic use, greatly favors the development of resistant bacteria which are transferred to human beings. In his book *Thar's gold in them thar pills*, Dr. Alan Klass, a Canadian physician, explains: "Some of us who are getting small amounts of animal feed antibiotics in our diets are becoming insensitive to the beneficial effects of antibiotics, generally. . . . The human consumer remains at risk, while the feeding of antibiotics to animals is permitted for economic reasons."

An FDA staff memorandum dated September 1972 acknowledges that many of our most essential "therapeutic" antibiotics, such as penicillin and streptomycin, are used in animal husbandry and are suspected of leaving illegal residues in edible portions of the animal.

27. For further DES information, write to the National Cancer Institute, Office of Cancer Communication, NIH, Bethesda, Maryland 20014. Ask for the following two booklets:

"Questions and Answers About DES Exposure Before Birth," DHEW Publications No. (NIH) 76-1118.

"Information For Physicians: DES Exposure in Utero," DHEW Publications No. (NIH) 76-1119.

"Women's Health Care: Resources, Writings, Bibliographies" by Belita Cowan. In addition to a comprehensive section called "Synthetic Estrogens, DES, and Cancer," this essential resource document also includes copious bibliographies on most of the other controversial issues in women's health care, including breast cancer treatment, women in psychotherapy, and rape prevention. It also has a complete directory of pertinent organizations. Send to: 556 2nd St., Ann Arbor, Mich. 48013. Price: $4.00. In addition to the discount available for bulk orders, "A 30% discount is available for those who are unemployed or otherwise do not have $4.00."

The National Cancer Institute has compiled the following list of "DES-Type Drugs That May Have Been Prescribed to Pregnant Women." This list is most important for it may help jog the memory of patients and physicians who are not sure whether DES exposure occurred.

Nonsteroidal Estrogens: Benzestrol, Chlorotrianisene, Comestrol, Cyren A., Cyren B., Delvinal, DES, DesPlex, Diestryl, Dibestril, Dienestrol, Dienoestrol, Diethylstilbestrol Diapalmitate, Diethylstilbestrol Diphosphate, Diethylstilbestrol Dipropionate, Diethlstilbenediol, Digestil, Domestrol, Estilben, Estrobene, Estrobene DP., Estrosyn, Fonatol, Gynben, Gyneben, Hexestrol, Hexoestrol, Hi-Bestrol, Menocrin, Meprane, Melstilbol,

Methallenestril, Microest, Mikarol, Mikarol forti, Milestrol, Monomestrol, Neo-Oestranol I, Neo-Oestranol II, Nulabort, Oestrogenine, Oestromenin, Oestromon, Orestol, Pabestrol D., Palestrol, Restrol, Stil-Rol, Stilbal, Stilbestrol, Stilbestronate, Stilbetin, Stilbinol, Stilboestroform, Stilboestrol, Stilboestrol DP., Stilestrate, Stilpalmitate, Stilphostrol, Stilronate, Stilrone, Stils, Synestrin, Synestrol, Synthoestrin, Tace, Vallestril, Willestrol.

Nonsteroidal Estrogen-Androgen Combinations: Amperone, Di-Erone, Estan, Metysil, Teserene, Tylandril, Tylosterone.

Nonsteroidal Estrogen-Progesterone Combination: Progravidium.

Vaginal Cream-Suppositories with Nonsteroidal Estrogens: AVC cream with Dienestrol, Dienestrol cream.

28. In 1977, FDA commissioner Donald Kennedy announced his intention to restrict penicillin, tetracyclines, and other antibiotics in animal feed, stating that the benefits (presumably economic benefits to animal breeders) clearly did not outweigh the risks to human meat and poultry consumers.

ORAL CONTRACEPTIVES: FROM THE WONDERFUL FOLKS WHO BROUGHT YOU THE PILL

Paragraph 1:
1. B. Seaman, "The dangers of oral contraception," *Playgirl,* June 1976, p. 64.
Paragraph 3:
2. Nora, 1973, pp. 941–942.
3. C. F. Westoff, "Coital frequency and contraception," *Family Planning Perspectives* 6:136–141 (1974).
Paragraph 4:
4. B. Seaman, "The dangers of sex hormones," *Playgirl,* July 1976, p. 70.
5. B. Seaman, "The new pill scare," *Ms.* 4:61 (1975).
6. B. Seaman, *Free and female* (N.Y.: Fawcett Crest, 1972), p. 253.
   This is a matter of public record information obtained from the FDA courtesy of Ben Gordon, staff economist in Senator Nelson's office.
Paragraph 5:
7. J. I. Mann et al., "Myocardial infarction in young women with special reference to oral contraceptive practice," *British Medical Journal* 2:241–245 (1975).
8. J. I. Mann, and W. H. W. Inman, "Oral contraceptives and death from myocardial infarctions," *British Medical Journal* 2:245–248 (1975).
9. Coronary Drug Research Group, "The coronary drug project: initial findings leading to modifications of its research protocol," *Journal of the American Medical Association* 214:1303–1313 (1976).

10. M. P. Stern et al., "Cardiovascular risk and use of estrogens or estrogen-progestogen combination: Stanford three-community study," *Journal of the American Medical Association* 235:811–815 (1976).

11. Veterans Administration Co-operative Urological Research Group, "Treatment and survival of patients in cancer of the prostate," *Surgery, Gynecology and Obstetrics* 124:1011–1017 (1967).

12. A. K. Jain, "Cigarette smoking, use of oral contraceptives, and myocardial infarction," *American Journal of Obstetrics and Gynecology* 126:301–307 (1976).

13. H. W. Ory, "A brief review of the association between oral contraceptive use and development of myocardial infarction," presented at the annual meeting of the American Public Health Association, Miami Beach, Oct. 17–21, 1976.

Paragraph 6:

14. B. Seaman, *The doctors' case against the pill* (N.Y.: Peter H. Wyden, 1969), p. 177.

Paragraph 7:

15. William Inman, personal interview, Apr. 1976.

Paragraph 8:

16. Seaman, *Free and female*, p. 247.

For example, Dr. Malcolm Potts of Planned Parenthood states: "Contraception is not merely a medical procedure. It is also a social convenience, and if a technique carried a mortality several hundreds of times greater than that now believed to be associated with the pill, its use might still be justified on social if not medical grounds." A mortality several hundreds of times greater! Healthy young women would be crippled or dying all over the place. As things stand, 1 in 100 to 1 in 300 pill users per year develop conditions severe enough to warrant hospitalization. If this figure were multiplied by "several hundreds of times," almost every pill user would be hospitalized each year. One cannot but ask whose social convenience Dr. Potts has in mind.

Paragraph 9:

17. Seaman, "The new pill scare."

Chapter 7: How the Pill Happened

Quotation:

1. Seaman, *The doctors' case against the pill*, p. 244.

Paragraph 2:

2. P. Vaughan, *The pill on trial* (N.Y.: Coward-McCann, 1970), p. 25.

Pincus, Chang, and Rock—paragraph 1:

3. E. C. Dodds et al., "Interruption of early pregnancy by means of orally active oestrogens," *British Medical Journal* 2:557 (1938).

4. L. Bascombe, "Do children suffer from the pill?" UPI story, Oct. 1975.
Pincus, Chang, and Rock—paragraph 3:
5. A. Lacassagne, "Apparition de cancers de la mamelle chez la souris male soumise à des injections de folliculine," *Comptes Rendus Hebdomadaires des Séances de l'Académie des Sciences* 195:630–632 (1932).
6. A. Lipschutz et al., "Granulosa-cell tumours induced in mice by progesterone," *British Journal of Cancer* 21:144–152 (1967).
7. E. C. Dodds, "Oral contraceptives: the past and future," *Clinical Pharmacology and Therapeutics* 10:147–161 (1969).
8. As Dr. Roy Hertz testified before the Senate Subcommittee on Health, Jan. 1976: "For over 30 years the ability of certain estrogenic substances to produce cancer in laboratory animals has been repeatedly demonstrated. Cumulative efforts in laboratories throughout the world have established that this class of substance will regularly produce malignant tumors of the breast, the neck and body of the womb, ovary, pituitary gland, testicle, kidney and bone marrow in either mice, rats, rabbits, hamsters, squirrel-monkeys or dogs." Kennedy hearings, 1976.
9. W. U. Gardner et al., "Hormonal factors in experimental carcinogenesis," in: R. Homburger and W. H. Dishmanc, eds., *Physiopathology of cancer*, 2nd ed. (N.Y.: Hoeber, 1959), p. 152.
10. A. Jabara, "Induction of canine ovarian tumors by diethylstilbestrol and progesterone," *Australian Journal of Experimental Biology and Medical Science* 40:139 (1962).
11. H. M. McClure and C. E. Graham, "Malignant uterine mesotheliomas in squirrel-monkeys following diethylstilbestrol administration," *Laboratory Animal Science* 23:493 (1973).
Pincus, Chang, and Rock—paragraph 6:
12. Vaughan, 1970, pp. 37–38.
Syntex, Searle, and Progestin—paragraph 4:
13. Dr. Victor Drill, professor of pharmacology at the University of Illinois College of Medicine, is former director of biological research at Searle, and author of a standard textbook, *Pharmacology in Medicine*. In his book Drill cautions against using insecticides while performing drug research with laboratory animals, for even low levels can produce "severe pathological changes in experimental animals." Yet, at the Searle laboratories, while Drill was in charge of research, an exterminating company sprayed the animal rooms twice monthly while the animals remained in their cages. See T. A. V. Haar and M. Miller, "Warning: your prescription may be dangerous to your health," *New York* magazine May 16, 1977, pp. 46–57. Drill continues to deny that the pill causes blood clots.
Syntex, Searle, and Progestin—paragraph 5:
14. Vaughan, 1970, p. 42.
The So-Called Tests—paragraph 1:

15. M. Mintz, *The Pill: an alarming report* (Boston: Beacon Press, 1970), pp. 24–25.

16. Seaman, *The doctors' case against the pill*, pp. 237–238.

17. "Birth control pills: health versus profits," *Dollars and Sense; A Monthly Bulletin of Economic Affairs*, No. 17, May 1976, pp. 10–11.

The So-Called Tests—paragraph 2:

18. Vaughan, 1972, pp. 34–35.

The Curious News Blackout—paragraph 2:

19. J. Rock, *The time has come* (N.Y.: Knopf, 1963). P. 167: "Today more than one million women of many countries are taking the pills, not simply because of their great effectiveness but also because they provide a natural means of fertility control such as nature uses after ovulation and during pregnancy." P. 169: "It must be emphasized that the pills, when properly taken, are not at all likely to disturb menstruation, nor do they mutilate any organ of the body, nor damage any natural process. They merely offer to the human intellect the means to regulate ovulation harmlessly, means which heretofore have come only from the ovary and, during pregnancy, from the placenta."

P. 167: "Sensational press reports during the summer of 1962 distorted the significance of what must be regarded, medically, as a relative handful of cases of thromboembolism—a blood clot in a vein—among women taking Enovid. Unfortunately these articles created doubts in the minds of some as to the drug's safety. I would reiterate here my own conviction that the pills are in no way the causal agent in these cases. Thromboembolism itself, as well as deaths from it, occurs in women who are taking no drugs at all, and many cases could certainly have been expected in as large a population sample as the million women taking Enovid. In fact the epidemiological evidence we have suggests strongly that instead of 150 cases, reported at this writing, one could expect something of the order of 700 or more cases."

The Curious News Blackout—paragraph 4:

20. Seaman, *The doctors' case against the pill*, p. 246.

The First Pill Conference—paragraph 1:

21. Seaman, *The doctors' case against the pill*, pp. 241–245.

The First Pill Conference—paragraph 14:

22. M. P. Vessey and R. Doll, "Investigation of relation between use of oral contraceptives and thromboembolic disease," *British Medical Journal* 2:199–205 (1968).

23. M. P. Vessey, "Oral contraceptives and thromboembolic disease," *British Medical Journal* 2:696 (1968).

Metabolic Effects of the Pill—paragraph 2:

24. Salhanick, 1969, p. ix.

Metabolic Effects of the Pill—paragraph 4:

25. Nelson hearings, 1970, Spellacy testimony.

26. See also Chap. 10, notes 38–46.
Metabolic Effects of the Pill—paragraph 6:
27. Seaman, "The new pill scare."
Metabolic Effects of the Pill—paragraph 8:
28. "The case of the unpublished report: cancer and the pill," *Sunday Times*, April 13, 1969.
29. "Text in Britain identical with one A.M.A. refused," *Medical Tribune*, Aug. 11, 1969.
Metabolic Effects of the Pill—paragraph 9:
30. Seaman, "The new pill scare."
31. "Research products funded at Southwest foundation," *Progress in Medical Research* 25:2–3 (1976).
32. "Scientists dispute 'the pill and blood clots theory,'" *Southwest Foundation Reporter* 10:1–2 (1976).
33. J. Griffiths, "Thromboembolism and the pill," *Medical Tribune*, May 5, 1976, pp. 32–35.
34. Goldzieher continues to deny any harmful effects of the pill and estrogens, stating in interview and articles—as recently as 1976—that he "disputes the blood clots theory."
35. Seaman, "The new pill scare," p. 102.
36. The AID contract, on the other hand, does support human investigations, and, all told, AID admits it has invested some one million dollars in Goldzieher.

Chapter 8: Where the Pill Is Now

Paragraph 1:

1. "Drug prescriptions declined last year, according to survey," *Wall Street Journal*, Mar. 17, 1976. 7.5 million fewer prescriptions were filled in 1975 than in 1974. However, the cost of an average prescription was $4.93 in 1975, or 3 cents more than in 1974.

Paragraph 2:

2. G. D. Searle and Co., *Annual report 1975* (Skokie, Ill.: G. D. Searle, 1976), p. 4.
3. G. D. Searle and Co., "Searle declares 106th consecutive dividend," press release, April 24, 1976.
4. G. D. Searle and Co., "Searle reports record sales and earnings in quarter and 1st half," press release, July 23, 1975.
5. C. Matthews, "Market gets high on drug industry," *New York Post*, April 20, 1976.

Paragraph 3:

6. Memorandum to Carlton Sharp, chairman, Searle Investigation Task Force, from Adrian Gross, Scientific Investigations Staff, dated March 15, 1976, distributed by FDA.
7. Memorandum from Searle Investigation Task Force to Searle Investigation Steering Committee, dated Mar. 24, 1976, distributed by FDA.

8. H. M. Schmeck, "FDA charges fraud in new-drug testing on research animals," *New York Times*, Nov. 15, 1976, p. 1.

9. "U.S. drug firms create blood money profits by using unethical promotions in Latin America," *Caveat Emptor*, June–July, 1976, p. 107.

10. "Searle concedes bribe payments," *New York Times*, Jan. 6, 1976.

11. "Drug research under question," *New York Times*, Jan. 21, 1976.

12. "Ten of the biggest spenders," *Newsweek*, Feb. 23, 1976.

13. M. Mintz, "Annals of commerce: selling the pill," *Washington Post*, Feb. 8, 1976.

The Pandora's Box of Adrian Gross—paragraph 1:

14. Adrian Gross, personal interview, 1976.

15. R. A. Lyons, "FDA broadens inquiry on testing of drugs," *New York Times*, Nov. 17, 1976, p. 24.

The Pandora's Box of Adrian Gross—paragraph 5:

16. Schmeck, Nov. 15, 1976.

17. H. M. Schmeck, "FDA to tighten rules on research," *New York Times*, Nov. 18, 1976, p. 21.

18. B. Rensberger, "Animal drug test guidelines," *New York Times*, Nov. 19, 1976, p. 18.

The Pandora's Box of Adrian Gross—paragraph 6:

19. On the other hand, in April 1977 the Senate released a 600-page study of FDA which concluded that the agency's "supervisory powers" were weighted too strongly *in favor* of industry. Employees who were *not* pro-business, the Senate investigators concluded, were likely to be harassed.

The Pandora's Box of Adrian Gross—paragraph 8:

20. FDA memorandum, Mar. 24, 1976, p. 51.

The Pandora's Box of Adrian Gross—paragraph 9:

21. H. M. Schmeck, "Drug unit seeks to check testing," *New York Times*, Apr. 9, 1976.

22. "FDA calls for grand jury investigation of G. D. Searle's drug-testing practices," *Wall Street Journal*, Apr. 9, 1976.

23. "Searle issues statement in response to FDA testimony," press release, Apr. 8, 1976.

24. S. Bangser, personal communication, Feb. 5, 1976.

The Pandora's Box of Adrian Gross—paragraph 11:

25. Searle's information center for the lay public was called the Women's Medical News Service, and was located at 3 West 57th St. in New York. It sent out undated information packets which mentioned in tiny print at the bottom that the Women's Medical News Service "Is operated by Interscience Information, Inc. through the support of G. D. Searle & Co.," but asked that Women's Medical News Service be credited if the story were used. (And many were, as filler items in newspapers.) This was in violation of the Code of Ethics of the Pharmaceutical

Manufacturers Association, which agrees not to promote prescription drugs directly to the lay public.

WMNS packet number 26 discusses how successful the pill is with ghetto patients. "No persuasion was exercised to keep patients on the oral contraceptive program," it states in reference to a Chicago study.

WMNS packet number 92 discusses how ideal the pill is for sexually active adolescents. "While a variety of birth control methods was offered, it became evident that the girls preferred the pills. It is the only form of contraception that is universally acceptable to these young people, according to the physicians."

Women's Medical News Service ceased operating after the Nelson pill hearings.

26. Letter to Mr. Geoffrey Wilff, book editor, *Washington Post*, from William W. Wicks, director of public relations at Searle, Nov. 3, 1969. The letter said, in part: "The public should at least know that the authors' generally negative position is contrary to authoritative medical and scientific knowledge. In effect, they are placing their own interpretation above the judgment of informed, unbiased and thoroughly qualified investigators for the medical profession. . . . The millions of women who rely on the Pill or any other prescription medicine deserve a fair presentation of the facts."

27. The Syntex Strategy letter prepared by Deltakos, a division of J. Walter Thompson, dated Apr. 22. 1969, says, in part: "The physician in 1968, was confronted with a rising tide of journal articles focused on morbidity and mortality associated with O.C.'s. It therefore should be assumed his attitude toward presently available products is undergoing rapid change. . . . Patients . . . are being exposed to lay press O.C. articles with increasing frequency The content of these articles is well designed to provoke consumer concern—even fear—regarding the use of O.C.'s . . . any extensive lay press coverage of new and purportedly safer innovations will send thousands of women back to their doctors' offices—with specific requests for the new product." The new Syntex product was Chlormadinone, a mini-pill, which the memo admits, in conclusion, to be a "tricky drug."

The Pandora's Box of Adrian Gross—paragraph 12:

28. Examples are Mead Johnson, a Bristol Myers Co. subsidiary; Wyeth Laboratories, a division of American Home Products (as is Ayerst); Ortho, a division of Johnson & Johnson; and Squibb.

Exaggerated Credit Given the Pill—paragraph 1:

29. Vaughan, p. 32.

The Good News—paragraph 2:

30. Seaman, *The doctors' case against the pill*, p. 65.

The Good News—paragraph 5:

31. V. Cohn, "Ley urges complete data to users on pill's defects," *Washington Post*, Dec. 1, 1969, p. 1.

32. American Medical Association, *What you should know about the pill*, Chicago, AMA.

33. U.S. Food and Drug Administration, "Birth control labeling," *FDA Talk Paper*, Oct. 16, 1975.

34. "More on the pill," *Off Our Backs*, 1970.

35. City of New York, Dept. of Consumer Affairs, "Commissioner Grant asks for hearing on FDA's 'new diluted' warning on oral contraceptives: Calls it a disgraceful way of sugar-coating the pill," news release, April 12, 1970.

36. "Bess charges sugar-coating of peril pill," *Sunday News*, Apr. 12, 1970.

37. "Text of the original proposed leaflet on birth control pills," *New York Times*, Mar. 5, 1970.

38. "Text of FDA's warning on oral contraceptives," *Federal Register*, Apr. 10, 1970, p. 5962.

The Good News—paragraph 6:

39. B. Seaman, "Forewarning on birth control," *New York Times*, July 25, 1975.

Types of Pill—paragraph 6:

40. U.S. Food and Drug Administration, "Sequential oral contraceptives," *FDA Talk Paper*, Dec. 22, 1975.

41. "Sequential pill taken off the market," *The Star Ledger* (Newark, N.J.), Feb. 24, 1976.

42. D. Henry, "Some birth pills face ban by FDA," *New York Times*, Dec. 29, 1975.

43. E. R. Frederich and H. F. S. Chellhas, "The endometrium of women on a sequential contraceptive regimen," unpublished paper.

44. "Sequential pills being withdrawn," *New York Times*, Feb. 26, 1976.

The Good News—paragraph 9:

45. U.S. Food and Drug Administration, "Labeling of prescription drugs for patients," *Federal Register* 40:52705–52706 (Nov. 7, 1975).

In the spring of 1977, FDA, continuing to hedge, announced that the matter of a complete patient package insert, containing all the information doctors see, was still "under study." The following commissioners, in succession, Ley in 1969, Edwards in 1970, and Schmidt in 1975, had all promised pill-consumers the insert, but failed to deliver. The new commissioner who approved the 1977 statement was Donald Kennedy.

The FDA As Consumer Adviser:

46. Information, on record at the FDA, supplied by Ben Gordon.

47. W. L. Pines, "Women and the pill," *FDA Consumer* 10:21 (1976).

48. At hearings before the Senate Subcommittee on Health on Jan. 21, 1976, Dr. Roy Hertz, one of the leading U.S. au-

thorities on carcinogenesis, stated: "Our official regulatory agencies and our health-directed official agencies have consistently defaulted in their undertakings (concerning such 'troubling and un-resolved' questions as the pill and cancer) and have too frequently been obliged to rely on findings abroad. The record is clearly one of inadequacy, if not inertia and neglect. Surely we can marshal a more effective and informed effort on a problem of such awesome importance to so many of us."

But experts from "abroad" are almost equally cynical. In his introduction to a 1975 textbook entitled *Neurological Complications of Oral Contraceptives* (Clarendon Press, 1975), Sir Edwin Bickerstaff, one of England's most esteemed neurologists, stated: "At first the tendency of official pronouncements was to play down the side effects, and figures were given to show that these did not exceed what might be expected in the reproductive age group any way. Gradually, however, the reports became too consistent to be ignored; the type and frequency of certain side effects, when carefully analyzed, were found not to correspond with the usual incidence in the appropriate age groups, and indeed were found to differ in many ways from the well-known adverse effects of multiple pregnancies."

49. The following exchange took place between Senator Gaylord Nelson, FDA Commissioner Alexander Schmidt, and Dr. Crout on Jan. 21, 1976, at Senate hearings on "Birth Control Pills and the Use of Estrogens in Menopause." It appears on pp. 100–103 of the unedited transcript by the Hoover Reporting Company of Washington, D.C.

Senator Nelson: "You know the history. You were not the commissioner, but you are aware, I am sure, of the original proposed package insert which was in considerable detail six years ago, and it came under heavy attack . . . from manufacturers and the American Medical Association."

Commissioner Schmidt: "I am aware of the belief by some people that the original patient package insert for oral contraceptives was watered down . . . it is my belief that patient labeling should be fully informative of the risks . . . it would be my intent that all this information is included in the patient package insert."

Senator Nelson: "Do you have an idea when the proposed new labeling will be prepared . . . ?"

Dr. Crout: "Senator, we had circulating for the past couple of months . . . a proposed . . . labeling . . . there will appear in the *Federal Register* within the month a formal proposal for physician's labeling aid . . . at the same time, patient labeling so that any person who wants to can see the two side by side . . . and . . . find out whether there has been a constructive and fair and honorable job of presenting to the patient what is also presented to the physician. . . . We are going to do that within the month."

(Authors' note: These proposed warnings did not appear in the *Federal Register* until December 7, 1976, almost a full year later.)

50. "The patient package insert," *Journal of the American Medical Association* 233:1089 (1975).

51. "The patient package insert," *Journal of the American Medical Association* 235:1003 (1976).

52. U.S. Dept. of Health, Education and Welfare, news release, Jan. 6, 1975. "The Nationwide survey was conducted among 1720 users and 949 former users of birth control pills to obtain information about the use of and need of patient labeling. Of the women who had both insert and booklets, 67 percent preferred the detailed booklet, while 18 percent believed the shorter insert was more helpful."

53. Harvey Kushner, personal communication, Dec. 6, 1976.

54. R. Kushner, *Breast cancer, a personal history and an investigative report* (N.Y.: Harcourt Brace Jovanovich, 1975).

55. "Drug companies update birth control information," *New York Times*, Dec. 6, 1976.

56. D. Rabin, "Cancer victim sues doc, drug-maker," *New York Daily News*, Dec. 16, 1976, p. 7.

The Weakness of the FDA—paragraph 1:
57. U.S. House of Representatives, Committee on Government Operations, 94th Congress, news release, Jan. 26, 1976.

The Weakness of the FDA—paragraph 2:
58. D. Greenberg, "Bitter testimony," *Medical Dimensions*, Nov. 1974, p. 9.

59. "FDA probe produces more heat than light," *Medical World News*, June 28, 1976, p. 23.

60. "Washington reports," *Private Practice*, Oct. 1976, p. 23.

The Weakness of the FDA—paragraph 4:
61. Seaman, *The doctors' case against the pill*, p. 2.

The Weakness of the FDA—paragraph 6:
62. Herbert Ley, press interview upon his retirement as FDA Commissioner, 1970.

The Weakness of the FDA—paragraph 8:
63. Morton Mintz, personal communication, 1976.

Chapter 9: Side Effects—Are They Rare?

Quotation:
1. Seaman, *The doctors' case against the pill*, p. 185.
Paragraph 1:
2. Royal College of General Practitioners, *Oral contraceptives and health* (London: Pittman Medical Pub., 1974).
3. A. Lake, "The pill: what we really know after 15 years of use," *McCalls*, Jan. 1975, p. 119.

Paragraph 2:
4. William Inman, interview, April 26, 1976.
Paragraph 3:
5. Seaman, "The new pill scare."
Paragraph 4:
6. V. Beral, "Oral contraceptives and health," *Lancet* 1:1280 (1974).
7. P. D. Stolley et al., "Thrombosis with low-estrogen oral contraceptives," *American Journal of Epidemiology* 102:197–208 (1975).
8. V. A. Drill and D. W. Calhoun, "Oral contraceptives and thromboembolic disease," *Journal of the American Medical Association* 206:77–84 (1968).
9. "The pill and myocardial infarction," *Medical World News,* Aug. 25, 1975.
10. W. H. W. Inman and M. P. Vessey, "Investigation of deaths from pulmonary, coronary and cerebral thrombosis and embolism of women of child-bearing age," *British Medical Journal* 2:193–199 (1968).
11. P. E. Sartwell et al., "Thromboembolism and oral contraceptives," *American Journal of Epidemiology* 90:365–380 (1969).
Paragraph 5:
12. V. Beral, "Cardiovascular disease mortality trends and oral contraceptive use in young women," *Lancet* 2:1047–1051 (1976).
Paragraph 6:
13. Seaman, *The doctors' case against the pill,* p. 194.
Paragraph 7:
14. "Diagnostic evaluation of a woman prior to beginning contraception," *Dialogues in Oral Contraception* 1:5 (1976).
Blood Clots—paragraph 1:
15. Nelson hearings, 1970, pp. 6156–6159.
16. J. E. Wood, "Oral contraceptives, pregnancy and the veins," *Circulation* 38:154 (1968).
17. S. M. Goodrich and J. E. Wood, "Effect of estradiol 17b on peripheral venous blood flow," *American Journal of Obstetrics and Gynecology* 96:407 (1966).
Blood Clots—paragraph 4:
18. Wessler, 1976.
Blood Clots—paragraph 5:
19. H. Jick et al., "Venous thromboembolic disease and ABO blood type," *Lancet* 1:539–542 (1969).
Blood Clots—paragraph 6:
20. L. Horwich et al., *Gut* 7:680 (1966).
21. M. J. S. Langman and R. Doll, *Gut* 6:270 (1965).
Blood Clots—paragraph 8:
22. William Spellacy, personal communication.

Blood Clots—paragraph 14:
23. F. Dinbar and M. E. Platts, "Intracranial venous thrombosis complicating oral contraception," *Canadian Medical Association Journal* 111:545 (1974).
Blood Clots—paragraph 17:
24. Collaborative Group for the Study of Stroke in Young Women, "Oral contraceptives and stroke in young women," *Journal of the American Medical Association* 231:718–722 (1975).
25. M. C. Cole, "Strokes in young women using oral contraceptives," *Archives of Internal Medicine* 120:551–555 (1967).
26. Nelson hearings, 1970, Vol. I, pp. 6135–6156.
Other Neurologic and Eye Disturbances:
27. W. F. Hughes; ed., *The yearbook of ophthalmology 1973* (Chicago: Year Book Medical Pub., 1973), p. 337.
28. E. R. Bickerstaff, *Neurological complications of oral contraceptives* (Oxford: Clarendon Press, 1975), pp. 1–93.
29. Seaman, *The doctors' case against the pill*, p. 126.
Liver Disease:
30. "Birth control linked to cancer of the liver," *New York Post*, Feb. 16, 1976, p. 4.
31. E. T. Mays et al., "Hepatic changes in young women ingesting contraceptive steroids: hepatic hemorrhage and primary hepatic tumors," *Journal of the American Medical Association* 235:730–732 (1976).
32. J. K. Baum et al., "Possible association between benign hepatomas and oral contraceptives," *Lancet* 2:926–929 (1973).
33. A. L. Jones and J. B. Emans, "The effects of progesterone administration on hepatic endoplasmic reticulum," in: Salhanick, 1969, pp. 68–85.
34. H. Wiendling and J. B. Henry, "Laboratory test results altered by the pill," *Journal of the American Medical Association* 229:1762–1768 (1974).
35. J. P. O'Sullivan and R. P. Wilding, "Liver hamartoma in patients on oral contraceptives," *British Medical Journal* 3:7–10 (1974).
36. J. A. Ameriks et al., "Hepatic cell adenomas, spontaneous liver rupture and oral contraceptives," *Archives of Surgery* 110:548–577 (1975).
37. J. K. Baum, "Liver tumors and oral contraceptives," *Journal of the American Medical Association* 232:1329 (1975).
38. W. M. Christopherson, E. T. Mays and G. H. Barrows, "Liver tumors in women on contraceptive steroids," *Obstetrics and Gynecology* 46:221–223 (1975).
39. B. Kramer, "Birth control pills may cause tumors, researchers suggest," *Wall Street Journal*, Feb. 17, 1976.
40. J. Randal, "Doctors link liver cancer to birth control pill," *New York Daily News*, Feb. 16, 1976, p. 13.
41. "Latest puzzle about the pill: can it cause a benign but

dangerous liver tumor?" *Medical World News*, 15:25–26 (1974).

42. "Progress report: hepatic adenomas and oral contraceptives," *Gut* 16:753–756 (1975).

43. J. E. Brody, "Oral pill linked to liver hazard," *New York Times*, Feb. 26, 1976.

44. "The pill: a new liver risk," *New York Post*, Feb. 26, 1976.

45. D. Neill, personal communication, July 25, 1976.

High Blood Pressure:

46. J. H. Laragh et al., "Oral contraceptives and high blood pressure: changes in plasma renin, renin substrate and aldosterone excretion," in: Salhanick, 1969, pp. 405–421.

47. J. H. Laragh, "Contraceptive hypertension: from 1967 on," *Hospital Practice* 10:13 (1975).

48. J. W. Woods, "Oral contraceptives and hypertension," *Lancet* 2:653–654 (1967).

49. Nelson hearings, 1970, Vol. 1, pp. 6161–6171.

50. M. H. Weinberger, "Oral contraceptives and hypertension," *Hospital Practice* 10:65–74 (1975).

51. A. J. Snider, "New alert on pill side effect," *New York Post*, Sept. 25, 1976.

Cancer:

52. W. U. Gardner, "Estrogens in carcinogenesis," *Archives of Pathology* 27:139–170 (1939).

53. L. Loeb, Significance of hormones in the origin of cancer," *Journal of the U.S. National Cancer Institute* 1:169–195 (1940).

54. R. Hertz, "The role of steroid hormones in the etiology and pathogenesis of cancer," *American Journal of Obstetrics and Gynecology* 98:1013–1019 (1967).

55. Nelson hearings, 1970, Vol. II, pp. 6022–6060.

56. Nelson hearings, 1970, Vol. II, pp. 6648–6654.

57. R. Hertz, W. W. Tullner and E. Raffelt, "Progestational activity of orally administered 17-alpha-ethinyl-19-nor-testosterone," *Endocrinology* 54:228 (1954).

58. R. Hertz, J. H. Waite and L. B. Thomas, "Progestational effectiveness of 19-norethinyl testosterone by oral route in women," *Proceedings of the Society of Experimental Biology and Medicine* 91:418 (1956).

59. S. W. Cook and E. C. Dodds, "Sex hormones and cancer producing compounds," *Nature* 131:205 (1933).

60. R. Hoover et al., "Cancer of the uterine corpus after hormonal treatment for breast cancer," *Lancet* 1:885–887 (1976).

61. M. Dolan, "New research links the pill and breast cancer," *Synapse* (U.C.S.F. Medical School), Nov. 13, 1975.

62. Statement by Heinz W. Berendes, Kennedy hearings, Jan. 21, 1976.

63. E. Fasal and R. S. Paffenbarger, "Oral contraceptives as related to cancer and benign lesions of the breast," *Journal of the National Cancer Institute* 55:4 (1975).

64. R. Hertz, "The problem of possible effects of oral con-

traceptives on cancer of the breast," *Cancer* 24:1140–1145 (1969).

65. A. R. Currie, *Endocrine aspects of breast cancer*. (Baltimore: Williams & Wilkins, 1958).

66. M. M. Black and H. Pleis, "Mammary carcinogenesis," *New York State Journal of Medicine* 72:1601–1605 (1972).

67. E. F. Lewison, "The pill, estrogens, and the breast," *Cancer* 28:1400 (1971).

68. H. M. Lemon, "Abnormal estrogen metabolism and tissue estrogen receptor proteins in breast cancer," *Cancer* 25:423 (1970).

69. Jahara, 1962.

70. T. B. Dunn, "Cancer of the uterine cervix in mice fed a liquid diet containing an anti-fertility drug," *Journal of the National Cancer Institute* 43:671 (1969).

71. P. Cole and B. MacMahon, "Oestrogen fractions during early reproductive life in the etiology of breast cancer," *Lancet* 1:604 (1969).

72. G. G. Wied et al., "Statistical evaluation of the effect of hormonal contraceptives on the cytologic smear pattern," *Obstetrics and Gynecology* 27:327 (1966).

73. M. Cutler, Nelson hearings, March 3, 1970.

74. E. F. Lewison, Nelson hearings, Feb. 25, 1970.

75. M. R. Melamed et al., "Prevalence rates of uterine cervical carcinoma in situ for women using the diaphragm or oral contraceptives," *British Medical Journal* 3:195 (1969).

76. H. B. Taylor, N. S. Irey and H. J. Morris, "Atypical endocervical hyperplasia in women taking oral contraceptives," *Journal of the American Medical Association* 202:637 (1967).

77. M. Candy and M. R. Abel, "Progestogen-induced adenomatous hyperplasia of the uterine cervix," *Journal of the American Medical Association* 203:323 (1968).

78. J. Wallach and P. H. Henneman, "Prolonged estrogen therapy in post-menopausal women," *Journal of the American Medical Association* 171:1637–1642 (1959).

79. P. Mustacchi and G. S. Gordon, *Frequency of cancer in estrogen-treated osteoporotic women* (St. Louis: Mosby, 1959). Pp. 163–169.

80. S. H. Geist et al., "Are estrogens carcinogenic in the human female?" *American Journal of Obstetrics and Gynecology* 41: 29–36 (1941).

81. Even as medical journals are publishing articles frankly stating the serious risks involved in estrogen therapy, usually responsible women's magazines still print favorable messages. Note the contrast in the following two passages:

A. E. Nourse, "Is hormone therapy right for you?" *Woman's Day*, Apr. 1976, p. 6:

"Ever since the female sex hormones were first identified in the early 1930's, these powerful chemical substances have been used to treat a wide variety of women's disorders. Estrogen, produced in the woman's ovaries and in lesser amounts in her adrenal glands, has proved particularly helpful in treating certain stubborn female health problems."

"More critics raise voices against estrogen therapy," *Journal of the American Medical Association* 235:787–788 (1976):

"The link between oral contraceptive use and an elevated risk of breast cancer in certain individuals was reported in last October's *Journal of the National Cancer Institute* (NCI) by Elfriede Fasal, M.D., Ph.D., and Ralph S. Paffenbarger, Jr., M.D., DPH, California State Department of Health."

The study involved 452 women with breast cancer and 446 women with benign breast disease. Analysis of the various subgroups showed increase to 2.5-fold in breast cancer incidence among women who had been taking oral contraceptives for a period of two to four years and were still doing so at the time of the study. Dr. Fasal found an increase to 11-fold in risk of breast cancer in women who had previously had a biopsy for benign breast disease. Commenting on these findings before a Senate subcommittee, Robert N. Hoover, M.D., head of the Environmental Studies Section of NCI, said, "The subgroups in this analysis that show evidence of excessive risk are clearly disturbing to those familiar with breast cancer epidemiology. Excesses are seen among long-term pill users with a history of benign breast disease and among those using the pill before having their first child. Since two variables—a history of benign breast disease and the age of the woman at birth of the first child—are related to a woman's risk of developing breast cancer, the appearance of an apparent adverse effect of the pill in these subgroups may be an important warning."

82. Actually cervical changes are the norm. In 1969 a study by Dr. S. A. Gall and others with 103 patients showed that 84 percent of the pill users showed cervical changes.

S. A. Gall, C. H. Bourgeois and R. McGuire, "The morphologic effects of oral contraceptive agents on the cervix," *Journal of the American Medical Association* 207:2243–2247 (1969).

83. W. P. Plate, "Foreword," in: B. Seaman, *De pil* (Rotterdam: Leminscat, 1970).

84. Seaman, *The doctors' case against the pill*, p. 159.

Infertility:

85. M. Vassey et al., "A long-term follow-up study of women using different methods of contraception—an interim report," *Journal of Biosocial Science* 8:373 (1976).

Diabetes:

86. Nelson hearings, 1970, Vol. I, pp. 6296–6344, 6426–6445.

87. H. Gershberg, H. Hulse and Z. Javier, "Hypertriglyceridemia during treatment with estrogen and oral contraceptives," *Obstetrics and Gynecology* 31:186–191 (1968).

88. "Editorial," *Lancet* 2:783–784 (1969).

89. W. N. Spellacy, "A review of carbohydrate metabolism and the oral contraceptives," *American Journal of Obstetrics and Gynecology* 104:448–460 (1969).

90. W. N. Spellacy, "Progesten and estrogen effects on carbohydrate metabolism," in: J. B. Josimovich, ed., *Uterine contraction: side effects of steroidal contraception* (N.Y.: Wiley, 1973), pp. 327–341.

91. W. N. Spellacy, "Metabolic effects of oral contraceptives," *Clinical Obstetrics and Gynecology* 17:53–64 (1974).

92. V. Wynn and J. W. H. Doar, "Some effects of oral contraceptives on carbohydrate metabolism," *Lancet* 2:715 (1966).

93. V. Wynn, J. W. H. Doar and G. L. Mills, "Some effects of oral contraceptives on serum lipid and lipoprotein levels," *Lancet* 2:720 (1966).

94. V. Wynn, "Some metabolic effects of oral contraceptives," *Clinical Trials Journal* 5:171 (1968).

95. J. W. H. Doar, V. Wynn and D. G. Cramp, "Blood pyruvate and plasma glucose levels during oral and intravenous glucose tolerance tests in obese and non-obese women," *Metabolism* 7:690 (1968).

96. V. Wynn and J. W. H. Doar, "Longitudinal studies of the effects of oral contraceptive therapy on plasma glucose, non-esterified fatty acid, insulin and blood pyruvate levels during oral and intravenous glucose tolerance tests," in H. A. Salhanick et al., 1969, pp. 157–177.

97. "Fasting serum triglyceride, cholesterol and lipoprotein levels during oral contraceptive therapy," *Lancet* 2:756–760 (1969).

98. W. N. Spellacy, "Carbohydrate metabolism in male infertility and female fertility-control patients," *Fertility and Sterility* 27:1132–1139 (1976). Spellacy now concludes that "the exacerbation of existing or borderline diabetes by oral contraceptives may be irreversible." He says that the following factors place women at "high risk for having significant carbohydrate metabolic abnormalities" while using the pill: (1) previously abnormal blood glucose values; (2) a strong family history of diabetes; (3) excessive weight gain while taking the pill, obesity, or both; (4) a history of high-birthweight infants (over nine pounds); (5) prior unexplained stillbirths or infants with congenital abnormalities; (6) older age or higher parity; and (7) early age at menarche. In addition, repeated or hard-to-cure monilial vaginitis may justify a blood glucose study.

Another Pill Side Effect—Pregnancy:

99. "Drug Interactions: plasma clearance—steroidal contraceptives (SOC)," *Drug Therapy*, Apr. 1976, p. 115.

100. J. L. Skolnick et al., "Rifampin, oral contraceptives and

pregnancy," *Journal of the American Medical Association* 236: 1382 (1976).

101. A partial listing of other drugs that have been implicated in blocking the contraceptive action of the pill includes: antihistamines, barbiturates (Amytal, Nembutal, phenobarbital, Seconal), Butazolidin, Dilantin, Equanil, Miltown, Rifadin, Rimactane, according to *The People's Pharmacy* by J. Gradeon (N.Y.: St. Martin's Press, 1976), p. 135.

Sex Drive:
102. Seaman, *The doctors' case against the pill*, pp. 127–144.
103. "Pill gets no credit for rise in female libido, study says," *Psychiatric News* 6:9 (1971).
104. "Find sexual pleasure abetted in only 39% of group on pill," *Medical Tribune*, Sept. 8, 1971.
105. Seaman, *Free and female*, p. 252.
106. R. P. Michael, "Hormones and sexual behavior in the female," *Hospital Practice* 10:69–76 (1976).

Depression:
107. A. Lewis and M. Hoghughi, "An evaluation of depression as a side effect of oral contraceptives," *British Journal of Psychiatry* 115:697–701 (1969).
108. M. Jefferies, "Three on pill tried suicide," *Evening Standard*, June 6, 1969.
109. Nelson hearings, 1970, Vol. II, pp. 6647–6648.
110. Nelson hearings, 1970, Vol. II, pp. 6492–6501.
111. E. C. G. Grant and H. Pryse-Davis, "Effects of oral contraceptives on depressive mood changes and on endometrial monoamine oxidase and phosphatases," *British Medical Journal* 3:777–780 (1968).
112. C. M. Idestrom, "Reaction to norethisterone withdrawal," *Lancet* 1:718 (1966).
113. F. J. Kane et al., "Emotional change associated with oral contraceptives in female psychiatric patients," *Comprehensive Psychiatry* 10:16–30 (1969).
114. F. J. Kane, "Psychosis associated with the use of oral contraceptive agents," *Southern Medical Journal* 62:190–192 (1969).
115. A. Nilsson and P. E. Almgren, "Psychiatric symptoms during the postpartum period as related to use of oral contraceptives," *British Medical Journal* 2:453–455 (1968).

116. It is of note that sensitive internists and gynecologists are fully as aware as psychiatrists of the pill's emotional side effects. At the Nelson hearings, Dr. John McCain, an Atlanta gynecologist, observed: "The emotional or psychiatric problems are the complications which seem to me to have the most serious potential danger. Three patients have stated that they were desperately afraid that they were going to kill themselves. Two of them had been on the pills 14 days or less. . . . If the

patients reported here were willing to discuss their problems without any invitation to do so, one is concerned regarding other patients who may not have discussed similar problems. It is disturbing to consider the patients on the pills whose depression may have ended in suicide and/or homicide with no recognition of any association with the contraceptive pills." Dr. McCain was somewhat unusual in that, starting in 1964, he maintained extremely careful records of every pill complication in all of his patients. Nelson hearings, 1970, Vol. II, pp. 6470–6492.

Newly Acknowledged Side Effects—paragraph 1:

117. L. J. Bennion et al., "Effects of oral contraceptives on the gallbladder bile of normal women," *New England Journal of Medicine* 294:189–192 (1976).

118. "Iatrogenic gallstones," *British Medical Journal* 1:859–60 (1976).

119. S. Cohen, "The pill linked to gallstones," *New York Post*, Jan. 23, 1976.

120. Boston Collaborative Drug Surveillance Program, "Oral contraceptives and venous thromboembolic disease, surgically confirmed gall bladder disease, and breast tumors," *Lancet* 1: 1399–1404 (1973).

121. Small, 1976.

Newly Acknowledged Side Effects—paragraph 3:

122. C. Dupont, "Herpes gestationis and the pill," *British Medical Journal* 2:699 (1968).

123. B. Gorden, "Herpes gestationis and the pill," *British Medical Journal* 1:51–52 (1967).

124. R. W. Lynch and R. J. Albrecht, "Hormonal factors in herpes gestationis," *Archives of Dermatology* 9:446–447 (1966).

125. D. M. Mitchell, "Herpes gestationis and the pill," *British Medical Journal* 4:1324 (1966).

126. W. B. Shelley, R. W. Preucell and S. S. Spoont, "Autoimmune progesterone dermatitis," *Journal of the American Medical Association* 190:35–38 (1964).

Newly Acknowledged Side Effects—paragraph 4:

127. M. Zahran, "Effects of contraceptive pills and intrauterine devices on urinary bladder," *Urology* 8:567 (1976).

Newly Acknowledged Side Effects—paragraph 5:

128. Nelson hearings, 1970, Vol. I. pp. 6086–6105.

129. E. M. Schleicher, "L.E. cells after oral contraceptives," *Lancet* 1:821–822 (1968).

130. E. L. Dubois et al., "L.E. cells after oral contraceptives," *Lancet* 2:679 (1968).

131. G. J. Gill, "Rheumatic complaints of women using antiovulatory drugs," *Journal of Chronic Disease* 21:435 (1968).

132. J. M. Dwyer et al., "Cell-mediated immunity in healthy women taking oral contraceptives," *Yale Journal of Biology and Medicine* 48:91–95 (1975).

133. E. W. Barnes et al., "Phytohaemagglutinin-induced lymphocyte transformation and circulating autoantibodies in women taking oral contraceptives," *Lancet* 1:898 (1974).

134. H. Speira and C. M. Plotz, "Rheumatic symptoms and oral contraceptives," *Lancet* 1:571–521 (1969).

135. G. G. Bole et al., "Rheumatic symptoms and serological abnormalities induced by oral contraception," *Lancet* 1:323 (1969).

Newly Acknowledged Side Effects—paragraph 10:

136. G. M. El-Ashiry et al., "Effects of oral contraceptives on the gingiva," *Journal of Periodontology* 42:273–275 (1971).

137. A. Y. Kaufman, "An oral contraceptive as an etiologic factor in producing hyperplastic gingivitis and a neoplasm of the pregnancy tumor type," *Oral Surgery* 28:666–670 (1969).

138. J. Lindhe and A. Bjorn, "Influence of hormonal contraceptives on the gingiva of women," *Journal of Periodontal Research* 2:1–6 (1967).

139. B. D. Lynn, "The pill as an etiologic agent in hypertrophic gingivitis," *Oral Surgery* 24:333–334 (1967).

Newly Acknowledged Side Effects—paragraph 11:

140. M. J. Brindle and I. N. Henderson, "Vascular occlusion of the colon associated with oral contraception," *Canadian Medical Association Journal* 100:681–682 (1969).

141. P. B. Cotton and M. L. Thomas, "Ischemic colitis and the contraceptive pill," *British Medical Journal* 3:27–28 (1971).

142. M. D. Gelfand, "Ischemic colitis associated with a depot synthetic progestogen," *American Journal of Digestive Disease* 17:275–277 (1972).

143. Z. M. Kilpatrick et al., "Vascular occlusion of the colon and oral contraceptives; possible relation," *New England Journal of Medicine* 278:438–440 (1968).

144. K. Sakaguchin and S. Shimomura, "Birth control pills and colitis," *Bulletin of the Hospital Pharmacy and the Drug Interaction Analysis Service* 23:1–2 (1975).

Newly Acknowledged Side Effects—paragraph 12:

145. C. J. Falliers, "Oral contraceptives and allergy," *Lancet* 2:515 (1974).

Birth Defects—paragraph 1:

146. Janerich, 1974.

147. Janerich, Kennedy hearings, Jan. 21, 1976.

148. Nelson hearings, 1970, Vol. II, pp. 600–609.

149. L. Wilkins, "Masculinization of the female fetus due to use of orally given progestins," *Journal of the American Medical Association* 172:1028–1032 (1960).

150. E. P. Levy et al., "Hormone treatment during pregnancy and congenital heart defects," *Lancet* 1:611 (1973).

151. Nora, 1973.

152. S. Harlap, R. Prywes and A. M. Davies, "Birth defects and

oestrogens and progesterones in pregnancy," *Lancet* 1:682–683 (1975).

153. M. M. Grumback et al., "On the fetal masculinizing action of certain oral progestins," *Journal of Clinical Endocrinology and Metabolism* 19:1369–1380 (1959).

154. D. H. Carr, "Chromosome anomalies as a cause of spontaneous abortion," *American Journal of Obstetrics and Gynecology* 97:283 (1967).

155. D. Siegal and P. Corfman, "Epidemiological problems associated with studies of the safety of oral contraceptives," *Journal of the American Medical Association* 203:950 (1968).

156. J. Robertson-Rintoul, "Oral contraception: potential hazards of hormone therapy during pregnancy," *Lancet* 2:1315 (1974).

157. J. M. Reinisch, "Effects of prenatal hormone exposure on physical and psychological development in humans and animals," in: E. J. Sachar, ed., *Hormones, behavior and psychopathology* (N.Y.: Raven, 1976).

157a. O. P. Heinonen et al., "Cardiovascular birth defects and antenatal exposure to female sex hormones," *New England Journal of Medicine* 296, Jan. 13, 1977.

Birth Defects—paragraph 3:

158. Bascombe, 1975.

159. M. Brenton, "How do hunger and nourishment affect the developing brain?" *Modern Medicine* 23:66–70 (1976).

Birth Defects—paragraph 12:

160. Seaman, *The doctors' case against the pill*, pp. 188–189.

161. Actually the effects of the pill on chromosomes was well established by 1969 as noted in the following reports:

"Do progestogens cause chromosomal damage?" *Medical World News*, Jan. 10, 1969.

"Growth anomalies in aborted fetuses of pill users," *Medical World News*, Dec. 28, 1969.

"Common breaks in chromosomes noted with pill," *Medical Tribune*, Oct. 10, 1971.

Birth Defects—paragraph 14:

162. Janerich, Kennedy hearings, Jan. 21, 1976.

Birth Defects—paragraph 15:

163. Harlap, 1975, pp. 682–683.

Birth Defects—paragraph 16:

164. Some of the women may have been given hormones in the first place because of conditions which in themselves might have caused an increase in birth defects.

Birth Defects—paragraph 17:

165. V. M. Barsivla and K. D. Virkar, "The effect of oral contraceptives on various components of human milk," *Contraception* 7:307 (1973).

166. S. J. Kora, "Effects of oral contraceptives on lactation," *Fertility and Sterility* 20:429 (1969).

167. V. S. Toddywalla, L. Joshi and K. Virkar, "Effect of contraceptive steroids on human lactation," *American Journal of Obstetrics and Gynecology* 127:245 (1977).
168. Both the quantity and quality of breast milk, including the fat and calcium content, can be markedly altered by the pill. Ovulen and Ovral are two of the brands reported to have serious detrimental effects. Lower-dose brands may be less harmful than others but this is not yet fully clarified.
Birth Defects—paragraph 33:
169. B. Seaman, "Pelvic autonomy: four proposals," *Social Policy* 6:43–47 (1975).

"Among the 16,500 Fellows of the American College of Obstetricians and Gynecologists, 978 are women. Yet, in 1974, out of 3,750 obstetrics-gynecology residents only 96 were women. Thus, while the ratio of women in the field is about one in 17, the ratio of women entering the field has declined to about one in 40."

Chapter 10: Recovering from the Pill

Paragraph 1:
1. M. Briggs and M. Briggs, "Vitamin C requirements and oral contraceptives," *Nature* 238:277 (1972).
2. M. Briggs and M. Briggs, "Vitamin C and colds," *Lancet* 1: 998 (1973).
3. F. McGinty and D. P. Rose, "Influence of androgens upon tryptophan metabolism in man," *Life Sciences* 8:1193 (1969).
4. D. P. Rose, "Aspects of tryptophan metabolism in health and disease," *Journal of Clinical Pathology* 25:17 (1972).
5. D. P. Rose, and I. P. Braidman, "Excretion of tryptophan metabolites as affected by pregnancy, contraceptive steroids and steroid hormones," *American Journal of Clinical Nutrition* 24:673 (1971).
Paragraph 2:
6. I. E. Jelinek, "Oral contraceptives and the skin," *American Family Physician* 4:68–74 (1971).
Paragraph 3:
7. Briggs, 1973, p. 998.
Paragraph 4:
8. A. M. Shojania, "Effect of oral contraceptives on vitamin B_{12} metabolism," *Lancet* 2:932 (1971).
9. A. M. Shojania and G. J. Hornady, "Oral contraceptive and folate absorption," *Journal of Laboratory and Clinical Medicine* 82:869–875 (1973).
10. J. E. Ryser et al., "Megaloblastic anemia due to folic acid deficiency in a young woman on oral contraceptives," *Acta Haematologica* 45:319–324 (1971).

11. A. S. Prasad et al., "Effect of oral contraceptive agents on nutrients: II. Vitamins," *American Journal of Clinical Nutrition* 28:385–391 (1975).

12. M. K. Horwitt, C. C. Harvey, C. H. Dahm, "Relationship between levels of blood lipids, vitamins C, A, and E, serum copper compounds, and urinary excretions of tryptophan metabolites in women taking oral contraceptive therapy," *American Journal of Clinical Nutrition* 28:403–412 (1975).

13. S. Margen, J. C. King, "Effect of oral contraceptive agents on the metabolism of some trace minerals," *American Journal of Clinical Nutrition* 28:392–402 (1975).

14. "The pill and changes in essential trace metals," *Medical World News* 15:32 (1974).

15. J. Lindenbaum, N. Whitehead and F. Reyner, "Oral contraceptive hormones, folate metabolism and the cervical epithelium," *American Journal of Clinical Nutrition* 28:346–352 (1975).

16. L. Boots, P. E. Cornwell and L. R. Beck, "Effect of ethynodiol diacetate and mestranol on serum folic acid and vitamin B_{12} levels and on tryptophan metabolism in baboons," *American Journal of Clinical Nutrition* 28:354–362 (1975).

17. A. M. Shojania, "Vitamins and oral contraceptive use," *Lancet* 1:1198 (1975).

18. C. C. Pfeiffer, *Mental and elemental nutrients* (New Canaan, Conn.: Keats, 1975).

19. *Medical World News*, 1974, p. 32.

20. M. Briggs and M. Briggs, "Oral contraceptives and vitamin requirements," *Medical Journal of Australia* 1:407 (1975).

Paragraph 6:

21. R. C. Theuer, "Effects of oral contraceptive agents on vitamin and mineral needs: a review," *Journal of Reproductive Medicine*, 8:13–19 (1972).

Paragraph 9:

22. "Feminins and other vitamin-mineral supplements for women taking oral contraceptives," *Medical Letter* 15:81–82 (1973).

Paragraph 10:

23. U. Larsson-Cohn, "Oral contraceptives and vitamins: a review," *American Journal of Obstetrics and Gynecology* 121:84–90 (1975).

24. Melamed, 1969.

25. Gall, 1969.

26. E. T. Tyler, "Current status of oral contraceptives," *Journal of the American Medical Association* 187:562 (1964).

27. F. B. Lewis, "Folate deficiency due to oral contraceptives," *Minnesota Medicine* 57:945–946 (1974).

28. Rosalind LaRoche, personal communication, 1976.

29. Wynn, 1975.

Paragraph 20:

30. L. Lacey, *Lunaception: A feminine odyssey into fertility and contraception* (N.Y.: Coward-McCann, 1974).

31. "Right now," *McCalls*, May 1976, pp. 61–62.

Vitamin B₆ (Pyridoxine):

32. A. L. Luhby et al., "Vitamin B₆ metabolism in users of oral contraceptive agents," *American Journal of Clinical Nutrition* 24:684 (1971).

33. P. Adams, V. Wynn and D. Rose, "Effects of pyridoxine hydrochloride (vitamin B₆) upon depression associated with oral contraception," *Lancet* 1:897 (1973).

34. Wynn, 1975.

35. J. Otte, "Oral contraceptives and depression," *Lancet* 2: 498 (1969).

36. Spain has been marketing an oral contraceptive containing pyridoxine (B₆) since 1967. It is sold under the proprietary name Ciclosequer.

37. See also chap. 9, notes 109–116.

38. W. N. Spellacy et al., "Carbohydrate and lipid studies during six months' treatment with megestrol acetate," *American Journal of Obstetrics and Gynecology* 116:1074–1078 (1973).

39. W. N. Spellacy et al., "Change in glucose and insulin after six months' treatment with the oral contraceptive Demulen," *American Journal of Obstetrics and Gynecology* 119:226–267 (1974).

40. W. N. Spellacy et al., "The effect of estrogens on carbohydrate metabolism," *American Journal of Obstetrics and Gynecology* 114:378–392 (1972).

41. W. N. Spellacy and S. A. Birk, "The effects of mechanical and steroid contraceptive methods on blood pressure in hypertensive women," *Fertility and Sterility* 25:467–470 (1974).

42. W. N. Spellacy, W. C. Buhi and S. A. Birk, "The effects of vitamin B₆ on carbohydrate metabolism in women taking steroid contraceptives," *Contraception* 6:265–273 (1972).

43. W. N. Spellacy, "Metabolic effects of oral contraceptives," *Clinical Obstetrics and Gynecology* 17:53–64 (1974).

44. W. N. Spellacy et al., "Metabolic studies on women taking norethindrone for 6 months' time (measurements of blood glucose, insulin and triglyceride concentrations)," *Fertility and Sterility* 24:419–425 (1973).

45. W. N. Spellacy et al., Vitamin B₆ treatment of gestational diabetes mellitus: studies of blood glucose and plasma insulin. Unpublished paper.

46. William Spellacy, personal communication, 1976.

47. Nelson hearings, 1970, Spellacy testimony.

Dietary Sources of Vitamin B₆—paragraph 4:

48. R. J. Williams, *Nutrition in a nutshell* (N.Y.: Doubleday, 1972).

49. R. J. Williams, *Nutrition against disease* (N.Y.: Bantam, 1973).

50. C. C. Fredericks, *Look younger, feel healthier* (N.Y.: Grosset & Dunlap, 1972), p. 116.
Dietary Sources of Vitamin B_6—paragraph 5:
51. Fredericks, 1972, p. 181.
Dietary Sources of Vitamin B_6—paragraph 6:
52. Pfeiffer, 1975.
Dietary Sources of Vitamin B_6—paragraph 7:
53. Pfeiffer, 1975, p. 151.
Dietary Sources of Vitamin B_6—paragraph 8:
54. Larsson-Cohn, 1975.
55. Wynn, 1975.
56. H. E. Aly et al., "Oral contraceptives and vitamin B_6 metabolism," *American Journal of Clinical Nutrition* 24:297–303 (1971).
57. I. L. Craft et al., "Oral contraceptives and amino acid utilization," *American Journal of Obstetrics and Gynecology* 108:1120 (1970).
58. D. P. Rose and D. G. Cramp, "Reduction of plasma tyrosine by oral contraceptives and oestrogens," *Clinica Chimica Acta* 29:49 (1970).
59. J. V. Levy and P. Bach-y-Rita, *Vitamins: their use and abuse* (N.Y.: Liveright, 1976), p. 90.
High C Problems—paragraph 1:
60. Pfeiffer, 1975, p. 137.
High C Problems—paragraph 3:
61. Levy, 1976, p. 32.
High C Problems—paragraph 5:
62. R. J. Kutsky, *Handbook of vitamins and hormones* (N.Y.: Van Nostrand Reinhold, 1973), pp. 71–78.
63. Levy, 1976, pp. 87–88.
High C Problems—paragraph 6:
64. A. B. Harris, M. Pillay and S. Hussein, "Vitamins and oral contraceptives," *Lancet* 2:83 (1975).
High C Problems—paragraph 8:
65. I. Horowitz, E. M. Fabry and C. D. Gerson, "Bioavailability of ascorbic acid in orange juice," *Journal of the American Medical Association* 235:2624–2625 (1976).
Folic Acid:
66. A. Paton, "Oral contraceptives and folate deficiency," *Lancet* 1:418 (1969).
67. R. Strief, "Folate deficiency and oral contraceptives," *Journal of the American Medical Association* 214:40 (1971).
68. R. Flury and W. Angehrn, "Folsaureman gelanamie infolge einnahme oraler kontrazeptiva," *Schweizerische Medizinische Wochenschrift* 102:1628–1629 (1972).
69. J. B. Alperin, "Folate metabolism in women using oral contraceptive agents," *American Journal of Clinical Nutrition* 26: xix (1973) (Abstract).

70. A. M. Shojania, G. J. Hornady and P. H. Barnes, "The effect of oral contraceptives on folate metabolism," *American Journal of Obstetrics and Gynecology* 111:782 (1971).

71. L. F. Wetalik et al., "Decreased serum B_{12} levels with oral contraceptive use," *Journal of the American Medical Association* 221:1371 (1972).

72. O. Martinez and D. A. Roe, "Diet and contraceptive steroids as determinants of folate status in pregnancy," *Federation Proceedings* 33:715 (1974) (Abstract).

73. Subnormal levels of serum folate are noted in 9 percent of women who have been on the pill for less than a year, according to Dr. Daphne Rose of Cornell University. After 4 years, the figure rises to 42 percent.

74. W. H. Hines, "Vitamins and birth control," *New York Post*, Oct. 3, 1973, p. 38.

75. Lewis, 1974, pp. 945–946.

76. Boston Collaborative Drug Surveillance Program, 1973.

Folic Acid, the Cervix, and the Pill—paragraph 1:

77. M. E. Atwood, "Cytology and the contraceptive pill," *Journal of Obstetrics and Gynecology* 73:662 (1966).

78. W. Liu et al., "Cytologic changes following the use of oral contraceptives," *Obstetrics and Gynecology* 30:228 (1967).

79. Melamed, 1969, p. 195.

80. Gall, 1969, p. 2243.

81. T. S. Kline, M. Holland and D. Wemple, "Atypical cytology with contraceptive hormone medication," *American Journal of Clinical Pathology* 53:215 (1970).

82. C. M. Dougherty, "Cervical cytology and sequential birth control pills," *Obstetrics and Gynecology* 36:741 (1970).

83. Taylor, 1967.

84. N. Whitehead, F. Reyner and J. Lindenbaum, "Megaloblastic changes in cervical epithelium. Association with oral contraceptive therapy and reversal with folic acid," *Journal of the American Medical Association* 226:1421 (1973).

85. D. A. Roe, "How the pill affects a woman's nutritional status," *Medical Opinion*, Sept. 1976, pp. 58–61.

Folic Acid, the Cervix, and the Pill—paragraph 4:

86. Lindenbaum, 1975.

87. Whitehead, 1973, p. 1421.

Folic Acid, the Cervix, and the Pill—paragraph 7:

88. L. G. Koss, "Megaloblastic changes in cervical epithelium," *Journal of the American Medical Association* 227:1262 (1974).

Folic Acid, the Cervix, and the Pill—paragraph 11:

89. Kutsky, 1973, pp. 87–95.

90. B_{12} deficiency anemia causes neurological and nervous system damage, as well as changes in the blood. Folic acid can cure the blood damage of B_{12} anemia, but not the problems with the nervous system. Thus if a B_{12}-deficient patient happens to take a gram a day of folic acid, his or her deceptively normal

blood tests may prevent doctors from identifying the true condition. The neurological symptoms will progress. But whether pill-users should have so much trouble getting folic acid in order to protect individuals with possible B_{12} anemia is a thorny question.

Zinc—paragraph 2:
91. R. A. Passwater, *Super-nutrition* (N.Y.: Pocket Books, 1976), p. 20.
Zinc—paragraph 3:
92. Pfeiffer, 1975, p. 219.
93. Levy, 1976, pp. 111–112.
Zinc—paragraph 4:
94. Pfeiffer, 1975, p. 328.
Zinc—paragraph 5:
95. Passwater, 1976, pp. 23–28.
Zinc—paragraph 9:
96. Levy, 1976, p. 112.
Copper—paragraph 1:
97. Pfeiffer, 1975, p. 337.
98. Pfeiffer, 1975, p. 328.
Copper—paragraph 2:
99. Pfeiffer, 1975, pp. 329–331.
100. Pfeiffer, 1975, p. 328.
Copper—paragraph 3:
101. *Medical World News* 15:32 (Sept, 1974).
Copper—paragraph 5:
102. Pfeiffer, 1975, p. 479. Excess copper has also been linked to mental disorders. Pfeiffer believes it is especially dangerous for a woman with a previous history of schizophrenia to take the pill.
Migraine—paragraph 2:
103. Seaman, *The doctors' case against the pill*, pp. 107–126.
104. See also chap. 9, notes 24–26.
Migraine—paragraph 3:
105. Pfeiffer, 1975, p. 440.
Other Trace Elements—paragraph 2:
106. *Medical World News* 15:32 (Sept. 1974).
Vitamin A—paragraph 2:
107. Wynn, 1975.
108. I. Gal, C. Parkinson and I. Craft, "Effects of oral contraceptives on human plasma vitamin-A levels," *British Medical Journal* 2:436–438 (1971).
Three B's—paragraph 2:
109. N. Sanpitak and L. Chayutimonkul, "Oral contraceptives and riboflavin nutrition," *Lancet* 1:836–837 (1974).
110. M. Briggs and M. Briggs, "Oral contraceptives and vitamin nutrition," *Lancet* 1:1234 (1974).
111. M. Briggs and M. Briggs, "Thiamin status and oral contraceptives," *Contraception* 11:151–154 (1975).

112. M. Briggs and M. Briggs, "Endocrine effects on serum vitamin B_{12}," *Lancet* 2:1037 (1972).

113. Wertalik, 1972, p. 1371.

114. L. Lumeng et al., "Effect of oral contraceptives on the plasma concentration of pyridoxal phosphate," *American Journal of Clinical Nutrition* 27:326 (1974).

115. L. T. Miller et al., "Vitamin B_6 metabolism in women using oral contraceptives," *American Journal of Clinical Nutrition* 27:797–805 (1974).

116. H. J. R. Coelingh and W. H. P. Schreurs, *Contraception* 9:347 (1974).

117. R. M. Salkeld et al., "Effect of oral contraceptives on vitamin B_6 status," *Clinica Chimica Acta* 49:195–199 (1973).

118. Shojania, *Lancet* 2:932 (1971).

119. National Institute of Nutrition, Hyderabad. Annual report, 1974, p. 107.

Three B's—paragraph 3:

120. Levy, 1976, p. 73.

121. Kutsky, 1973, pp. 7–15.

Three B's—paragraph 4:

122. Levy, 1976, p. 73.

Three B's—paragraph 6:

123. Kutsky, 1973, pp. 46–53.

Three B's—paragraph 7:

124. Wynn, 1975, p. 563.

Two Case Histories—paragraph 6:

125. Lacey, 1974, pp. 15–18.

After-care for Skin—paragraph 4:

126. Jelinek, 1971, pp. 68–74.

After-care for Skin—paragraph 6:

127. Georgette Klinger, the skin care authority, notes that she is seeing "a tremendous increase" in acne in adult women, often "when they are going on and off the birth control pill." Her advice is:
    —Don't squeeze
    —Don't use lanolin-based or mineral oil products
    —Avoid make-up, or use a water-based foundation
    —Have your skin professionally steamed and cleaned at a skin-care salon if you can.
G. Klinger, "Pimples are not just for teenagers: a look at adult skin acne," press release.

After-care for Skin—paragraph 10:

128. Jelinek, 1971, pp. 68–74.

129. W. C. Ellerbroek, "Oral contraceptives and malignant melanoma," *Journal of the American Medical Association* 206:649–650 (1968).

After-care for Skin—paragraph 14:

130. H. Balin, "Oral contraceptives," *American Family Physician* 13:109–116 (1976).

131. D. E. D. Jones, and D. R. Halbert, "Oral contraceptives: clinical problems and choices," *American Family Practice* 12: 115–123 (1975).

132. "Oral contraceptives," *Medical Letter* 16:37–39 (1974).

133. R. A. Pattillo, "Drug and patient matching for safer oral contraception," *Drug Therapy*, Apr. 1975, pp. 105–112.

134. "Side effect profile may guide many women on pill," *Medical Tribune*, Feb. 2, 1977, p. 6.

NUTRITION AND THE PILL—ADDITIONAL READINGS

135. J. E. Leklem et al., "Metabolism of tryptophan and niacin in oral contraceptive users receiving controlled intakes of vitamin B_6," *American Journal of Clinical Nutrition* 28:146–156 (1975).

136. B. Luke, "Think 'nutrition' if she's on the pill," *R N Magazine*, Mar. 1976, pp. 33–38.

137. B. Shane and S. F. Contractor, "Assessment of vitamin B_6 status, studies on pregnant women and oral contraceptive users," *American Journal of Clinical Nutrition* 28:729–747 (1975).

138. Shojania, 1975, p. 1198.

139. J. L. Smith et al., "Effects of oral contraceptive steroids on vitamin and lipid levels in serum," *American Journal of Clinical Nutrition* 28:371–376 (1975).

140. V. Wynn and J. W. H. Doar, "Some effects of oral contraceptives on carbohydrate metabolism," *Lancet*, Oct. 11, 1969, pp. 761–765.

141. V. Wynn et al., "Fasting serum triglyceride, cholesterol, and lipo-protein levels during oral-contraceptive therapy," *Lancet*, Oct. 11, 1969, pp. 756–760.

142. P. W. Adams et al., "Vitamin B_6, depression and oral contraception," *Lancet* 2:516–517 (1974).

143. P. Corfman, Metabolic effects of oral contraceptives. Unpublished paper.

Chapter 11: Help for Post-Pill Menstrual Problems

Paragraph 1:

1. Rock, 1963.

2. J. Rock, *Contraceptive methods for global control of population.* Presented at Tufts-New England Medical Center, Jan. 31, 1967.

3. J. Rock, "Let's be honest about the pill," *Journal of the American Medical Association* 192:401 (1965).

4. M. J. Whitelaw, V. F. Nola and C. F. Kalman, "Irregular menses, amenorrhea and infertility following synthetic progestational agents," *Journal of the American Medical Association* 195:780–782 (1966).

5. Nelson hearings, 1970, Vol. I, pp. 6013–6015.

Paragraph 5:
6. D. C. Marcourt, "A new synthetic agent for the induction of ovulation," *Medical Journal of Australia*, Apr. 1974, pp. 631–632.
7. R. P. Shearman, "Progress in the investigation and treatment of anovulation," *American Journal of Obstetrics and Gynecology* 103:444 (1969).
8. R. P. Shearman, *Induction of ovulation* (Springfield, Ill.: Charles C. Thomas, 1969).
9. J. C. Marshall, P. I. Reed and H. Gordon, "Luteinizing hormone secretion in patients presenting with post-oral contraceptive amenorrhea," *Clinical Endocrinology* 5:131–143 (1976).
10. R. E. Evrand et al., "Amenorrhea following oral contraception," *American Journal of Obstetrics and Gynecology* 124:88 (1976).
11. D. T. Janerich et al., "Fertility patterns after discontinuation of use of oral contraceptives," *Lancet* 1:1051–1053 (1976).
Paragraph 6:
12. R. P. Rankin, "Prolonged anovulation subsequent to oral progestins," *American Journal of Obstetrics and Gynecology* 103:919–924 (1969).
Paragraph 8:
13. R. Jewelewicz, "Management of infertility resulting from anovulation," *American Journal of Obstetrics and Gynecology* 122:909–920 (1975).
14. J. E. Tyson et al., "Neuroendocrine dysfunction in galactorrhea-amenorrhea after oral contraceptive use," *Obstetrics and Gynecology* 46:1–11 (1975).
Nutritional Aids for Amenorrhea—paragraph 16:
15. G. G. Brooks and M. R. Butcalis, "Amenorrhea following oral contraception," *American Journal of Obstetrics and Gynecology* 124:88–91 (1976).
16. M. E. Lane, "Contraception for adolescents," *Family Planning Perspectives* 5:19–20 (1973).
17. R. B. Shearin, "Contraception for adolescents," *American Family Physician* 13:117–122 (1976).

Dr. Shearin lays out the following specific guidelines for prescribing oral contraceptives:

1. There should be evidence of a mature hypothalamic-pituitary-ovarian axis (regular cycles for two years).

2. Complete blood count, liver/thyroid function tests, chemical profile and glucose tolerance tests should be obtained.

3. A low-estrogen pill should be chosen.

4. The patient should be followed at one, three, six and twelve months for the first year: if problems develop, the oral contraceptive should be discontinued.

Nutritional Aids for Amenorrhea—paragraph 17:
18. Vessey, 1976.

Nutritional Aids for Amenorrhea—paragraph 21:

19. R. W. Kistner, "Sequential use of clomiphene citrate and human menopausal gonadotropin in ovulation induction," *Fertility and Sterility* 27:72–82 (1976).

Post-pill Menstrual Cramps—paragraph 5:

20. J. E. Jelinek, "Cutaneous side effects of oral contraceptives," *Archives of Dermatology* 101:181–186 (1970).

Post-pill Menstrual Cramps—paragraph 9:

21. E. R. Novak, G. S. Jones and H. W. Jones, *Novak's Textbook of Gynecology,* 9th ed. (Baltimore: Williams & Wilkins, 1975), pp. 725–726.

Post-pill Menstrual Cramps—paragraph 10:

22. Novak, 1975, p. 724.

Post-pill Menstrual Cramps—paragraph 13:

23. Novak, 1975, p. 722.

Calcium—paragraph 1:

24. J. Prensky, *Healing yourself* (Seattle, Wash.: Healing Yourself Press, 1976).

Calcium—paragraph 6:

25. H. L. Snider and D. F. Dietman, "Pyridoxine therapy for premenstrual acne," *Archives of Dermatology* 110:130 (1974).

Calcium—paragraph 7:

26. *Ob/Gyn News,* Dec. 1976.

Patent Medicines, Herbal Teas, and Ginseng—paragraph 2:

27. D. McCarthy, "Staying loose with menstrual cramps," *Wellbeing: a healing magazine* # 7, Dec. 1975, pp. 35–36.

28. But as *Consumers' Research Magazine* warns in its issue for March 1977, herb teas should at best be reserved for sparing and infrequent use. Three hundred and ninety-six herbs and spices are available in the United States. Many have pharmaceutical properties, but these are little understood. With regular and repeated consumption they involve some risk of injury to the stomach and intestinal and urinary tracts, and perhaps even to the nerve centers of the brain. Diuretic teas, including juniper berries, dog grass, watermelon seed, dandelion root, bearberries, buchu and cranberries, can irritate the kidneys if used in excess, according to botanist Julia Morton at the University of Miami.

Forty-three common herbs and spices, including nutmeg, contain mind-altering agents, according to Dr. Ronald Siegel of the Los Angeles School of Medicine, University of California. Another investigator, pharmacognosist Alvin Segelman at Rutgers, urges caution in the use of sassafras, watermelon seeds, juniper berries, trailing arbutus, yellow dock, alfalfa and blueberry leaves.

So-called terpenes, which include valerian, fennel, camomile, eucalyptus, mint, and rosemary, may cause irritation of the kidneys and bladder, act as depressants or induce abortion. Pennyroyal, savin, rue, tansy and nutmeg may all have abortion-inducing properties at dose levels high enough to also produce vomiting, pain and diarrhea.

All told, many of the so-called menstrual teas do have properties which either sedate or unblock the uterus, and some cause abortion at high dosages. Some have soothing or stimulating effects on the nervous system as well. In short they are drugs, and should not be taken regularly.

It's not a good idea to get hooked on a lot of herbal tea. More than four to six cups daily of ordinary tea is also inadvisable, for it may deplete thiamine, causing weakness and lassitude.

Exercise and Body Care—paragraph 1:
29. Boston Women's Health Book Collective, *Our bodies, ourselves,* 2nd ed. (N.Y.: Simon & Schuster, 1976), p. 119.
Exercise and Body Care—paragraph 3:
30. Craig, *Miss Craig's 21-day shape-up program* (N.Y.: Random House, 1968).
31. H. Kraus, *Backache, stress and tension* (N.Y.: Pocket Books, 1969).
Exercise and Body Care—paragraph 4:
32. A. Michele, *Orthotherapy* (N.Y.: Evans, 1971).
Exercise and Body Care—paragraph 6:
33. Kraus, 1969, p. 41.
Exercise and Body Care—paragraph 7:
34. Kraus, 1969, p. 23.
Physician Remedies for Premenstrual Tension and Edema—paragraph 1:
35. Novak, 1975, p. 727.
Physician Remedies for Premenstrual Tension and Edema—paragraph 2:
36. J. F. Kuhl et al., "Circadian and lower frequency rhythms in male grip strength and body weight," in: M. Ferin et al., eds., *Biorhythms and human reproduction* (N.Y.: Wiley, 1974), pp. 529–548.
37. G. G. Luce, *Biological rhythms in human and animal physiology* (N.Y.: Dover, 1971).
38. M. H. Smolensky et al., "Secondary rhythms related to hormonal changes in the menstrual cycle: special reference to allergology," in: Ferin, 1974, pp. 287–306.
39. R. A. Harkness, "Variations in testosterone excretion by man," in: Ferin, 1974, pp. 469–478.
Physician Remedies for Premenstrual Tension and Edema—paragraph 5:
40. Novak, 1975, p. 728.

BIRTH CONTROL: ALTERNATIVES TO THE PILL

1. C. Tietze and S. Lewit, "Mortality and fertility control," presented at the 1st National Medical Conference on the Safety of Fertility Control, Chicago, Illinois, March 7–9, 1977.

2. "Palaver over patient package inserts," *Patient Care*, Feb. 1, 1977, p. 22.

3. Christopher Tietze, personal communication, Feb. 1977.

Chapter 12: Pain and Perforation: The Inside Story of the IUD

Paragraph 2:

1. H. J. Davis, *Intrauterine devices for contraception: the IUD* (Baltimore: Williams & Wilkins, 1971).

2. A. L. Southam, "Historical review of intra-uterine devices," in: S. J. Segal, A. L. Southam and D. Shaffer, eds., *Intrauterine contraception. Proceedings of the 2nd International Conference, New York, Oct 2–3, 1964* (Amsterdam: Excerpta Medica, 1965), pp. 3–5.

3. A. L. Southam, "Scale of use, safety and impact of birth control methods," *Contraception* 8:1–11 (1973).

How It Works:

4. H. W. Hawk, "Investigations of the anti-fertility effect of intra-uterine devices in the ewe," *Journal of Reproductive Fertility* 14:49–59 (1967).

5. H. W. Hawk, H. H. Conley and T. H. Brinsfield, "Studies on the antifertility effect of intra-uterine devices in the cow," *Fertility and Sterility* 19:411–418 (1968).

6. R. J. Gerrits, H. W. Hawk and F. Stromshak, "Fertility and corpus luteum characteristics in pigs with plastic devices in the uterine lumen," *Journal of Reproductive Fertility* 17:501–508 (1968).

7. A. Cuadros et al., Scanning electron microscopy of the human endometrium under the effect of intrauterine devices. Paper presented at the 3rd International Conference on Intrauterine Contraception, Cairo, Egypt, Dec. 12–14, 1974 (Abstract).

8. D. N. Morese, W. F. Peterson and S. T. Allen, "Endometrial effects of an intrauterine contraceptive device," *Obstetrics and Gynecology* 28:323–328 (1966).

9. D. Moyer and D. Mishell, "Reactions of human endometrium to the intra-uterine foreign body. II. Long-term effects on the endometrial histology and cytology," *American Journal of Obstetrics and Gynecology* 111:66–80 (1971).

10. N. Sagiroglu and E. Sagiroglu, "Biologic mode of action of the Lippes Loop in intrauterine contraception," *American Journal of Obstetrics and Gynecology* 106:506–515 (1970).

11. N. Sagiroglu, Local effects of polyethylene IUDs in women. Paper presented at the 3rd International Conference on Intrauterine Contraception, Cairo, Egypt, Dec. 12–14, 1974 (Abstract).

Reliability—paragraph 1:
12. S. C. Huber et al., "IUDs reassessed: a decade of experience," *Population Reports: Intrauterine Devices*, Series B, No. 2, 1975, p. B-32.
13. G. P. Cernada, ed., *Taiwan family planning reader* (Taichung, Taiwan: Chinese Center for International Training in Family Planning, 1970), p. 381.
14. C. Tietze, "Evaluation of intrauterine devices. Ninth progress report of the cooperative statistical program," *Studies in Family Planning* 1:1–40 (1970).
Reliability—paragraph 2:
15. R. P. Bernard, "Factors governing IUD performance," *American Journal of Public Health* 61:559–567 (1971).
Reliability—paragraph 4:
16. Huber, 1975, p. B-33.
Reliability—paragraph 5:
17. M. E. Lane, R. Arceo and A. J. Sobrero, "Successful use of the diaphragm and jelly by a young population: report of a clinical study," *Family Planning Perspectives* 8:81–86 (1976).
Safety:
18. Huber, 1975, p. B-38.
19. L. Andolesk, "The 'M'-IUD: a four-year follow-up study at Ljubljana," presented at the 101st Annual Meeting of the American Public Health Association, San Francisco, California, Nov. 4–8, 1973.
20. Pathfinder Fund, International IUD Programme (Report of the special meeting of the medical advisory committee held May 26, 1970), Nov. 12, 1970.
21. P. Snowden, P. Eckstein and D. Hawkins, "Social and medical factors in the use and effectiveness of IUDs," *Journal of Biomedical Science* 5:31–49 (1973).
22. J. Jennings, "Report of the safety and efficacy of the Dalkon Shield and other IUDs." Prepared by the ad hoc Obstetric-Gynecology Advisory Committee to the United States Food and Drug Administration, Oct. 29–30, 1974 (Mimeo).
23. United States Department of Health, Education and Welfare. Center for Disease Control, "IUD safety: report of a nationwide physician survey," *Morbidity and Mortality* 23:226–231 (1974).
24. Mortality rates associated with the pill have been revised substantially upward since the date of the FDA's 1974 report, primarily because new conditions such as fatal liver tumors, heart attacks and cardiovascular disease have now been recognized as pill side-effects.

According to Valerie Beral's analysis of the World Health Organization's statistics for 1958–1975:

"The actual excess annual mortality from all non-rheumatic cardio-vascular disease may be 20 per 100,000 women [pill-

users] aged 15–44. This excess is substantial when compared with mortality rates of 70 per 100,000 of all causes, and 1 per 100,000 of all causes associated with child-bearing . . ."
Beral, 1976, p. 1051.

25. S. M. Keeny and G. P. Cernada, "Taiwan," *Country Profiles,* 1970.

26. S. S. Ratnam and J. C. K. Yin, "Translocation of Lippes Loop: the missing loop," *British Medical Journal* 1:612–614 (1968).

27. Tietze, 1970, pp. 1–40.

28. D. R. Mishell, "Current status of contraceptive steroids and intrauterine device," *Clinical Obstetrics and Gynecology* 17: 35–51 (1974).

29. S. S. Ratnam and S. S. Tow, "Translocation of the loop," in: D. Wolfers, ed., *Post-partum intra-uterine contraception in Singapore* (Amsterdam: Excerpta Medica, 1970), pp. 134–157.

30. A. W. Rudel, F. A. Kincl and M. R. Henzl, *Birth control: contraception and abortion* (N.Y.: Macmillan, 1973), pp. 154–185.

31. F. D. Scutchfield and N. W. Long, "Perforation of the uterus with the Lippes Loop: epidemiological analysis," *Journal of the American Medical Association* 208:2335–2336 (1969).

32. Rudel, 1973, pp. 154–185.

33. S. Koetswang, "Laparoscopic removal of a perforated Copper T IUD: a case report," *Contraception* 7:327–332 (1973).

34. G. Oster and M. P. Salgo, "The copper intrauterine device and its mode of action," *New England Journal of Medicine* 293:432–438 (1975).

Pregnant with an IUD—paragraph 1:

35. Huber, 1975, p. B-33.

Pregnant with an IUD—paragraph 9:

36. M. P. Vessey et al., "Outcome of pregnancy in women using intrauterine device," *Lancet* 1:495–498 (1974).

Pregnant with an IUD—paragraph 10:

37. R. M. Shine and J. F. Thompson, "The in situ IUD and pregnancy outcome," *American Journal of Obstetrics and Gynecology* 119:124–130 (1974).

Pregnant with an IUD—paragraph 11:

38. J. Lippes and S. S. Ogra, "The loop, age 7: with five significant years of observation," *International Journal of Fertility* 13:444–452 (1965).

39. A. J. Sobrero, "Intrauterine devices in clinical practice," *Family Planning Perspectives* 3:16–24 (1971).

40. World Health Organization, *Intra-uterine devices: physiological and clinical aspects* (Geneva: World Health Organization, 1968) (Technical Reports Series, No. 397).

41. L. B. Tyrer, "The intrauterine device—a technical bulletin

prepared by the American College of Obstetricians and Gynecologists," presented at the United States Food and Drug Administration hearing regarding the Dalkon Shield and other intrauterine devices, Rockville, Maryland, August 22, 1974.

Pregnant with an IUD—paragraph 13:

42. H. J. Tatum, "Contraceptive practices and extrauterine pregnancy: a realistic perspective," presented at the First National Medical Conference on the Safety of Fertility Control, Chicago, Illinois, March 6–9, 1977.

The Lippes Loop and the Dalkon Shield—paragraph 1:

43. Jennings, 1974.

44. P. B. Mead, J. S. Beecham and J. V. S. Maeck, "Incidence of infections associated with the intrauterine contraceptive device in an isolated community," *American Journal of Obstetrics and Gynecology* 125:79–82 (1976).

The Lippes Loop and the Dalkon Shield—paragraph 4:

45. "Bringing birth control to millions," *Medical World News*, Oct. 21, 1966, p. 103.

The Lippes Loop and the Dalkon Shield—paragraph 6:

46. Seaman, *The doctors' case against the pill*, p. 29.

The Lippes Loop and the Dalkon Shield—paragraph 9:

47. L. Wan, paper presented at the IUD conference held at the New York Academy of Medicine, March 17, 1974.

48. C. C. Chang and H. J. Tatum, "Effect of intrauterine copper wire on resorption of fetuses in rats," *Contraception* 11:79–84 (1975).

49. C. C. Chang, "A study of the antifertility effect of intrauterine copper," *Contraception* 1:265–270 (1970).

50. H. Tatum, "The 'T' intrauterine contraceptive device and recent advances in hormonal anticonceptional therapy," presented at the 4th Northeastern Obstetrics and Gynecology Congress, Bahia, Brazil, Oct. 4–9, 1968.

51. H. Timonen, "Hysterographic studies with the copper T (TCu 200) in situ," *Contraception* 6:513–521 (1972).

52. Christopher Tietze and Howard Tatum, personal communication, 1976.

The IUD and Infection—paragraph 2:

53. Tietze, 1970, pp. 1–40.

The IUD and Infection—paragraph 3:

54. N. H. Wright, "Acute pelvic inflammatory disease in an indigent population: an estimate of its incidence and relationship to methods of contraception," *American Journal of Obstetrics and Gynecology* 101:976–990 (1968).

The IUD and Infection—paragraph 4:

55. W. I. Faulkner and H. W. Ory, "Intrauterine devices and acute pelvic inflammatory disease," *Journal of the American Medical Association* 237:1851–1853 (1976).

56. S. D. Targum and N. H. Wright, "Association of the intrauterine device and pelvic inflammatory disease: a retrospective pilot study," *American Journal of Epidemiology* 100: 262–271 (1974).

57. "Turbo-ovarian abscesses seen increasing in women with IUDs," *Medical Tribune*, Jan. 12, 1977, p. 31.

The IUD and Infection—paragraph 8:

58. Novak, 1975, pp. 404–405.

59. Boston Women's Health Book Collective, 1976, p. 141.

Pelvic Inflammatory Disease (PID)—paragraph 7:

60. H. J. Tatum et al., "The Dalkon Shield controversy: structural and bacteriological studies of IUD tails," *Journal of the American Medical Association* 231:711–717 (1975).

Pelvic Inflammatory Disease (PID)—paragraph 10:

61. Novak, 1975, p. 405.

Pelvic Inflammatory Disease (PID)—paragraph 15:

62. Novak, 1975, p. 404.

The IUD and Perforations—paragraph 6:

63. Charles Debrovner, personal communication, 1976.

Who Should Not Get an IUD—paragraph 2:

64. Boston Women's Health Book Collective, 1976, p. 199.

When to Get an IUD—paragraph 1:

65. M. Zuckerman, "The IUD in family planning," *The Female Patient*, July 1976, pp. 17–19.

When to Get an IUD—paragraph 4:

66. Huber, 1975, p. B-29.

When to Get an IUD—paragraph 5:

67. G. I. Zatuchni, "Overview of program: two-year experience," in: G. I. Zatuchni, ed., *Post-partum family planning: a report on the international program.* (N.Y.: McGraw-Hill, 1970), pp. 30–88.

New Models—paragraph 3:

68. IUD conference held at the New York Academy of Medicine, 1974.

New Models—paragraph 4:

69. R. L. Kleinman, ed., *Intrauterine contraception.* 3rd ed. (London: International Planned Parenthood Federation, 1973).

New Models—paragraph 5:

70. "Differences in IUD data by parity vanish when 'confidence levels' are reconciled," *Ob/Gyn News* 9:2, 60–61 (1974).

How Long Can an IUD Be Kept?—paragraph 4:

71. "Pathologic changes reported in study of women using IUDs," *Medical Tribune*, Oct. 14, 1968, p. 12.

How Long Can an IUD Be Kept?—paragraph 10:

72. IUD conference held at the New York Academy of Medicine, 1974.

Two Women's Experiences—paragraph 1:

73. A. Clark, "Me and my diaphragm: love at third sight," *Country Women*, No. 19, March 1976, pp. 50–51.

Chapter 13: The Diaphragm: Queen of Contraception

Paragraph 1:
1. R. S. Ebenstein, "The diaphragm is back in town," *Cosmopolitan*, June 1976, pp. 148–150.
2. Clark, 1976, pp. 50–51.
3. B. K. Rothman and M. L. Storch, "Update on birth control," *Woman's Day*, June 1976, pp. 36–38, 132.
The Sanger Research Bureau Study—paragraph 4:
4. Lane, 1976.
5. J. Wortman, "The diaphragm and other intravaginal barriers —a review," *Population Reports: Barrier Methods*, Series H, No. 4, Jan. 1976.
Getting a Diaphragm—paragraph 2:
6. M. Vessey and P. Wiggins, "Use-effectiveness of the diaphragm in a selected family planning clinic in the United Kingdom," *Contraception* 9:15–21 (1974).
Getting a Diaphragm—paragraph 3:
7. N. S. Greenfield, *First do no harm* (N.Y.: Sun River Press, 1976).
Getting a Diaphragm—paragraph 7:
8. Boston Women's Health Book Collective, 1976, p. 200.
Types of Diaphragm—paragraph 4:
9. D. P. Swartz and R. L. Vande Wiele, *Methods of conception control: a programmed instruction course* (Raritan, N.J.: Ortho Pharmaceutical Corp., 1972), frames 100–124.
10. S. Okrent, *A clinical guide to the intrauterine device and vaginal diaphragm* (Wantagh, N.Y.: pub. by author, 1974).
Types of Diaphragm—paragraph 5:
11. Clark, 1976, p. 50.
Types of Diaphragm—paragraph 10:
12. Wortman, 1976, pp. H-58–60.
Use of the Diaphragm—paragraph 2:
13. N. E. Himes, *Medical history of contraception* (N.Y.: Schocken Books, 1970), pp. 170–185, 249, 252, 305, 391.
Use of the Diaphragm—paragraph 3:
14. S. Lobel, *Conception, contraception: a new look* (N.Y.: McGraw-Hill, 1974), pp. 25, 26, 121, 141.
Use of the Diaphragm—paragraph 4:
15. V. E. Johnson and W. H. Masters, "Intravaginal contraceptive study. Phase I. Anatomy," *Western Journal of Obstetrics and Gynecology* 70:202–207 (1962).
Use of the Diaphragm—paragraph 6:
16. Lane, 1976, p. 84.
Health Advantages and Drawbacks:
17. D. W. Beacham and W. D. Beacham, "Contraception," in D. W. Beacham and W. D. Beacham, *Synopsis of gynecology* (St. Louis: Mosby, 1972), pp. 351–366.

18. Melamed, 1969.
The Sanger Clinic Success Story—paragraph 2:
19. Lane, 1976, p. 81.
Multiple Intercourse and the Diaphragm—paragraph 2:
20. Aquiles J. Sobrero, interview, May 31, 1976.
Multiple Intercourse and the Diaphragm—paragraph 9:
21. Ames Women's Community Health Project, "The Diaphragm method: responsible birth control," unpublished draft.
Diaphragms Used Without Spermicides—paragraph 1:
22. R. Menninger, "Further follow-up on the jellyless diaphragm," *CoEvolution Quarterly*, No. 10, June 1976, p. 107.
23. On May 6, 1977, FDA announced the recall of 86,000
Koro-Flex Arcing diaphragms because of a defect wherein the
central disc is apt to separate from the rim. All sizes produced
from June through September 1976 were recalled. Lot numbers
are F-6, G-6, H-6, and I-6, printed on the edge. The manufacturer, Holland-Rantos in Piscataway, New Jersey, is further
asking that *any* apparently defective Koro-Flex Arcing diaphragm be returned, at the point of purchase, for refund or
replacement. The diaphragms were distributed nationwide
through Planned Parenthood clinics (70%); surgical supply
dealers (10%); pharmacies and doctors (10%); and hospitals
(10%). Aside from the recalled lots, you can figure out when
your diaphragm from Holland-Rantos was manufactured. The
months are assigned letters from A to L (January-A, February-B,
etc.), and the year is indicated by the digit (1975-5, 1976-6,
etc.).
Diaphragm Insertion—paragraph 1:
24. Wortman, 1976, p. H-63.
Diaphragm Insertion—paragraph 3:
25. Ames Women's Community Health Project.
Diaphragm Care—paragraph 1:
26. V. H. Parker, *The illustrated birth control manual* (N.Y.:
Cadillac, 1957), pp. 189–229.
27. J. Peel, "The Hull family survey," *Journal of Biosocial
Science* 4:333–346 (1972).
28. J. Peel and M. Potts, "Diaphragms and caps," in: J. Peel
and M. Potts, *Textbook of contraceptive practice* (Cambridge:
Cambridge University Press, 1969), pp. 63–73.
29. H. Wright, *Contraceptive technique* (London: J. and A.
Churchill, 1968).
Diaphragm Care—paragraph 6:
30. Vessey and Wiggins, 1974, pp. 15–21.
Diaphragm Care—paragraph 7:
31. Lane, 1976, p. 86.
Diaphragm Care—paragraph 8:
32. H. Burkhalter of the Ames Women's Community Health
Project.

Chapter 14: Gone but Not Forgotten: The Cervical Cap

Paragraph 10:
1. Lady R.B. is correct. The U.S. product is called Tassaways.
The Cap Then and Now—paragraph 1:
2. Wortman, 1976, p. H-70.
3. B. E. Finch, "Balls, feathers and caps," in: B. E. Finch and H. Green. *Contraception through the ages* (Springfield, Ill.: Charles C. Thomas, 1963), pp. 38–45.
4. A. F. Guttmacher, *Pregnancy, birth and family planning* (N.Y.: Viking, 1973), pp. 287–289.
5. Himes, 1970, pp. 170–185, 249, 252, 305, 391.
6. Finch, 1963, pp. 38–45.
7. Himes, 1970.
8. L. L. Langley, *Contraception* (Stroudsburg, Pennsylvania: Dowden, Hutchinson and Ross, 1973), pp. 244–245.
9. Peel, 1969, pp. 62–73.
The Cap Then and Now—paragraph 6:
10. Wortman, 1976, pp. H-71 and 72.
The Cap Then and Now—paragraph 7:
11. Wortman, 1976, p. H-70.
The Cap Then and Now—paragraph 8:
12. C. Tietze, H. Lehfeldt and H. G. Liebmann, "The effectiveness of the cervical cap as a contraceptive method," *American Journal of Obstetrics and Gynecology* 66:904–908 (1953).
The Cap Then and Now—paragraph 10:
13. E. Grafenberg and R. L. Dickinson, "Conception controlled by plastic cervical cap," *Western Journal of Surgery* 52:335 (1944).
The Cap Then and Now—paragraph 12:
14. Planned Parenthood Federation of America. Medical Committee. *Methods of birth control in the United States* (N.Y.: Planned Parenthood Federation of America, 1972).
The Cap Versus the Diaphragm—paragraph 1:
15. M. Sein, "Flexible plastic contraceptive cervical caps: an ideal contraceptive for developing countries," unpublished, 1975.
The Cap Versus the Diaphragm—paragraph 13:
16. H. Lehfeldt, "Cervical cap," in: M. S. Calderone, *Manual of family planning and contraceptive practice* (Baltimore: Williams and Wilkins, 1970), pp. 368–375.
17. Hans Lehfeldt, personal communication, 1976.
The Cap Versus the Diaphragm—paragraph 18:
18. Wortman, 1976, p. H-72.

Chapter 15: Vaginal Spermicides: The Contraceptive That Improves Vaginal Health

Paragraph 1:
1. Himes, 1970.

2. J. R. Baker, *The chemical control of contraception* (London: Chapman and Hall, 1935).

Mary Ware Dennett and Margaret Sanger—paragraph 1:

3. L. Cisler, "A campaign to repeal legal restrictions on non-prescription contraceptives: the case of New York," in: M. H. Redford, G. W. Duncan and D. J. Prager, eds., *The condom: increasing utilization in the United States* (San Francisco: San Francisco Press, 1974), p. 83.

Contraception for Teen-agers—paragraph 1:

4. Faulkner, 1976.

Contraception for Teen-agers—paragraph 5:

5. R. Gilbert and V. G. Matthews, "Young males' attitudes toward condom use," in: Redford, 1974, pp. 164–172.

6. W. W. Darrow, "Attitudes toward condom use and the acceptance of venereal disease prophylactics," in: Redford, 1974, pp. 173–185.

7. P. G. Veerhusen, "The role of the condom in Planned Parenthood programs," in: Redford, 1974, pp. 186–193.

8. D. S. Solomon and R. J. Pion, "Pharmacists and condoms: a preliminary view from Hawaii," in: Redford, 1974, pp. 194–198.

9. M. Lubin-Finkel and D. Finkel, "Sexual and contraceptive knowledge, attitudes and behavior of male adolescents," *Family Planning Perspectives* 7:256–260 (1975).

Contraceptive Advertising—paragraph 1:

10. S. A. Baker, "Advertising male contraceptives," in: Redford, 1974, pp. 115–130.

11. L. R. Brenner, "Condommunications," in: Redford, 1974, pp. 131–145.

12. T. Knightlinger, "The problem of condom ads on radio and TV," in: Redford, 1974, pp. 146–157.

Contraceptive Advertising—paragraph 3:

13. R. J. Cook, "State laws regulating condoms," in: Redford, 1974, p. 67.

14. Cisler, 1974, p. 84.

15. Solomon, 1976, pp. 194–198.

Foam Compared to Other Contraceptives—paragraph 2:

16. R. Belsky, "Vaginal contraceptives: a time for reappraisal," *Population Reports: Barrier Methods*, Series H, No. 3, p. H-40, Jan. 1975.

Foam Compared to Other Contraceptives—paragraph 3:

17. L. F. Bushnell, "Aerosol foam: a practical and effective method of contraception," *Pacific Medicine and Surgery* 73: 353–355 (1965).

18. R. K. Kleppinger, "A vaginal contraceptive foam," *Pennsylvania Medical Journal* 63:31–34 (1965).

19. C. Tietze and S. Lewit, "Comparison of three contraceptive methods: diaphragm with jelly or cream, vaginal foam, and jelly/cream alone," *Journal of Sex Research* 3:295–311 (1967).

20. M. E. Panizgua, H. W. Valiant and C. J. Gamble, "Field

trial of contraceptive foam in Puerto Rico," *Journal of the American Medical Association* 177:125–129 (1961).

21. A. J. Sobrero, "Evaluation of a new contraceptive," *Fertility and Sterility* 11:518–524 (1960).

Foam Compared to Other Contraceptives—paragraph 4:

22. J. B. Martin, "Tolerance to repeated application of a foam contraceptive in the human vagina," *Clinical Medicine* 69(9) (Sept. 1962).

Foam Compared to Other Contraceptives—paragraph 5:

23. V. E. Johnson and W. H. Masters, "Intravaginal contraceptive study. Phase II: Physiology (a direct test for protective potential)," *Western Journal of Surgery, Obstetrics and Gynecology* 71:144–153 (1963).

Foam Compared to Other Contraceptives—paragraph 10:

24. V. E. Johnson, W. H. Masters and K. C. Lewis, "The physiology of intravaginal contraceptive behavior," in: Calderone, 1970, pp. 232–245.

25. Johnson, 1963.

Recent Studies of Foam—paragraph 1:

26. Howard Osofsky, personal communication, 1974.

Recent Studies of Foam—paragraph 3:

27. G. S. Bernstein, "Physiological aspects of vaginal contraception: a review," *Contraception* 9:333–345 (1974).

28. G. S. Bernstein, "Clinical effectiveness of an aerosol contraceptive foam," *Contraception* 3:37–43 (1971).

29. G. S. Bernstein, "Conventional methods of contraception: condom, diaphragm and vaginal foam," *Clinical Obstetrics and Gynecology* 17:21–33 (1974).

30. Bushnell, 1965.

31. Kleppinger, 1965.

32. G. Carpenter and J. B. Martin, "Clinical evaluation of a vaginal contraceptive foam," in: A. J. Sobrero and C. McKee, eds., *Advances in planned parenthood*, Vol. 5. *Proceedings of the Seventh Annual Meeting of the American Association of Planned Parenthood Physicians, San Francisco, California, Apr. 9–10, 1969* (N.Y.: Excerpta Medica, 1970) (International Congress Series No. 207), pp. 170–175.

Recent Studies of Foam—paragraph 5:

33. N. B. Ryder, "Contraceptive failure in the United States," *Family Planning Perspectives* 5:133–142 and Table 6, p. 140 (1973).

The Effects of Spermicides—paragraph 4:

34. V. Miller, P. A. Klavano and E. Csonka, "Absorption, distribution and excretion of phenylmercuric acetate," *Toxicology and Applied Pharmacology* 2:344–352 (1960).

35. N. Nelson et al., "Hazards of mercury: special report to the Secretary's Pesticide Advisory Committee, U.S. Department of Health, Education and Welfare, Nov. 1970," *Environmental Research* 4:1–69 (1971).

36. J. M. Stryker, S. B. Sparber and A. M. Goldberg, "Subtle consequences of methylmercury exposure: behavioral deviations in offspring of treated mothers," *Science* 177:621–623 (1972).

37. J. Wilson, *Birth defects and the environment* (N.Y.: Academic Press, 1973).

38. U. Murakami, Y. Kameyama and T. Kato, "Effects of a vaginally applied contraceptive with phenylmercuric acetate upon developing embryos and their mother animals," in: *Annual Report of the Research Institute of Environmental Medicine* (Japan: Nagoya University, 1955), pp. 88–89.

39. U.S. Food and Drug Administration, "Procedures for classification of over-the-counter drugs," *Federal Register* 37:9464–9475 (May 11, 1972).

40. U.S. Food and Drug Administration, "Over-the-counter contraceptives and other vaginal drug products," *Federal Register* 38:12840–12842 (May 16, 1974).

41. U.S. Food and Drug Administration, Advisory Committee, *Proceedings*, Jan. 1975.

42. *The Spokeswoman*, Oct. 15, 1973.

The Effects of Spermicides—paragraph 6:

43. Transcript of testimony by Dr. Elizabeth Connell, Nelson hearings, Feb. 24, 1970.

Foam, VD, and Vaginitis—paragraph 1:

44. J. B. Lucas, "The national venereal disease problem," *Medical Clinics of North America* 56:1073–1086 (1972).

45. W. H. Smartt and A. G. Lighter, "The gonorrhea epidemic and its control," *Medical Aspects of Human Sexuality* 5:96–115 (1971).

46. P. F. Sparling, "Antibiotic resistance in Neisseria gonorrhea," *Medical Clinics of North America* 56:1133–1144 (1972).

47. P. F. Sparling, "Penicillin," in: *Epidemic venereal disease. Proceedings of the Second International Venereal Disease Symposium, St. Louis, Missouri, 1972.* (N.Y.: Pfizer, Inc., 1973), pp. 58–63.

Foam, VD, and Vaginitis—paragraph 5:

48. O. H. Bolch, Jr. and J. C. Warren, "In vitro effects of Emko on Neisseria gonorrheae and Trichomonas vaginalis," *American Journal of Obstetrics and Gynecology* 115:1145–1148 (1973).

49. M. E. Cowan and G. E. Cree, "A note on the susceptibility of N. Gonorrhoeae to contraceptive agent Nonyl-P," *British Journal of Venereal Diseases* 49:65–66 (1973).

50. M. E. Cowan, "Prophylaxis in the venereal diseases," *Medical Clinics of North America* 56:1211–1216 (1972).

51. M. E. Cowan, C. J. Nickens and H. Balisky, "Pro-con vaginal contraceptives as venereal disease prophylactic agents," presented at the Eleventh Annual Meeting of the American

Association of Planned Parenthood Physicians, Houston, Texas, April 11–13, 1973.

52. M. E. Cowan et al., "Studies on development of a vaginal preparation providing both prophylaxis against venereal disease, other genital infections and contraception. I. Venereal disease prophylaxis, past experience, present status and plans for future studies," *Military Medicine* 138:88–91 (1973).

53. T. Y. Lee et al., "The potential impact of chemical prophylaxis on the incidence of gonorrhoeae," *British Journal of Venereal Diseases* 48:376–380 (1972).

54. B. Singh, "Anti-VD effect of spermicides. [Response to Letter to the Editor]," *Medical Aspects of Human Sexuality* 7:268 (1973).

55. B. Singh, J. C. Cutler and H. M. D. Utidjian, "Studies on the development of a vaginal preparation providing both prophylaxis against venereal disease and other genital infections and contraception. II: Effect in vitro of vaginal contraceptive and noncontraceptive preparations on Treponema pallidum and Neisseria gonorrhoeae," *British Journal of Venereal Diseases* 48:57–64 (1972).

56. B. Singh, J. C. Cutler and H. M. D. Utidjian, "Studies of the development of a vaginal preparation providing both prophylaxis against venereal disease and other genital infections and contraception. III: In vitro effect of vaginal contraceptive and selected vaginal preparations on Candida albicans and Trichomonas vaginalis," *Contraception* 5:401–411 (1972).

Foam, VD, and Vaginitis—paragraph 6:
57. E. M. Brecher, "Women-victims of the VD rip-off," *Viva* 1:29 (1973).

Foam, VD, and Vaginitis—paragraph 8:
58. Belsky, 1975, p. H-50.

59. Balwant Singh, personal interview, Feb. 2, 1977.

Foam, VD, and Vaginitis—paragraph 9:
60. B. Singh, B. Postic and J. C. Cutler, "Virucidal effect of certain chemical contraceptives on Type 2 herpes virus," *American Journal of Obstetrics and Gynecology* 126:422–425 (1976).

Chapter 16: Working With Nature: Organic Birth Control

Paragraph 3:
1. B. Malinowski, *The sexual life of savages in north-western Melanesia* (N.Y.: Harcourt, Brace & World, 1929), pp. 168–197.

Paragraph 6:
2. I. Oyle, *The healing mind* (Milbrae, Cal.: Celestial Arts, 1974).

Making Rhythm Work—paragraph 1:
3. Soranus, *Gynaeciorum*, ed. by V. Rose (Lipsae: B. G. Teubneri, 1882).

Making Rhythm Work—paragraph 2:
4. H. Knaus, "Die periodische frucht- und unfruchtbarkeit des weibes (Periodic fertility and infertility in women)," *Zentralblatt fur Gynäkologie* 57:1393 (1933).
5. K. Ogino, "Ovulationstermin und konzeptionstermin (Ovulation day and conception day)," *Zentralblatt fur Gynäkologie* 54:464–479 (1930).

Making Rhythm Work—paragraph 3:
6. J. T. Noonan, *Contraception: a history of its treatment by the Catholic theologians and canonists* (Cambridge: Harvard Univ. Press, 1966).

Making Rhythm Work—paragraph 4:
7. L. J. Latz, *The rhythm of sterility and fertility in women* (Chicago: L. J. Latz, 1932).

Making Rhythm Work—paragraph 5:
8. C. Ross and P. T. Piotrow, "Birth control without contraceptives," *Population Report: Periodic Abstinence* Series I, No. 1, 1974, p. I-5.

The Calendar Method—paragraph 2:
9. R. G. Potter et al., "Long cycles, late ovulation, and calendar rhythm," *International Journal of Fertility* 12:127–140 (1967).

The Calendar Method—paragraph 3:
10. Ross, 1974, p. I-2.
11. "Rhythm: I. Periodic abstinence," *Child and Family* 7:290 (1968).

The Calendar Method—paragraph 4:
12. "U.S. backing rhythm test," *New York Post*, Feb. 2, 1976.

The Temperature Method, or BBT (Basal Body Temperature) —paragraph 1:
13. W. Squire, "Puerperal temperatures," *Transactions of the Obstetrical Society* (London) 9:129 (1868).
14. I. Habrecht, "Ovarian function and body temperature," *Lancet* 2:668–669 (1945).
15. P. L. Martin, "Detection of ovulation by basal temperature curve with correlating endometrial studies," *American Journal of Obstetrics and Gynecology* 46:53–62 (1943).
16. B. B. Rubenstein, "The relation of cyclic changes in human vaginal smears to body temperature and BMR," *American Journal of Physiology* 119:635–641 (1937).

The Temperature Method, or BBT (Basal Body Temperature) —paragraph 2:
17. T. T. Zuck, "The relation of basal body temperature to fertility and sterility in women," *American Journal of Obstetrics and Gynecology* 36:998–1005 (1938).
18. J. Ferin, "Détermination de la période stérile prémenstruelle par la courbe thermique (Determination of the premenstrual sterile period by means of the thermal curve)," *Bruxelles Medical* 27:2786–2793 (1947).
19. Ross, 1974, p. I-5.

The Temperature Method, or BBT (Basal Body Temperature) —paragraph 4:
20. Ross, 1974, p. I-6.
The Temperature Method, or BBT (Basal Body Temperature) —paragraph 5:
21. Ross, 1974, p. I-8.
The Cervical Mucus (Billings) Method—paragraph 4:
22. J. J. Billings, *The ovulation method* (Melbourne, Aust.: Advocate Press, 1970).
23. J. J. Billings, *Natural family planning: the ovulation method* (Collegeville, Minn.: Liturgical Press, 1973).
24. J. J. Billings and E. L. Billings, "Determination of fertile and unfertile days by the mucus pattern," in: W. A. Uricchio, ed., *Proceedings of a Research Conference on Natural Family Planning* (Wash., D.C.: Human Life Foundation, 1973).
25. "Vatican OKs a birth control test," *New York Daily News*, Feb. 16, 1976.
26. M. C. Weissmann, "A trial of the ovulation method of family planning in Tonga," *Lancet* 2:813–816 (1972).
The Cervical Mucus (Billings) Method—paragraph 5:
27. Ross, 1974, p. I-7.
Not for the Squeamish—paragraph 4:
28. A. Rosenblum and L. Jackson, *The natural birth control book* (Boston: Tao Publications, 1974).
Kosasky's Ovutimer—paragraph 1:
29. Harold Kosasky, personal communication, 1976.
Kosasky's Ovutimer—paragraph 8:
30. "Ovulation predictable within one hour in office and home," *Medical Tribune*, July 1976.
31. "Researchers claim instrument to detect time of ovulation," *Wall Street Journal*, July 13, 1976.
Lunaception—paragraph 1:
32. Lacey, 1974.
Lunaception—paragraph 3:
33. I. E. Treloar, "Variations of the human menstrual cycle through reproductive life," *International Journal of Fertility* 12:77–126 (1967).
34. Ross, 1974, p. I-3.
Lunaception—paragraph 4:
35. R. Dubos, *Man adapting* (New Haven, Conn.: Yale Univ. Press, 1965).
Lunaception—paragraph 5:
36. E. M. Dewan, "On the possibility of a perfect rhythm method of birth control by periodic light stimulation," *American Journal of Obstetrics and Gynecology* 99:1016–1019 (1967).
Lunaception—paragraph 6:
37. G. G. Luce, *Body time* (N.Y.: Pocket Books, 1976).
Lunaception—paragraph 7:
38. Lacey, 1974, p. 113.

Cosmic Birth Control—paragraph 3:
39. Rosenblum, 1974, p. 87.
40. S. Ostrander and L. Schroeder, *Psychic discoveries behind the iron curtain* (N.Y.: Prentice-Hall, 1971).
Self-observation—paragraph 4:
41. *New women's survival sourcebook* (N.Y.: Knopf, 1975).
Body Aware—paragraph 1:
42. G. Oster and S. Oster, "Self-test for ovulation and its implications in family planning," presented at the Centre Medical, Port-au-Prince, Haiti, Jan. 28, 1976.
43. G. Oster et al., "Cyclic variation of sialic acid content in saliva," *American Journal of Obstetrics and Gynecology* 114: 190–193 (1972).

Chapter 17: Sterilization: The Ultimate Control

Quotation:
1. Committee of the American Neurological Association for the Investigation of Eugenical Sterilization. *Eugenic sterilization: a reorientation of the problem* (N.Y.: Macmillan, 1936).
Paragraph 2:
2. E. T. Anderson, "Peritoneoscopy," *American Journal of Surgery* 35:36–39 (1937).
3. M. R. Cohen, *Laparoscopy, culdoscopy and gynecology technique and atlas* (Philadelphia: Saunders, 1970).
4. F. H. Power and A. C. Barnes, "Sterilization by means of peritoneoscopic tubal fulguration," *American Journal of Obstetrics and Gynecology* 41:1038–1043 (1941).
Paragraph 4:
5. J. Wortman and P. T. Piotrow, "Laparoscopic sterilization. II. What are the problems?" *Population Reports: Sterilization*, Series C, No. 2, 1973, p. C-17.
Paragraph 5:
6. J. Wortman and P. T. Piotrow, "Colpotomy—the vaginal approach," *Population Reports: Sterilization*, Series C, No. 3, 1973, p. C-29.
Paragraph 6:
7. R. A. Leonardo, *History of gynecology* (N.Y.: Froben Press, 1944).
8. R. W. Cali, "Operations for sterilization of the female," *Surgical Clinics of North America* 53:495–510 (1973).
Paragraph 7:
9. A. E. Garb, "A review of tubal sterilization failures," *Obstetrical and Gynecological Survey* 12:291–305 (1957).
10. K. E. Huang et al., "Experience with endoscopic tubal sterilization," in: Association for Voluntary Sterilization of the Republic of China, *Proceedings of the Asian Regional Conference on Voluntary Sterilization*, May 10–12, 1975 (Taipei, Taiwan: 1975), pp. 134–135.

11. W. Merz, "Sterilization," in: International Planned Parenthood Federation (IPPF), *Preventive Medicine and Family Planning: Proceedings of the Sixth Conference of the Europe and Middle East Region of IPPF, Copenhagen, July 1966* (London: IPPF, 1967), pp. 80–92.

12. C. A. White, "Tubal sterilization," *American Journal of Obstetrics and Gynecology* 95:38 (1966).

13. Wortman, 1973, No. 3, p. C-17.

Paragraph 8:

14. "Reversible sterilization by spring clip," *Medical Tribune,* July 7, 1976, p. 33.

15. T. Kumarasamy et al., "Spring clip tubal occlusion: a report of the first 400 cases," *Fertility and Sterility,* 26:1122–1131 (1975).

16. J. F. Hulka et al., "Conplications Committee of the American Association of Gynecological Laparoscopists, First Annual Report," *Journal of Reproductive Medicine* 10:301–306 (1973).

17. C. W. Porter and J. F. Hulka, "Female sterilization in current clinical practice," *Family Planning Perspectives* 6:30–38 (1974).

Paragraph 9:

18. Wortman, 1973, No. 2, pp. C-20 and C-21.

19. White, 1966.

20. R. L. Mueller, C. S. Scott and A. P. Bukeavich, "Puerperal laparoscopic sterilization," *Journal of Reproductive Medicine* 16:307–309 (1976).

Paragraph 15:

21. R. Wadhwa and R. McKenzie, "Complications of band-aid surgery for sterilization," *Journal of the American Medical Association* 222:1558 (1972).

22. J. Wortman, "Tubal sterilization—review of methods," *Population Reports: Sterilization,* Series C, No. 7, 1973, p. C-73.

23. E. L. Williams et al., "Subsequent course of patients sterilized by tubal ligation; consideration of hysterectomy for sterilization," *American Journal of Obstetrics and Gynecology* 1:423 (1951).

Paragraph 17:

24. P. Barglow and M. Eisner, "An evaluation of tubal ligation in Switzerland," *American Journal of Obstetrics and Gynecology* 95:1090 (1966).

25. Barglow, 1966, p. 1091.

Paragraph 18:

26. Barglow, 1966, p. 1088.

27. P. Barglow, "Pseudocyesis and psychiatric sequelae of sterilization," *Archives of General Psychiatry* 11:571–580 (1964).

Paragraph 24:

28. C. F. Westoff, "Trends in contraceptive practice: 1965–1973," *Family Planning Perspectives* 8:54 (1976).

28a. "Pill may take second place," *New York Daily News*, May 20, 1976, p. 96.
Paragraph 25:
29. J. Herman, "Controlling third world populations: forced sterilization," *Sister Courage*, Feb. 1976.
Paragraph 26:
30. J. E. Brody, "Sterilization: for women, an easier way," *New York Times*, March 24, 1976.
Paragraph 28:
31. C. Dreifus, "Sterilizing the poor," *The Progressive* 39:13–18 (1975).
Paragraph 29:
32. Dreifus, 1975, pp. 15–16.
Paragraph 31:
33. Herman, 1976, p. 2.
Paragraph 32:
34. Dreifus, 1975, p. 16.
Paragraph 35:
35. Herman, 1976.
Paragraph 38:
36. Herman, 1976.
Paragraph 40:
37. "U.S. AID sterilization program for foreign doctors: St. Louis, Pittsburgh, Baltimore," *Off Our Backs*, July/Aug. 1976, p. 24.
Paragraph 46:
38. Dreifus, 1975, p. 14.
Paragraph 49:
39. Herman, 1976.

Chapter 18: Abortion: Relief if Not Pleasure

Quotation:
1. "Columnist raps priests' claim," *Abortion Trends*, No. 12, Sept. 1976, p. 2.
Whose Right to Life?—paragraph 1:
2. J. C. Smith, "The complexity of compiling abortion statistics," *Public Health Reports* 90:502–523 (1975).
3. C. Tietze and M. C. Murstein, "Induced abortion: 1975 fact book," *Reports on Population/Family Planning*, No. 14, 1975, pp. 1–76.
Whose Right to Life?—paragraph 2:
4. International Planned Parenthood Federation, *Survey of world needs in family planning* (London: IPPF, 1974).
5. A. Klinger, "Demographic aspects of abortion," in: *International Planned Population Conference, London, Sept. 2–11, 1969*, vol. 2 (London: International Union for the Scientific Study of Population, 1969), pp. 1153–1164.

Whose Right to Life?—paragraph 3:
6. D. Fisher, "Whose 'right to life'?" *Hospital Practice* 10:11 (1975).
Definitions—paragraph 6:
7. C. C. Means, "The phoenix of abortion freedom: is a penumbral or ninth-amendment right about to rise from the nineteenth-century legislative ashes of a fourteenth-century common law liberty?" *New York Law Forum* 17:335–410 (1971).
8. H. J. Osofsky and J. D. Osofsky, eds., *The abortion experience* (Hagerstown, Maryland: Harper and Row, 1973).
9. D. Callahan, *Abortion: law, choice and morality* (N.Y.: Macmillan, 1970).
10. G. Hardin, *Mandatory motherhood* (Boston: Beacon Press, 1974).
11. L. Lader, *Abortion* (Boston: Beacon Press, 1974).
12. D. Schulder and F. Kennedy, *Abortion rap* (N.Y.: McGraw-Hill, 1971).
Definitions—paragraph 7:
13. Rae Blomberg, personal communication, 1976.
Definitions—paragraph 8:
14. J. Pakter, F. Nelson, M. S. Vigir, "Legal abortion: a half-decade of experience," *Family Planning Perspectives* 7:248–255 (1975).
15. J. Pakter, director, Bureau of Maternity Services, New York City Department of Health, cited in *Effects of New York State's liberalized abortion law*, pamphlet prepared and issued by Abortion Rights Association, Inc. (National Abortion Rights Action League).
16. Joint Program for Study of Abortion reports can be found in *Studies in Family Planning*, a periodical of The Population Council.
Definitions—paragraph 10:
17. Tietze, 1975, p. 3.
Abortion Methods—paragraph 1:
18. Tietze, 1975, p. 46.
Abortion Methods—paragraph 9:
19. S. Polgar and E. S. Fried, "The bad old days: clandestine abortion among the poor in New York City before liberalization of the abortion law," *Family Planning Perspectives* 8:125–127 (1976).
Abortion Methods—paragraph 17:
20. Malinowski, 1929, p. 197.
Abortion Methods—paragraph 19:
21. C. J. Eaton et al., "Laminaria tent as a cervical dilator prior to aspiration-type therapeutic abortion," *Obstetrics and Gynecology* 39:533–537 (1973).
22. I. M. Golditch and M. H. Glasser, "The use of laminaria tents for cervical dilation prior to vacuum aspiration abortion,"

American Journal of Obstetrics and Gynecology 119:481–485 (1974).

23. K. R. Niswander, "Laminaria tents as an aid in suction abortion," *California Medicine* 119:11–14 (1973).

24. *Consumers' Research Magazine*, March 1977, pp. 35–36. See also chap. 11, note 28, for discussion of some specific abortion-producing herbs.

Abortion Methods—paragraph 23:

25. Tietze, 1975, p. 46.

Abortion Methods—paragraph 27:

26. M. Bygdeman and S. Bergstrom, "Clinical use of prostaglandins for pregnancy termination," *Population Reports: Prostaglandins*, Series G, No. 7, 1976, p. G-65.

27. M. Bygdeman et al., "Induction of first and second trimester abortion by vaginal administration of 15-methyl-PGF₂ a methyl ester," *Obstetrics and Gynecology*, in press.

28. M. Bygdeman et al., "Outpatient postconceptional fertility control with vaginally administered 15-methyl-PGF₂ a methyl ester," *American Journal of Obstetrics and Gynecology* 124: 495–498 (1976).

29. A. L. Leader et al., "Induced abortion in the 8th–9th week of pregnancy with vaginally administered 15-methyl-PGF₂ a methyl ester," *Prostaglandins* 12:631–638 (1976).

Abortion Methods—paragraph 32:

30. Surgical abortion (dilation and evacuation) was "significantly safer" than saline or prostaglandin in the 13th to 20th weeks of pregnancy. Dilation and evacuation was 1st in safety, saline 2nd, and prostaglandin 3rd, according to a report, "Comparative risks of three methods of 3rd trimester abortion," *Morbidity and Mortality Weekly Report*, Nov. 26, 1976.

Safety and Current Techniques:

31. J. F. Williford and R. G. Wheeler, "Advances in non-electric vacuum equipment for uterine aspiration," *Advances in Planned Parenthood* 9:74–83 (1975).

32. Tietze, 1975, p. 44.

33. J. E. Hodgson et al., "Menstrual extraction: putting it and all its synonyms into proper perspective as pseudonyms," *Journal of the American Medical Association* 228:849–850 (1974).

34. United States Center for Disease Control (CDC), *Abortion surveillance—annual summary 1974* (Atlanta, Ga.: CDC, 1976).

35. I. S. Burnett et al., "An evaluation of abortion: techniques and protocols," *Hospital Practice* 10:97–105 (1975).

36. Burnett, 1975, p. 98.

37. Tietze, 1975, pp. 44–45.

38. Tietze, 1975, p. 52.

39. Tietze, 1975, p. 57.

40. S. Harlap and A. M. Davies, "Late sequelae of induced abortion: complications and outcome of pregnancy and labor," *American Journal of Epidemiology* 102:217–224 (1975).

41. Hungary, Central Statistical Office, *Perinatalis halalozas* (Budapest: Central Statistical Office, 1972).

42. R. L. Kleinman, ed., *Induced abortion* (London: International Planned Parenthood Federation, 1972).

43. Y. Moriyama and O. Hirokawa, "The relationship between artificial termination of pregnancy and abortion or premature birth," in: Y. Moriyama, ed., *Harmful effects of induced abortion* (Tokyo: Family Planning Federation of Japan, 1966), pp. 64–73.

44. J. K. Russell, "Sexual activity and its consequences in the teenager," *Clinics in Obstetrics and Gynecology* 1:683–698 (1974).

45. C. S. W. Wright et al., "Second-trimester abortion after vaginal termination of pregnancy," *Lancet* 1:1278–1279 (1972).

46. J. R. Darling and I. Emanuel, "Induced abortion and subsequent outcome of pregnancy," *Lancet* 1:170–172 (1975).

47. L. H. Roht and H. Aoyama, "Induced abortion and its sequelae: prematurity and spontaneous abortion," *American Journal of Obstetrics and Gynecology* 120:868–874 (1974).

48. H. P. David, "Psychological studies in abortion," in: J. T. Fawcett, ed., *Psychological perspectives on population* (N.Y.: Basic Books, 1973), pp. 241–273.

49. Osofsky, 1973.

50. C. Tietze and S. Lewit, "Joint program for the study of abortion: early medical complications of legal abortion," *Studies in Family Planning* 3:97–122 (1972).

51. United States National Academy of Sciences, Institute of Medicine, *Legalized abortion and the public health: report of a study by a committee of the Institute of Medicine, May, 1975* (Washington, D.C.: National Academy of Sciences, 1975).

52. World Health Organization, *Spontaneous and induced abortion* (Geneva: World Health Organization, 1970) (Technical Report No. 461).

Abortion and M.D. Mismanagement—paragraph 2:

53. J. Robins, "Failure of contraceptive practice," *New York State Journal of Medicine* 76:361 (1976).

Abortion and M.D. Mismanagement—paragraph 5:

54. W. B. Miller, "Psychological antecedents to conception among abortion seekers," *Western Journal of Medicine* 122:12 (1975).

His Turn? Methods of Contraception For Men

Chapter 19: King Condom

Paragraph 1:

1. "Condom sales rise in Sweden, VD falls," *Ob./Gyn. News* 8:9 (1973).

2. "La contraception au Japon (Contraception in Japan)," *Population* 28:691–692 (1973).

Paragraph 2:

3. I. A. Dalsimer, P. T. Piotrow and J. J. Dumm, "Condom: an old method meets a special new need," *Population Reports: Barrier Methods*, Series H, No. 1, 1973, p. H-1.

Paragraph 3:

4. L. Ajax, "How to market a nonmedical contraceptive: a case study from Sweden," in: Redford, 1974, pp. 5–22.

Paragraph 4:

5. Dalsimer, 1973, p. H-3.

The Advertising Blackout—paragraph 1:

6. D. W. Hastings and G. E. Provol, "Pharmacists' attitudes and practices toward contraceptives," *Journal of the American Pharmaceutical Association* 12:74–81 (1972).

The Advertising Blackout—paragraph 3:

7. Hastings, 1972.

The Advertising Blackout—paragraph 6:

8. Brenner, 1974, pp. 131–145.

The Matter of Size—paragraph 1:

9. N. R. Hardy, "Condom testing," in: Redford, 1974, p. 222.

10. Hardy, 1974, pp. 210–223.

11. *International Planned Parenthood Federation, Europe Region, Proceedings of IPPF working group on condom*, London, April 27–28, 1972.

12. P. Kestelman, "Condom testing: part 1," *IPPF Europe Regional Information Bulletin* 2:5–7 (1973).

13. Natural Rubber Producers' Research Association, *Natural rubber: the manufacture of prophylactics* (Welwyn Garden City, Herts, England: Natural Rubber Producers' Research Association, Dec. 1967) (Technical Information Sheet No. 109).

14. A. D. Sollins and R. L. Belsky, "Commercial production and distribution of contraceptives," *Reports on Population/ Family Planning* 4:1–23 (1970).

15. Himes, 1963.

16. C. Tietze, *The condom as a contraceptive* (N.Y.: National Committee on Maternal Health, 1960) (Publication No. 5).

17. United Nations Industrial Development Organization, 1971.

18. United States General Services Administration, Federal Supply Service, Standardization Division. *Interim federal specification: condom, rubber contraceptive, ZZ-C-0001597 (GSA-FSS), includes Amendment 1, dated Feb. 20, 1971* (Washington, D.C.: Government Printing Office, Feb. 10, 1970).

The Matter of Size—paragraph 3:

19. Editorial, "Condoms of the wrong size," *Prachathipatai*, Apr. 1, 1973, in: Redford, 1974, pp. 289–290.

Advantages and Disadvantages—paragraph 6:

20. M. Finkel and D. Finkel, "Sexual and contraceptive knowl-

edge, attitudes and behavior of male adolescents," *Family Planning Perspectives* 7:256–260 (1975).
Packaging and Selling—paragraph 1:
21. Consumer Reports, *Family planning guide*, 1970.
Packaging and Selling—paragraph 3:
22. P. D. Harvey, "Condoms—a new look," *Family Planning Perspectives* 4:27–30 (1972).
23. International Planned Parenthood Federation, 1972.
24. International Standardization Organization, Proposal for undertaking the preparation of international standards in a new field: contraceptives, originated by Sveriges Standardiseringskomission (SIS) (Swedish Standardization Commission), dated Aug. 30, 1972. Reference No. ISO/TS/P 118. Geneva, International Standardization Organization, Nov. 9, 1972.
25. Harvey, 1972, p. 29.
26. Kestelman, 1973.
27. P. Kestelman, "Condom testing: Part 2," *IPPF Europe Regional Information Bulletin* 3:4–6 (1974).
28. I. Koyama and N. Oato, "Review of condom use in Japan," in Redford, 1974, pp. 23–35.
29. J. J. Dumm, P. T. Piotrow and I. A. Dalsimer, "The modern condom—a quality product for effective contraception," *Population Report: Barrier Methods*, Series H, No. 2, 1974, p. H-28.
How to Select American Condoms—paragraph 4:
30. Harvey, 1972, p. 28.

Chapter 20: *Vasectomy: The Myths and the Facts*

Paragraph 1:
1. R. L. Kleinman, ed., *Male and female sterilization, a report of the meeting of the IPPF Panel of Experts on Sterilization held in Bombay, Jan. 11–14, 1973* (London: International Planned Parenthood Federation, 1973).
2. J. Wortman, "Vasectomy—what are the problems?" *Population Reports: Sterilization*, Series D, No. 2, 1975, p. D-25.
Paragraph 2:
3. B. B. Cooper, ed., *Observations on the structure and disease of the testis: a collection of lectures of A. C. Cooper*, 2nd ed. (London: Churchill, 1941).
4. R. E. Hackett and K. Waterhouse, "Vasectomy—reviewed," *American Journal of Obstetrics and Gynecology* 116:438–455 (1973).
5. H. C. Sharpe, "Vasectomy as a means of preventing procreation in defectives," *Journal of the American Medical Association* 53:1897–1902 (1909).
Paragraph 3:
6. E. Steinach, *Sex and life: forty years of biological and medical experiments* (N.Y.: Viking Press, 1940).

Paragraph 5:

7. J. Wortman and P. T. Piotrow, "Vasectomy—old and new techniques," *Population Reports: Sterilization*, Series D, No. 1, 1973, p. D-2.

Paragraph 6:

8. Wortman, 1973, p. D-3.

Paragraph 7:

9. Westoff, 1976.

Reliability and Safety—paragraph 1:

10. J. P. Blandy, "Vasectomy," in: J. D. Ferguson and J. P. Williams, eds., *Operative Surgery*, vol. 12 (Philadelphia: Lippincott, 1970), pp. 388–392.

11. J. E. Davis, "Vasectomy," *American Journal of Nursing*, 72:509–513 (1972).

12. B. Seaman, "Dangers of birth-control operations," *Ladies' Home Journal* 84:50 (July 1967).

Reliability and Safety—paragraph 2:

13. Battelle Memorial Institute. Population Study Programs, New and improved approaches to reversible sterilization of the male. Fourth Progress Report, Contract AID/csd-3152, Seattle, Wash., July 15, 1973.

14. K. B. Benjamin, "Vasectomy as an office procedure," in: L. Lader, ed., *Foolproof birth control* (Boston: Beacon Press, 1972), pp. 82–89.

15. T. Bruce, "Vasectomy, a survey of 98 men," *Medical Journal of Australia* 1:17–19 (1972).

16. G. C. Denniston, *Vasectomy technique* (Seattle, Wash.: Population Dynamics, 1972).

17. D. J. Dodds, "Description of an in-office operation," in: L. Lader, ed., *Foolproof birth control* (Boston: Beacon Press, 1972), pp. 90–96.

18. I. Gersh, "Vasectomy," *Rocky Mountain Medical Journal* 69:67–70 (1972).

19. P. J. Howard and L. P. James, "Immunological implications of vasectomy," *Journal of Urology* 109:76–78 (1973).

20. A. J. Leader, "The structure of a large-scale vasectomy clinic," in: A. J. Sobrero and R. M. Harvey, eds., *Advances in Planned Parenthood. Vol. 7. Proceedings of the Ninth Annual Meeting of the American Association of Planned Parenthood Physicians, Kansas City, Missouri, April 5–6, 1971* (Princeton: Excerpta Medica, 1972), pp. 203–206.

21. S. S. Schmidt, "Prevention of failure in vasectomy," *Journal of Urology* 109:296–297 (1973).

22. S. S. Schmidt, "Technique of vasectomy [Letter to the editor]," *British Medical Journal* 2:524–525 (1971).

Reliability and Safety—paragraph 3:

23. Wortman, 1973, pp. D-11–D-13.

Reliability and Safety—paragraph 4:

24. H. E. Carlson, "Vasectomy of election," *Southern Medical Journal* 63:766–770 (1970).

25. H. J. Klapproth and I. S. Young, "Vasectomy, vas ligation and vas occlusion," *Urology* 1:292–300 (1973).

26. S. Marshall and R. P. Lyon, "Variability of sperm disappearance from the ejaculate after vasectomy," *Journal of Urology* 107:815–817 (1972).

Possible Side Effects—paragraph 1:

27. S. Kase and M. Goldfarb, "Office vasectomy—review of 500 cases," *Urology* 1:60–62 (1973).

28. G. Kasirsky, "After the vasectomy," in: G. Kasirsky, *Vasectomy, manhood and sex* (N.Y.: Springer, 1972), pp. 57–67.

29. Simon Population Trust, *Vasectomy: follow-up of a thousand cases* (Cambridge: Simon Population Trust, 1969).

30. N. N. Wig, D. Pershad and R. P. Isaac, "A prospective study of symptom and non-symptom groups following vasectomy," *Indian Journal of Medical Research* 61:621–626 (1973).

31. J. R. Blandy, "Male sterilization," in A. J. Smith, ed., *Contraception today* (London: Family Planning Association, 1971), pp. 101–107.

32. *Social Biology* 20:303–307 (1973).

33. Margaret Pyke Center, "One thousand vasectomies," *British Medical Journal* 4:216–221 (1973).

34. R. E. Morgan, "Vasectomy," *Pennsylvania Medicine* 75: 38–40 (1972).

35. J. McEwan et al., "Hospital family planning: a vasectomy service," *Contraception* 9:177–192 (1974).

36. J. P. Blandy, "Vasectomy as a method of family limitation," *Midwife and Health Visitor* 8:161–165 (1973).

37. H. Edey, "Psychological aspects of vasectomy," *Medical Counterpoint* 4:19–24 (1972).

38. K. H. Kohli and A. J. Sobrero, "Vasectomy: a study of psychosexual and general reactions," *Social Biology* 20:298–302 (1973).

Possible Side Effects—paragraph 9:

39. "Antibody risk after vasectomies is rare," *Ob./Gyn. News* 8:3 (1973), p. 3.

40. R. Ansbacher, "Vasectomy: sperm antibodies," *Fertility and Sterility* 24:788–792 (1973).

41. Kleinman (London: International Planned Parenthood Federation, 1973).

42. R. I. Kleinman, ed., *Vasectomy* (London: International Planned Parenthood Federation, 1972).

43. M. D. Nickell et al., "Long-term effect of vasectomy on reproduction and liver function," *Federation Proceedings* 33: 531 (1974).

44. A. M. Phadke and K. Padukone, "Presence and significance of the auto-antibodies against spermatozoa in the blood of men

with obstructed vas deferens," *Journal of Reproduction and Fertility* 7:163–170 (1964).

45. I. S. Puvan, "Complications and long-term effects of sexual sterilization," in: R. A. Esmundo and K. C. Arun, eds., *Proceedings of the First Meeting of the IGCC Expert Group Working Committee on Sterilization and Abortion, Penang, Malaysia, Jan. 3–5, 1973*, Intergovernmental Coordinating Committee, 1973, pp. 24–27.

46. H. J. Roberts, "Delayed thrombophlebitis and systemic complications after vasectomy: possible role of diabetogenic hyperinsulinism," *Journal of the American Geriatrics Society* 16:267–280 (1968).

47. H. J. Roberts, "Is vasectomy innocuous?" *Medical Counterpoint* 3:13–16 (1971).

48. H. J. Roberts, "Thrombophlebitis after vasectomy. [Letter to the editor]," *New England Journal of Medicine* 284:1330 (1971).

49. H. J. Roberts, "Vasectomy problems [Letter to the editor]," *Family Planning Perspectives* 5:6 (1973).

50. P. Rumke, "Sperm antibodies and their action upon human spermatozoa," *Annales de l'Institut Pasteur* 118:525–528 (1970).

51. N. J. Alexander, "Immunologic effects of vasectomy in Rhesus monkeys," in: J. J. Sciarra, C. Markland, and J. J. Speidel, eds., *Control of male fertility: Proceedings of the workshop, San Francisco, June 19–21, 1974* (Hagerstown, Maryland: Harper and Row, 1975).

52. J. E. Davis, "The consequences of vasectomy," *Medical Counterpoint* 3:50–51 (1971).

53. M. Freund and W. Ventura, "Male sterilization: basic science aspects," in: M. E. Schima et al., eds., *Advances in voluntary sterilization, Proceedings of the Second International Conference, Geneva, Feb. 25–Mar. 1, 1973* (N.Y.: Elsevier, 1974), pp. 235–247.

53a. A. Halim and D. Antoniou, "Autoantibodies to spermatozoa in relation to male infertility and vasectomy," *British Journal of Urology* 45:559–562 (1973).

54. H. B. Presser, "Voluntary sterilization: a world view," *Reports on Population/Family Planning*, No. 5, July 1970.

Attitudes Toward Vasectomy—paragraph 2:

55. Arthur Godfrey, personal communication.

Attitudes Toward Vasectomy—paragraph 3:

56. M. H. Johnson, "Social and psychological effects of vasectomy," *American Journal of Psychiatry* 121:482–486 (1964).

57. Jim Bouton, personal communication.

58. J. Bouton with L. Shecter, "Why we adopted an interracial child," *Family Circle*, May 1971.

59. J. Bouton, "One man's family planning," *New York Magazine*, April 10, 1972.

Attitudes Toward Vasectomy—paragraph 11:

60. A. S. Ferber, C. Tietze and S. Lewit, "Men with vasectomies: a study of medical, sexual and psychosocial changes," *Psychosomatic Medicine* 29:354–366 (1967).
61. D. A. Rogers and F. J. Ziegler, "Effects of surgical contraception on sexual behavior," in: M. E. Schima et al., eds., *Advances in voluntary sterilization. Proceedings of the Second International Conference, Geneva, Feb. 25–Mar. 1, 1973* (N.Y.: Elsevier, 1974), pp. 277–282.
62. D. A. Rogers and F. J. Ziegler, "Psychological reactions to surgical contraception," in: J. T. Fawcett, ed., *Psychological perspectives on population* (N.Y.: Basic Books, 1973), pp. 303–326.
63. D. A. Rogers, "Vasectomy," *Alaska Medicine* 12:60–61 (1970).

Attitudes Toward Vasectomy—paragraph 12:

64. R. G. Burnight, V. Muangmun and M. J. Cook, "Male sterilization in Thailand: a follow-up study," Apr. 1974 (unpublished).
65. H. Wolfers, "Psychological aspects of vasectomy," *British Medical Journal* 4:297–300 (1970).
66. H. Wolfers, N. Subbiah and A. Mazurka, "Psychological aspects of vasectomy in Malaysia," *Social Biology* 20:315–322 (1973).

Attitudes Toward Vasectomy—paragraph 15:

67. John Gagnon, personal communication, Aug. 1976.

Chapter 21: A Pill for Men

Quotation:

1. "The pill," *Consumer Reports*, 35:314 and 35:429 (1970).

Paragraph 5:

2. S. J. Segal, "Contraceptive research: a male chauvinist plot?" *Family Planning Perspectives* 4:21–25 (1972).

Early Work on a Male Pill—paragraph 1:

3. Seaman, *The doctors' case against the pill*, p. 128.

Early Work on a Male Pill—paragraph 2:

4. B. Yuncker, "The pill for men—when?" *New York Post Magazine*, Feb. 23, 1974, p. 3.

Early Work on a Male Pill—paragraph 4:

5. Vaughan, 1970, p. 38.

Early Work on a Male Pill—paragraph 8:

6. Segal, 1972, p. 23.
7. W. J. Bremner and D. M. de'Kretser, "Contraceptives for males," *Signs* 1:387–396 (1975).
8. W. J. Bremner and C. A. Paulsen, "Colchicine and testicular function in man," *New England Journal of Medicine* 294:1384–1385 (1976).

A Male Pill That's Already Here:

9. "Sex hormone combo proposed for male pill," *Medical Tribune*, Feb. 5, 1975, p. 8.

10. M. Briggs and M. Briggs, "Oral contraceptive for men," *Nature* 252:585–586 (1974).

His Safety or Hers?—paragraph 3:

11. J. S. Lubin, "The man's turn," *Wall Street Journal*, Sept. 29, 1975, p. 1.

His Safety or Hers?—paragraph 6:

12. S. J. Segal, "Male fertility studies," *Contraception* 8:187–189 (1973).

13. E. M. Coutinho and J. F. Melo, "Successful inhibition of spermatogenesis in man without loss of libido," *Contraception* 8:119 (1973).

14. J. Frick, "Control of spermatogenesis in men by combined administration of progestin and androgen," *Contraception* 8:103 (1973).

15. C. G. Heller et al., "Effects of progestational compounds on the reproductive processes of the human male," *Annals of the New York Academy of Science* 71:649 (1958).

16. C. G. Heller et al., "Improvement in spermatogenesis following depression of the human testis with testosterone," *Fertility and Sterility* 1:415 (1950).

17. E. D. B. Johansson and K. C. Nygren, "Depression of plasma testosterone levels in men with norethindrone," *Contraception* 8:131 (1973).

18. G. Terner and J. MacLaughlin, "Effect of sex hormones in germinal cells of the rat testes," *Journal of Reproductive Fertility* 32:453–464 (1973).

Other Sperm Inhibitors—paragraph 4:

19. Segal, 1972.

Other Sperm Inhibitors—paragraph 7:

20. G. Corea, *The Hidden Malpractice* (N.Y.: William Morrow, 1977), pp. 160–165.

Other Sperm Inhibitors—paragraph 13:

21. "Treatment with ultrasound blocks spermatogenesis," *Medical Tribune* 17:1 (1976).

22. Corea, 1977, pp. 167–169.

Sperm Switches, Sperm Banks—paragraph 6:

23. T. Mann, *The biochemistry of semen and of the male reproductive tract* (London: Methuen, 1964).

24. Philip Corfman, personal communication.

ERT: PROMISE HER ANYTHING, BUT GIVE HER . . . CANCER

1. United States Food and Drug Administration, "Estrogens and endometrial cancer," *FDA Drug Bulletin*, Feb./March, 1976, p. 18.

2. H. K. Ziel and W. D. Finkle, "Increased risk of endometrial

carcinomas among users of conjugated estrogens," *New England Journal of Medicine* 293:1167–1170 (1975).

3. J. P. Bunker, "Surgical manpower," *New England Journal of Medicine*, Jan. 15, 1970, pp. 135–143.

4. *FDA Drug Bulletin*, 1976, p. 18.

5. S. Sturgis, "Hormone therapy in menopause: indications and contraindications," *Medical Aspects of Human Sexuality*, May 1969.

6. K. Ryan and D. Gibson, eds., *Menopause and aging. Summary report and selected papers from a research conference on menopause and aging, May 23–23, 1971*, Hot Springs, Arkansas, U.S. National Institutes of Health (Washington, D. C.: Government Printing Office, 1971).

7. "Estrogens and the menopausal patient," *Medical Letter* 15: 6–8 (1973).

8. *FDA Drug Bulletin*, 1976.

Chapter 22: Menopause, Money, and Depression

Quotation:

1. H. Osofsky and R. Seidenberg, "Is female menopausal depression inevitable?" *Obstetrics and Gynecology* 36:611–615 (1970).

Paragraph 3:

2. P. Weidegar, *Menstruation and menopause* (N.Y.: Alfred Knopf, 1975), p. 194.

Paragraph 4:

3. Boston Women's Health Book Collective, 1976.

Paragraph 6:

4. Advertisement, *Medical World News* 17:56 (1976).

Paragraph 7:

5. Emotions and the menopausal woman. A background paper from the Information Center on the Mature Woman, 3 West 57th St., N.Y., N.Y. 10019—"a service of Multidiscipline Research, Inc., through the support of Ayerst Laboratories."

Paragraph 8:

6. Advertisement, *American Family Physician*, 12:9 (1975).

Depressed—Or Just Blue?—paragraph 1:

7. B. Neugarten and R. J. Kraines, "Menopausal symptoms in women of various ages," *Psychosomatic Medicine* 27:266–273 (1965).

8. Novak, 1975, p. 178.

Depressed—Or Just Blue?—paragraph 2:

9. Neugarten, 1965, p. 272.

Depressed—Or Just Blue?—paragraph 10:

10. G. Winokur, "Depression in the menopause," *American Journal of Psychiatry* 130:92–93 (1973).

Depressed—Or Just Blue?—paragraph 12:

11. Novak, 1975, p. 718.

Depressed—Or Just Blue?—paragraph 13:
12. See a description of this in A. Klass, *Thar's gold in them thar pills: an inquiry into the medical industrial complex* (N.Y.: Penguin, 1975).
Not a True Antidepressant—paragraph 3:
13. *Medical Letter* 15:6–8 (1973).
Attitudes Toward Menopause—paragraph 3:
14. P. Bart, "Mother Portnoy's complaint," *Trans-Action* 8:69–74 (1970).
15. P. Bart, "Depression in middle-aged women," in: V. Gornick and B. K. Moran, eds., *Woman in a sexist society* (N.Y.: New American Library, 1972).
Attitudes Toward Menopause—paragraph 6:
16. It is commendable that some institutions, such as the College of New Rochelle in Westchester, N.Y., now give credit for "life experience" to returning housewives so they can obtain degrees and qualify for jobs more quickly.
The Menopausal Women's Image—paragraph 2:
17. B. Seaman, "The mother knot," *Washington Post Review*, April 1, 1976.
The Menopausal Woman's Image—paragraph 3:
18. M. Mannes, "Of time and the woman," *Psychosomatics* 9:9 (1968).
The Menopausal Woman's Image—paragraph 4:
19. M. Flint, "The menopause: reward or punishment?" *Psychosomatics* 16:161–163 (1975).
20. M. Flint, "Menarche and menopause of Rajput women," unpublished Ph.D. dissertation, City University of New York Graduate Center, 1974.
Menopause and Psychotherapy—paragraph 1:
21. Osofsky, 1970, p. 614.
Menopause and Psychotherapy—paragraph 2:
22. R. Seidenberg, *Corporate wives—corporate casualties?* (N.Y.: Anchor, 1975), p. 149.
Menopause and Psychotherapy—paragraph 3:
23. Osofsky, 1970, p. 64.

Chapter 23: The Selling of ERT

Paragraph 2:
1. Advertisement, *American Journal of Obstetrics and Gynecology* 54:17 (1947).
2. Advertisement, *American Journal of Obstetrics and Gynecology* 54:7 (1947).
Gusberg's Warnings—paragraph 1:
3. S. B. Gusberg, "Precursors of corpus carcinoma: estrogens and adenomatous hyperplasia," *American Journal of Obstetrics and Gynecology* 54:905–926 (1947).

Gusberg's Warnings—paragraph 3:
4. Gusberg, 1947, p. 910.
Gusberg's Warnings—paragraph 5:
5. R. Wilson, *Feminine forever* (N.Y.: M. Evans, 1966).
Wilson versus Living Decay—paragraph 2:
6. J. Kinderlehrer, "Can you sail through menopause without synthetic estrogen?" *New Woman*, June 1971, p. 69.
Wilson versus Living Decay—paragraph 3:
7. Sturgis, 1969, p. 70.
Wilson versus Living Decay—paragraph 4:
8. R. Wilson, "A key to staying young," *Look*, Jan. 1966, p. 66.
Wilson versus Living Decay—paragraph 5:
9. M. Mintz, *The pill: an alarming report* (N.Y.: Fawcett, 1969), pp. 30–31.
Wilson versus Living Decay—paragraph 8:
10. Mintz, 1969, pp. 30–31.
Wilson versus Living Decay—paragraph 9:
11. Barbara Yuncker, interview, May 5, 1976.
Wilson versus Living Decay—paragraph 10:
12. *FDA Drug Bulletin*, Feb./Mar. 1976.
Wilson versus Living Decay—paragraph 11:
13. Robert Wilson, interview, 1976.
The Service for Media—paragraph 1:
14. S. Gorney and C. Cox, *After forty* (N.Y.: Dial, 1973), pp. 36–37.
The Service for Media—paragraph 5:
15. Seaman, *Free and female*, pp. 87–90.
The Service for Media—paragraph 7:
16. "Emotions and the menopausal women," background paper from the Information Center on the Mature Woman.
Clouds on the Horizon—paragraph 4:
17. Ryan, 1971.
Clouds on the Horizon—paragraph 5:
18. Novak, 1975, pp. 717–718.
The Bubble Bursts—paragraph 2:
19. Marcia Storch, personal interview.
The Bubble Bursts—paragraph 4:
20. Kennedy hearings, 1975, p. 130.
The Bubble Bursts—paragraph 6:
21. J. Brody, "Physicians' views unchanged on use of estrogen therapy," *New York Times*, Dec. 5, 1975.
The Bubble Bursts—paragraph 7:
22. Brody, 1975.

Chapter 24: The Flash and the Flesh

Paragraph 1:
1. R. Frisch et al., "Critical weights, a critical body composition, menarche and the maintenance of menstrual cycles," in: *Bio-*

social Interrelation In Population Adaptation (The Hague: Mouton, 1976).
Paragraph 4:
2. J. Bernard, *The future of motherhood* (N.Y.: Dial, 1974).
3. Weideger, 1975.
The Anatomy of Flashes—paragraph 2:
4. G. W. Molnar, "Body temperatures during menopausal hot flashes," *Journal of Applied Physiology*, 35:463 (1975).
The Anatomy of Flashes—paragraph 4:
5. Boston Women's Health Book Collective, 1976, p. 329.
The Anatomy of Flashes—paragraph 5:
6. B. L. Neugarten, *Personality in middle and later years* (N.Y.: Atherton, 1964).
7. Boston Women's Health Book Collective, 1976, p. 335.
Severe Flashes—paragraph 1:
8. Boston Women's Health Book Collective, 1976, p. 330.
Severe Flashes—paragraph 6:
9. Neugarten, 1965.
Severe Flashes—paragraph 9:
10. Boston Women's Health Book Collective, 1976, p. 334.
Severe Flashes—paragraph 10:
11. S. H. Cherry, *The menopause myth* (N.Y.: Ballantine, 1976), p. 20.
Early Studies of Flashes—paragraph 4:
12. J. T. King, "Observations on the menopause. I. The basal metabolism after the artificial menopause," *Bulletin, Johns Hopkins Hospital* 39:281–303 (1926).
Early Studies of Flashes—paragraph 5:
13. S. R. M. Reynolds, "Dermovascular action of estrogen, the ovarian follicular hormone," *Journal of Investigative Dermatology* 4:7–22 (1941).
Early Studies of Flashes—paragraph 6:
14. E. M. Klaften, "Utero-thermometry: a study of uterine temperature during reproductive life, menopause and amenorrhea," *Journal of Clinical Endocrinology and Metabolism* 4: 159–165 (1944).
15. M. Aubeaux-Fernet and J. Deribreux, "La bouffée de chaleur symptome majeur du ménopause," *Semaine Hospital Paris* 22:1500–1502 (1946).
16. M. E. Collett, "Basal metabolism at the menopause," *Journal of Applied Physiology* 1:629–636 (1949).
Molnar's Unique Study:
17. Molnar, 1975.
Flesh Effects—paragraph 10:
18. Novak, 1975. (We suspect that B-complex deficiencies or malabsorption may contribute to menopausal weight gain. Women who take B supplements seem to control their weight more easily.)

Flesh Effects—paragraph 12:
19. "Dangers in eternal youth," *Lancet* 2:1135 (1975).

Chapter 25: *The Ovary Explained*

Paragraph 6:
1. M. McClintock, "Menstrual synchrony and suppression," *Nature* 229:244–245 (1971).
Follicle Stimulating Hormone—paragraph 2:
2. R. Frisch, R. Roger and C. Sole, "Components of weight at menarche and the initiation of adolescent growth spurt in girls," *Human Biology* 45:469 (1973).
Follicle Stimulating Hormone—paragraph 5:
3. Seaman, *The doctors' case against the pill*, p. 146.
Follicle Stimulating Hormone—paragraph 10:
4. Cherry, 1976, p. 18.
ERT Proponents—paragraph 1:
5. R. Greenblatt and N. Stahl, "Sex hormone therapy of menopausal women," *Drug Therapy*, Apr. 1972, pp. 38–51.
6. H. Kupperman, The climacteric syndrome," *Medical Folio* 15:1–4 (1972).
7. H. Jern, "Hormone therapy of the menopause," *Journal of the American Medical Women's Association* 30:491–492 (1975).
ERT Proponents—paragraph 2:
8. Greenblatt, 1972, p. 44.
Ziel and Finkle and the Youth Pill Fantasy—paragraph 1:
9. Ziel, 1975.
10. H. Ziel and W. Finkel, "Association of estrone with the development of endometrial cancer," *American Journal of Obstetrics and Gynecology* 124:735 (1976).
Ziel and Finkle and the Youth Pill Fantasy—paragraph 3:
11. Ziel, 1976.
Ovaries and Hysterectomy—paragraph 1:
12. Cherry, 1976, p. 63.
Ovaries and Hysterectomy—paragraph 2:
13. B. MacMahon and J. Worcester, *Age at menopause, United States—1960–1962* (Washington, D.C.: Government Printing Office, 1966).
14. P. Braun and E. Druckman, "Public health rounds at the Harvard School of Public Health, elective hysterectomy—pro and con," *New England Journal of Medicine* 295:1–3 (1976).
15. *FDA Drug Bulletin*, Feb./Mar. 1976.
16. J. Money and A. Ehrhardt, *Man, woman, boy and girl* (Baltimore: Johns Hopkins Univ. Press, 1972).
Ovaries and Hysterectomy—paragraph 3:
17. "How much unnecessary surgery: a hard look at the evidence," *Medical World News* 17:23 (1976).

Ovaries and Hysterectomy—paragraph 4:
18. W. Miller and A. Forrest, "Oestradiol synthesis from C19 steroids by human breast cancer," *British Journal of Cancer* 33:116 (1976).
Ovaries and Hysterectomy—paragraph 6:
19. *Medical World News* 17:23 (1976).
David Reuben's Old Tune—paragraph 1:
20. D. Reuben, *Everything you always wanted to know about sex but were afraid to ask* (N.Y.: McKay, 1969).
David Reuben's Old Tune—paragraph 3:
21. D. Reuben, *How to get more out of sex . . . than you ever thought you could* (N.Y.: McKay, 1974).
David Reuben's Old Tune—paragraph 5:
22. Reuben, 1974.
David Reuben's Old Tune—paragraph 7:
23. Reuben, 1974.
Vermeulen's Research—paragraph 1:
24. A. Vermeulen, "The hormonal activity of the post-menopausal ovary," *Journal of Clinical Endocrinology and Metabolism* 42:247–253 (1976).
Vermeulen's Research—paragraph 4:
25. P. K. Siiteri et al., "Estrogen binding in the rat and human," *Advances in Experimental Biology* 36:97–112 (1973).
26. P. K. Siiteri, *Journal of Endocrinology and Metabolism* (1967).
27. P. K. Siiteri, in: *Handbook of physiology*, Section 7, Endocrinology (Washington: American Physiological Society, 1973).
Vermeulen's Research—paragraph 6:
28. H. Judd et al., "Endocrine function of the post-menopausal ovary," *Journal of Clinical Endocrinology and Metabolism* 39: 1020 (1974).
Vermeulen's Research—paragraph 7:
29. P. K. Siiteri and P. C. MacDonald, "Estrogen receptors and the estrone hypothesis in relation to endometrial and breast cancer," *Gynecological Oncology* 2:228–238 (1974).

There is a growing body of evidence that excessive levels of circulating estrogens in the later years, whether natural or from a bottle, are involved in the development of certain cancers. In 1974, Siiteri, MacDonald and their colleagues reported that, for example, patients with endometrial cancer have "excess peripheral conversion of andristone to estrone."

Chapter 26: The Vagina and Sexuality

Paragraph 1:
1. W. H. Masters and V. E. Johnson, *Human sexual inadequacy* (Boston: Little, Brown, 1970), p. 342.
2. For an excellent discussion of sex and the older woman, see

pages 507–524 of *The Hite Report* by Shere Hite (N.Y.: Dell, 1976). One of Ms. Hite's respondents stated: "I thought that menopause was the leading factor in my dry and irritable vaginal tract. My doctors thought that it was lack of hormones . . . but with my new lover, I am reborn. Plenty of lubrication, no irritation!" (p. 509).

Paragraph 2:

3. Masters, 1970.

4. S. Kent, "Balancing the pluses and the minuses of the menopause," *Geriatrics* 30:160 (1975).

Absorption Through the Vagina—paragraph 2:

5. G. Bernstein, statement at FDA metting, Jan. 1975.

Absorption Through the Vagina—paragraph 3:

6. Staples, statement at FDA meeting, Jan. 1975.

Better Sex After Menopause—paragraph 2:

7. Boston Women's Health Book Collective, 1976, p. 328.

Better Sex After Menopause—paragraph 3:

8. Boston Women's Health Book Collective, 1976, p. 328.

Better Sex After Menopause—paragraph 5:

9. Neugarten, 1964, p. 82.

Better Sex After Menopause—paragraph 6:

10. M. Sherfy, "The evolution and nature of female sexuality in relation to psychoanalytic theory," *Journal of the American Psychoanalytic Association* 14:50 (1966).

The Older Woman As Sexual Leader—paragraph 1:

11. June Nash, personal comunication with Brooke G. Schoepf.

The Older Woman As Sexual Leader—paragraph 3:

12. D. S. Marshall and R. Suggs, ed., *Human sexual behavior* (N.Y.: Basic Books, 1971), p. 188.

The Menopausal Husband—paragraph 2:

13. Ongoing studies of Drs. Eric Pfeiffer, Adrian Verwoerdt and their associates in the psychiatry department at Duke University.

14. Seaman, *Free and female*, p. 76.

The Menopausal Husband—paragraph 4:

15. Cherry, 1976, pp. 78–79.

The Menopausal Husband—paragraph 5:

16. Cherry, 1976, p. 84.

Chapter 27: Osteoporosis: Another ERT Target

Paragraph 2:

1. S. M. Garn, *The earlier gain and later loss of cortical bone in nutritional perspective* (Springfield, Ill.: Charles C. Thomas, 1970).

2. P. A. Alffram, "An epidemiologic study of cervical and intertrochanteric fractures of the femur in an urban population," *Acta Orthopaedica Scandivica.* Supplement 65 (1964).

3. G. C. H. Bauer, "Epidemiology of fractures," in: U.S. Barzel, ed., *Osteoporosis* (N.Y.: Grune & Stratton, 1970).

4. J. Stevens et al., "The incidence of osteoporosis in patients with femoral neck fracture," *Journal of Bone and Joint Surgery* 44B:520 (1962).

5. M. R. Urist, "Observations bearing on the problem of osteoporosis," in: K. Rodahl et al., eds., *Bone as a tissue* (N.Y.: McGraw-Hill, 1960).

6. H. F. Newton-John and D. B. Morgan, "The loss of bone with age, osteoporosis, and fractures," *Clinical Orthopaedics and Related Research* #71, July–Aug. 1970.

7. R. P. Heaney, "Estrogen effects on the skeleton," in Salhanick, 1969, pp. 493–502.

Possible Causes and Cures—paragraph 1:

8. J. Jowsey, "Osteoporosis: etiology and treatment," *Contemporary Surgery* 6:13–16 (1975).

Possible Causes and Cures—paragraph 2:

9. J. Chalmers and K. C. Ho, "Geographical variations in senile osteoporosis: the association with physical activity," *Journal of Bone and Joint Surgery* 52B:667 (1970).

10. Heaney, 1969.

Possible Causes and Cures—paragraph 3:

11. A. A. McBeath, "The aging skeleton: osteoporosis and degenerative arthritis," *Postgraduate Medicine* 57:171–175 (1975).

12. Jowsey, 1975.

13. Jowsey, "Prevention and treatment of osteoporosis," in: M. Winick, ed., *Nutrition and aging* (N.Y.: Wiley, 1976), pp. 131–144.

Possible Causes and Cures—paragraph 4:

14. McBeath, 1975, p. 173.

15. J. Jowsey et al., "Effect of combined therapy with sodium fluoride, vitamin D and calcium in osteoporosis," *American Journal of Medicine* 53:43–49 (1972).

Possible Causes and Cures—paragraph 5:

16. L. V. Avioli, paper presented at Symposium on Nutritional Disorders of Women, held at Columbia University, New York, N.Y., 1975.

17. J. R. Shapiro, "Osteoporosis: evaluation of diagnosis and therapy," *Archives of Internal Medicine* 135:563–567 (1975).

Albright's Theory—paragraph 1:

18. F. Albright and E. C. Reifenstein, *The parathyroid glands and metabolic bone disease* (Baltimore: Williams & Wilkins, 1958).

19. F. Albright, P. Smith and R. Richardson, "Postmenopausal osteoporosis, its clinical features," *Journal of the American Medical Association* 117:2473–2476 (1941). (We are thankful to Dr. Fred Bartter of the National Institutes of Health for

pointing out the enormous historical significance of this report, which we might easily have missed.)

Albright's Theory—paragraph 7:
20. L. F. Hawkinson, "The menopausal syndrome: one thousand consecutive patients with estrogen," *Journal of the American Medical Association* 111:390–393 (1938).
21. H. Weisbader and Kurzork, "The menopause: a consideration of the symptoms, etiology, and treatment by means of estrogens," *Endocrinology* 23:32–38 (1938).
Albright's Theory—paragraph 8:
22. Albright, 1941, p. 2474.
Efficacy Still Uncertain—paragraph 2:
23. *Medical Letter* 15:6–8 (1973).
Efficacy Still Uncertain—paragraph 4:
24. Lila Nachtigall, personal communication, Feb. 14, 1977.
Efficacy Still Uncertain—paragraph 5:
25. Merrill Lynch Pierce Fenner & Smith, Inc., *Institutional Report*, Sept. 16, 1976.
Efficacy Still Uncertain—paragraph 6:
26. Transcript of Endocrinology and Metabolism Advisory Committee, FDA, Feb. 18, 1977.
27. F. Moira, "'Estrogens forever': marketing youth and death," *Off Our Backs*, March, 1977, p. 12.
Efficacy Still Uncertain—paragraph 11:
28. E. N. Todhunter, "Good Nutrition and Menopause," speech reported in *OB/GYN News*, Vol. 2, No. 3.

Chapter 28: The Reckoning

Paragraph 2:
1. N. Hicks, "Doctors strong, patients weak, costs up," *New York Times*, April 28, 1976.
Hooked on ERT—paragraph 2:
2. J. Coope, J. M. Thompson and L. Poller, "Effects of 'natural oestrogen' replacement therapy on menopausal symptoms and blood clotting," *British Medical Journal* 4:139–143 (1975). Dr. Coope has stated that the judgment to administer estrogen "should not depend solely on relief of pain, since placebos have been shown to be as effective as estrogens in this regard."
3. See also subsequent follow-up of Coope's patients concerning blood clotting factors in: L. Poller, J. M. Thomson and J. Coope, "Conjugated equine oestrogens and blood clotting: a follow-up report," *British Medical Journal* 1:935–936 (1977).
4. C. Proudfit, "Estrogens and menopause," *Journal of the American Medical Association* 236:940 (1976).
Warnings to Doctors:
5. *P.D.R.* 1976, pp. 1522–1528.

Gall-Bladder Disease:

6. Boston Collaborative Drug Surveillance Program, "Surgically confirmed gall bladder disease, venous thromboembolism, and breast tumors in relation to postmenopausal estrogen therapy," *New England Journal of Medicine* 290:15–19 (1974).

7. G. N. Weiss and E. B. Weiss, "Hormonal therapy and cholelithiasis," *International Surgery* 61:472–474 (1976).

Depletion of Vitamins:

8. Spellacy, *American Journal of Obstetrics and Gynecology* 114:378–392 (1972).

9. Kutsky, 1973.

10. See also notes for chap. 10: "Recovering from the Pill."

Facial Scars:

11. "Estrogens," *Clin-Alert* #267, Dec. 9, 1971.

Hysterectomy Risks, 4. Hematometra:

12. "Estrogens—elderly women," *Clin-Alert* #48, 1971.

Chapter 29: ERT and Cancer

Paragraph 1:

1. "Estrogens: do they increase the risk of cancer?" *Science* 191: 838–840 (1976).

Paragraph 3:

2. K. J. Ryan, "Cancer risk and estrogen use in menopause," *New England Journal of Medicine* 293:1199–1200 (1975).

3. D. C. Smith et al., "Association of exogenous estrogen and endometrial carcinoma," *New England Journal of Medicine* 293: 1164–1167 (1975).

4. N. S. Weiss, "Risks and benefits of estrogen use," *New England Journal of Medicine* 293:1200–1201 (1975).

5. Ziel, 1975, pp. 1167–1170.

6. *FDA Drug Bulletin*, Feb./Mar. 1976.

Pentti Siiteri—paragraph 2:

7. Ryan, 1975, p. 1199.

8. Editorial, *Science* 191:23 (1976).

Donald Austin—paragraph 1:

9. D. W. Cramer, S. J. Cutler and B. Christine, "Trends in the incidence of endometrial cancer in the United States," *Gynecologic Oncology* 2:130–143 (1974).

Donald Austin—paragraph 2:

10. D. Austin, *Journal of the American Medical Association* 235:788 (1976).

Donald Austin—paragraph 5:

11. J. R. Crout, *FDA Consumer*, Apr. 1976, p. 6.

Bruce Stadel—paragraph 1:

12. B. Stadel and N. Weiss, "Characteristics of menopausal women: a survey of King and Pierce counties in Washington, 1973–1974," *Journal of Epidemiology* 102:215 (1975).

Bruce Stadel—paragraph 6:
13. Stadel, 1975, p. 215.
Cancer of the Uterus—paragraph 2:
14. Weiss, 1975, p. 1201.
Cancer of the Uterus—paragraph 3:
15. T. Mack, "Estrogens and endometrial cancer in a retirement community," *New England Journal of Medicine* 294:1262–1267 (1976).
Cancer of the Uterus—paragraph 4:
16. American Cancer Society.
Cancer of the Uterus—paragraph 6:
17. "The course of carcinoma and how to change it," *Emergency Medicine*, March, 1976, p. 194.
Cancer of the Uterus—paragraph 8:
18. *Emergency Medicine*, Mar. 1976, p. 194.
Cancer of the Uterus—paragraph 10:
19. *Emergency Medicine*, Mar. 1976, p. 196.
Breast Cancer—paragraph 1:
20. F. D. Moore et al., "Carcinoma of the breast," *New England Journal of Medicine* 277:293 (1967).
Breast Cancer—paragraph 23:
21. R. Hoover et al., "Menopausal estrogens and breast cancer," *New England Journal of Medicine* 295:401–405 (1976).

Chapter 30: Products and Dosages

Monitoring of ERT Patients—paragraph 4:
1. Novak, 1975, p. 713.
2. H. P. Kupperman, "The menopausal woman and hormones," *Medical Aspects of Human Sexuality*, 1967, pp. 64–68.
"One cannot use the vaginal smear as the sole diagnostic criterion for determining whether or not the patient needs estrogen replacement. For example, the menstruating woman in whom ovulation may still be occurring may show an estrogen-deficient smear despite her remoteness in age from the climacteric. The progesterone from the ovary will induce shedding of the vaginal epithelium, preventing it from reaching its fully mature or cornified state. The vaginal smear will then yield a picture not unlike that of an estrogen deficiency despite more than adequate estrogen levels."
The ERT Products:
3. *P.D.R.*, 1976.
How These Products Are Used: The Pills—paragraph 1:
4. Novak, 1975, p. 712.
How These Products Are Used: The Pills—paragraph 3:
5. Debrovner, personal communication, 1976.
How These Products Are Used: The Pills—paragraph 4:
6. Kupperman, 1972, pp. 1–4.

How These Products Are Used: The Pills—paragraph 5:
7. Kupperman, 1967, pp. 64–68.
How These Products Are Used: The Pills—paragraph 6:
8. "Oestrogens as a cause of endometrial carcinoma," *British Medical Journal* 1:6013 (1976).
How These Products Are Used: The Injections—paragraph 3:
9. Greenblatt, 1972, p. 45.
How These Products Are Used: The Pellets—paragraph 1:
10. Greenblatt, 1972, p. 50.

MENOPAUSE: WHOLESOME REMEDIES

Paragraph 4:
1. Text of interview with Dr. Theodore Cooper by Dr. Arthur M. Sackler, *Medical Tribune*, Nov. 3, 1976, p. 24.
Paragraph 6:
2. M. Winick, "Rx for nutritional ignorance: humble pie?" *Modern Medicine*, March 15, 1977, p. 41.
Paragraph 8:
3. L. Pauling, "Q & A from interviews with Dr. Pauling," *Medical Tribune*, April 6, 1977, p. 7.
Paragraph 9:
4. L. Pauling, *Vitamin C, the common cold, and the flu* (San Francisco: W. H. Freeman, 1976).
Paragraph 13:
5. M. Jacobson, "The real problem with food additives," *Caveat Emptor*, Feb. 1977.
6. R. Everdell and M. Jacobson, "The baby food industry—who benefits?" *Nutrition Action*, Dec. 1976.
Paragraph 15:
7. "Oh what's so rare as invocation of Delaney Clause?" *Medical Tribune*, May 4, 1977, p. 1.
8. "Top medical experts question carcinogenicity studies," *Medical Tribune*, May 4, 1977, p. 1.

In an interview with Dr. Arthur Sackler, former FDA Commissioner Dr. Charles Edwards admitted: "I don't believe FDA has such standards [for carcinogenicity], just a hodge-podge of ideas."

Paragraph 16:
9. G. O. Barney, ed., *The unfinished agenda* (New York: Thomas Y. Crowell, 1977).
Paragraph 17:
10. "Infants on formula + zinc grow more," *Medical World News*, Dec. 27, 1976, p. 45. Also see *Medical World News*, July 12, 1976, p. 54.

Chapter 31: Ginseng: A Natural Remedy from the Orient

Paragraph 1:
1. C. P. Li and R. C. Li, "An introductory note to ginseng," *American Journal of Chinese Medicine* 1:249–261 (1973).

Studies of Ginseng—paragraph 1:
2. L. Lasagna, "Herbal pharmacology and medical therapy in the People's Republic of China," *Annals of Internal Medicine* 83:887–893 (1975).
Studies of Ginseng—paragraph 3:
3. Norman Farnsworth, personal interview, June 24, 1976.
Studies of Ginseng—paragraph 5:
4. Li, 1973, pp. 249–261.
Studies of Ginseng—paragraph 6:
5. I. I. Brekhman and I. V. Dardymov, "Pharmacological investigation of glycosides from ginseng and eleutherococcus," *Lloydia* 32:46 (1969).
Studies of Ginseng—paragraph 7:
6. I. I. Brekhman and I. V. Dardymov, "New substances of plant origin which increase nonspecific resistance," in: *Annual Review of Pharmacology* (Palo Alto, Cal.: Annual Review Co., 1969), p. 419.
7. I. I. Brekhman, *Zhen-shen* (*Panax ginseng*) (Leningrad: Medgiz, 1957).
8. I. I. Brekhman, "Panax ginseng," *Medical Science Service* (India), 4:17–25 (1967).
9. I. I. Brekhman, "Eleutherococcus senticosus—a new medicinal herb of the Araliaceae family," *Proceedings of the second international pharmacology meeting, Prague, 1963* (Pergamon; Oxford; Czechoslovak Medical Press; 1965), vol. 7, pp. 97–102.
10. N. K. Fruentov, "Materialy k izucheniju schen-shenja: limonnika (Materials for the study of Panax ginseng and Shizandra chinesis)," *Izdanic Akad. Nauk SSSR* 3:133–40 (1958).
11. A. S. Saratikov, *Stimulatori centralnoy nervony sistemi (Stimulators of central nervous system)* (Tomsk: Izdatelstov Tomskago University, 1966), pp. 3–23.
12. C. Kim, C. C. Kim, M. S. Kim, C. Y. Hu and J. S. Rhe, "Influence of ginseng on the stress mechanism," *Lloydia* 33: 43–48 (1970).
Studies of Ginseng—paragraph 8:
13. I. I. Brekhman, "Ginseng in the U.S.S.R.," *Indian Journal of Public Health* 9:148–149 (1965).
Studies of Ginseng—paragraph 10:
14. M. A. Medvedev, "The effects of ginseng on the working performance of radio operators," *Papers on the Study of Ginseng and Other Medicinal Plants of the Far East*, Issue N. 5, 1963.
15. I. M. Popov et al., "A review of the proporties and clinical effects of ginseng," *American Journal of Chinese Medicine* 1: 263–270 (1973).
Ginseng and Hot Flashes—paragraph 2:
16. Robert Atkins, personal communication, Mar. 1976.

Ginseng and Hot Flashes—paragraph 4:
17. B. Goldstein, "Ginseng: its history, dispersion, and folk tradition," *American Journal of Chinese Medicine* 3:223–234 (1975).
Farnsworth's Opinions—paragraph 1:
18. Lasagna, 1975, p. 888.
19. Farnsworth, personal interview, 1976.
Farnsworth's Opinions—paragraph 7:
20. W. H. Park et al., *Journal of the Catholic Medical College* (Korea) 19:83 (1970).
21. K. Shida et al., *Japanese Journal of Fertility and Sterility* 15:113 (1970).
22. C. Choi et al., *Journal of the Catholic Medical College* (Korea) 21:211 (1971).
23. V. Petkov et al., *Biochemical Pharmacology* 12:48 (1963).
Farnsworth's Opinions—paragraph 10:
24. Lasagna, 1975, p. 892.
Farnsworth's Opinions—paragraph 16:
25. Sarah Roshan, personal communication, 1976.
Dosages for Menopause—paragraph 2:
26. Farnsworth, personal interview, 1976.
Buying Ginseng, Taking Ginseng—paragraph 12:
27. Farnsworth, personal interview, 1976.
Buying Ginseng, Taking Ginseng—paragraph 13:
28. J. S. Massey, "Ginseng, folklore cure-all, is being regarded seriously," *Smithsonian*, Feb. 1976, pp. 104–111.

Chapter 32: Vitamin E and Other Helps for Menopause Symptoms

Paragraph 1:
1. Novak, 1975, p. 712.
Paragraph 2:
2. R. A. Passwater, *Prevention*, Aug. 1974.
Paragraph 4:
3. C. J. Christy, "Vitamin E in menopause," *American Journal of Obstetrics and Gynecology* 50:84–87 (1945).
Paragraph 5:
4. R. S. Finkler, "The effect of Vitamin E in the menopause," *Journal of Clinical Endocrinology* 9:89–94 (1949).
Paragraph 6:
5. E. Shute, "Wheat germ oil therapy: dosage-idiosyncrasy," *American Journal of Obstetrics and Gynecology* 35:249 (1938).
Paragraph 7:
6. H. C. McLaren, "Vitamin E in the menopause," *British Medical Journal* 1:1378–1382 (1949).
Why Was E Abandoned by Most Gynecologists?—paragraph 1:
7. E. Shute, "Notes on menopause," *Canadian Medical Association Journal* 37:350 (1937).

Why Was E Abandoned by Most Gynecologists?—paragraph 4:
8. W. E. Shute, *Vitamin E for ailing and healthy hearts* (N.Y.: Pyramid, 1969).
Dosages of E—paragraph 1:
9. B. T. Hunter, "The case of vitamin E," *Consumers' Research Magazine,* August 1973, p. 28.
Dosages of E—paragraph 5:
10. "Studies firm up some metals' role in cancer," *Chemical and Engineering News,* Jan. 17, 1977, p. 35.

Some scientists now urge that to protect against cancer, Americans increase the dietary intake of selenium to the average Asian level. Currently the average United States selenium intake is about half that. A high selenium diet involves reducing sugar intake to about one-tenth its present level, fat and oil to about one-third, and eating more cereal and fish. Too much zinc may offset the protective effect of selenium; therefore, high dosages of zinc should probably not be taken over long periods of many months or years unless medically indicated.

Chapter 33: The Real Keys to Osteoporosis

Nutrition Therapy—paragraph 1:
1. "Osteoporosis," *Medical Letter* 18:99–100 (1976).
Nutrition Therapy—paragraph 5:
2. Jowsey, in: M. Winick, 1976.
Nutrition Therapy—paragraph 12:
3. A. A. Albanese, *New York State Journal of Medicine,* Feb. 1975.
4. D. H. Marshall, *Proceedings of the Nutrition Society,* Sept. 1976.
Nutrition Therapy—paragraph 13:
5. Jowsey, 1975.
6. Jowsey, 1976, pp. 131–144.
7. G. M. Berlyne et al., "The aetiology of senile osteoporosis," *Quarterly Journal of Medicine* 64:505–521 (1975).
Exercise and Bones—paragraph 2:
8. Jowsey, 1975, pp. 13–16.
9. Chalmers, 1970.
Exercise and Bones—paragraph 3:
10. Chalmers, 1970, p. 673.
Exercise and Bones—paragraph 5:
11. A. Adams, "Effect of exercise upon ligament strength," *Research Quarterly of the American Association for Health, Physical Education, and Recreation* 37:163–167 (1966).
Exercise, Health, and Longevity—paragraph 3:
12. E. V. Beverley, "The mechanics of putting those little-used muscles in motion," *Geriatrics* 31:132–134 (1976).
Oh, My Aching Back—paragraph 1:
13. R. P. Heaney, "The osteoporoses," in: P. B. Beeson and W.

McDermott, eds., *Cecil-Loeb textbook of medicine*, 13th ed. (Philadelphia: Saunders, 1971), pp. 1826–1830.
Osteoarthritis and Diet—paragraph 1:
14. "On the arthritis mystery," *Executive Health* 11:1 (1975).
Osteoarthritis and Diet—paragraph 2:
15. Williams, 1971.
Osteoarthritis and Diet—paragraph 3:
16. W. Kaufman, *The common form of joint dysfunction: its incidence and treatment* (Brattleboro: E. L. Hildrith, 1949).
17. *Executive Health*, 1975, p. 2.
Osteoarthritis and Diet—paragraph 4:
18. J. M. Ellis, *The doctor who looked at his hands* (N.Y.: ARC, 1966).
19. J. M. Ellis, *Vitamin B₆: the doctor's report* (N.Y.: Harper & Row, 1973).

ADDITIONAL READINGS
20. L. W. Friedman and L. Galton, *Freedom from backaches* (N.Y.: Pocket Books, 1976).
21. H. Kraus, *Backache, stress and tension* (N.Y.: Pocket Books, 1969).

Chapter 34: Healthy Skin at Menopause

Paragraph 5:
1. Kutsky, 1973, p. 263.
Estrogen and Facial Skin—paragraph 1:
2. "Patient skin changes may be indication for discontinuing OC," *Ob/Gyn News*, Apr. 15, 1976.
Estrogen and Facial Skin—paragraph 3:
3. Kutsky, 1973, p. 262.
Estrogen and Facial Skin—paragraph 6:
4. D. Chase, *The medically based no-nonsense beauty book* (N.Y.: Pocket Books, 1976), pp. 91–92.
Vitamins and Skin—paragraph 1:
5. Kutsky, 1973, p. 263.
Vitamins and Skin—paragraph 3:
6. Kutsky, 1973, p. 58.
Vitamins and Skin—paragraph 13:
7. Georgette Klinger, personal communication, Nov. 11, 1976.

ADDITIONAL READINGS
8. D. D. Buchman, *The complete herbal guide to natural health and beauty* (N.Y.: Doubleday, 1973).
9. D. D. Buchman, *How to look good and feel great* (N.Y.: Scholastic Book Services, 1976).
10. B. Traven, *The complete book of natural cosmetics* (N.Y.: Pocket Books, 1976).

Chapter 35: Vitamins and Minerals That All Women Need

Supplements—paragraph 2:
1. J. Wright, in: "A frank talk about nerves, marriage, and menopause," *Prevention*, March 1977, p. 91.
Supplements—paragraph 5:
2. In 1977, the American Academy of Pediatrics defined megavitamins for children as ten or more times the recommended daily allowances, except for vitamins A and D, where the Academy states that no multiples should be given. The Academy states that the mega range is potentially dangerous for children.
Supplements—paragraph 9:
3. T. Brewer, "Consequences of malnutrition in human pregnancy," *CIBA Review: Perinatal Medicine* (1975), pp. 5–6.
General Advice—paragraph 2:
4. As reported on Physicians Radio Network on May 15, 1977, research performed at the University of Texas demonstrates that a diet excessively high in fiber may induce zinc deficiency. Thus, observers of high fiber diets are advised to add moderate zinc supplements.
Essential Minerals and Trace Elements:
5. For those who are interested in naturopathic medicine, Dr. Kurt Donsbach at the International Institute of Health Sciences in Huntington Beach, California, maintains that the most beneficial form of E to take at menopause is one that contains both raw wheat germ oil and lecithin. He advocates 600 units as a minimum dosage. The adrenals, which apparently help produce estrogen after menopause, can be stimulated by pantothenic acid, he contends. In deficiency cases, massive doses of up to 3 g may stimulate adrenal function within 24 hours, according to Donsbach. Some menopausal women require 5 g daily of C, in Donsbach's opinion, and 1,200 mg is the minimum he advocates. Concerning minerals, about which there is little scientific agreement on menopause and postmenopause requirements, Donsbach proposes the following supplements: calcium, 1 g; magnesium, 400 mg; phosphorus, 150 mg; potassium, 99 mg; iron, 15 mg; iodine, 225 mcg; copper, 2 mg; chromium, 500 mcg; manganese, 15 mg; zinc, 15 mg.

Donsbach urges that white sugar, alcohol, cigarettes, coffee and conventional teas be eliminated from the diet, and that raw fruits, especially tomatoes and cabbage, be eaten daily. In addition to ginseng, the menopause herbs he deems useful are: red raspberry, cramp bark, sarsaparilla, licorice, damiana, squaw vine and black cohosh. Herbs should of course be used with extreme caution, as they *are drugs*, but interested readers may wish to investigate these traditional remedies further. Most of these herbs have been much less studied, by modern pharmacologists, than ginseng, and their properties are less understood. In some cases, toxicity has been reported when large dosages are used.

See also chap. 11, note 28.

RECOMMENDED READINGS: See under chap. 36.

Chapter 36: A Personal Nutritional Profile

RECOMMENDED READINGS

1. R. Ashley and H. Duggal, *Dictionary of nutrition* (N.Y.: Pocket Books, 1976).
2. M. Bricklin, *The practical encyclopedia of natural healing* (Emmaus, Pa.: Rodale Press, 1976).
3. E. Cheraskin and W. M. Ringsdorf with A. Brecher, *Psychodietetics* (N.Y.: Stein & Day, 1974).
4. A. Davis, *Let's eat right to keep fit* (N.Y.: New American Library, 1970).
5. A. Davis, *Let's get well* (N.Y.: New American Library, 1965).
6. W. Dufty, *Sugar blues* (Radnor, Pa.: Chilton, 1975).
7. M. Ebon, *The essential vitamin counter* (N.Y.: Bantam, 1974).
8. M. Ebon, *Which vitamins do you need?* (N.Y.: Bantam, 1974).
9. E. B. Ewald, *Recipes for a small planet* (N.Y.: Ballantine Books, 1974).
10. R. Fermes and O. Sabry, *Nutriscore: the rate-yourself plan for better nutrition* (N.Y.: Methuen, 1976).
11. C. Fredericks, *Carlton Fredericks' calorie and carbohydrate guide* (N.Y.: Pocket Books, 1977).
12. C. Fredericks, *Look younger, feel healthier* (N.Y.: Grosset & Dunlap, 1972).
13. C. Fredericks, *The nutrition handbook: your key to good health* (Chatsworth, Cal.: Major, 1964).
14. B. C. Harris, *Kitchen medicines* (N.Y.: Pocket Books, 1970).
15. B. T. Hunter, *Consumer beware! your food and what's been done to it* (N.Y.: Bantam, 1971).
16. B. T. Hunter, *Food additives and federal policy: the mirage of safety* (N.Y.: Scribner's, 1975).
17. B. T. Hunter, *The natural foods primer* (N.Y.: Simon and Schuster, 1972).
18. M. F. Jacobson, *Nutrition scoreboard: your guide to better eating* (N.Y.: Avon, 1974).
19. N. Jolliffe, *The prudent diet* (N.Y.: Simon and Schuster, 1963).
20. B. Kraus, *The Barbara Kraus guide to fiber in foods* (N.Y.: New American Library, 1975).
21. R. J. Kutsky, *Handbook of vitamins and hormones* (N.Y.: Van Nostrand Reinhold, 1973).

22. F. M. Lappe, *Diet for a small planet,* revised edition (N.Y.: Ballantine Books, 1976).

23. C. Lerza and M. Jacobson, *Food for people, not for profit* (N.Y.: Ballantine, 1975).

24. J. V. Levy and P. Bach-y-Rita, *Vitamins: their use and abuse* (N.Y.: Liveright, 1976).

25. J. Mayer, *A diet for living* (N.Y.: Pocket Books, 1977).

26. R. A. Passwater, *Super-nutrition* (N.Y.: Pocket Books, 1976).

27. L. Pauling, *Vitamin C, the common cold, and the flu* (San Francisco: W. H. Freeman, 1976).

28. C. C. Pfeiffer, *Mental and elemental nutrients: a physician's guide to nutrition and health care* (New Canaan, Conn.: Keats, 1975).

29. N. S. Schrimshaw, C. E. Taylor and J. E. Gordon, *Interactions of nutrition and infection* (Geneva: World Health Organization, 1968) Monograph Series No. 57.

30. R. Searcy, *Diagnostic biochemistry* (N.Y.: McGraw-Hill, 1969).

31. R. J. Williams, *Nutrition against disease: environmental prevention* (N.Y.: Pitman, 1971).

32. R. J. Williams, *Nutrition in a nutshell* (N.Y.: Dolphin, 1962).

R. J. Williams (technical works):

33. (With R. E. Eakin, E. Beerstecher, W. Shire), *The biochemistry of B vitamins, 1950.*

34. *Nutrition and alcoholism, 1951.*

35. *Free and unequal, 1953.*

36. *Biochemical individuality, 1956.*

37. *Alcoholism: the nutritional approach, 1959.*

38. *You are extraordinary, 1967.*

39. *Physicians' handbook of nutritional science, 1975.*

40. S. R. Williams, *Nutrition and diet therapy,* 3rd ed. (St. Louis: Mosby, 1977).

41. H. Verret and J. Carper, *Eating may be hazardous to your health* (N.Y.: Anchor, 1975).

Epilogue: The Grotesque Limits of Sex Hormones

Quotation:
1. D. Schaap, "The breakfast of champions ain't Wheaties," *The Village Voice,* July 26, 1976, p. 23.

Athletes, Nutrition, and Hormones—paragraph 1:
2. "Crackdown on drugs at the Olympics," *Medical World News* 17:50 (1976).

Athletes, Nutrition, and Hormones—paragraph 3:
3. J. Rodda, "Steroids test catches three," *Manchester Guardian,* Aug. 8, 1976, p. 24.

4. Coronary Drug Research Group, "The coronary drug project: findings leading to the discontinuation of the 2.5 mg/day estrogen groups," *Journal of the American Medical Association* 226: 652–657 (1973).

5. Mann, 1975.

6. "Testosterone and estrogen both linked to cardiovascular disease," *Medical Tribune*, Sept. 1, 1976, p. 3.

Athletes, Nutrition, and Hormones—paragraph 7:

7. *Medical World News* 17:50 (1976).

The Sign of the Yellow Cross—paragraph 1:

8. Rodda, 1976, p. 24.

Will Frank Shorter Keep It Clean?—paragraph 2:

9. Schaap, 1976, p. 23.

Will Frank Shorter Keep It Clean?—paragraph 4:

10. "Effects of drugs to aid athletes studied by U.S.," *New York Times*, Aug. 22, 1976, p. 51.

The Search for the Double X Chromosome—paragraph 2:

11. "MD tennis star's sex surgery spotlights transsexualism," *Medical World News* 17:26–27 (1976).

12. "Experts say competitive advantage holds for MD tennis star despite sex change," *Medical Tribune*, Sept. 22, 1976, p. 37.

A Tragic Case—paragraph 1:

13. K. L. Lehrman, "Pulmonary embolism in a transsexual man taking diethylstilbestrol," *Journal of the American Medical Association* 235:532–533 (1976).

More Tragic Cases—paragraph 1:

14. "Estrogen in the air is called a hazard to makers of pills," *New York Times*, April 2, 1977, p. 46.

Tall Daughters and Short Sons:

15. "Too short or too tall," *Medical World News* 17:55–75 (1976).

16. N. Brozan, "The use of estrogen as a growth inhibitor in over-tall girls is being questioned," *New York Times*, Feb. 11, 1976, p. 55.

Which Twin Has the High-C Vitamin?—paragraph 1:

17. J. Z. Miller et al., "Therapeutic effect of vitamin C: a co-twin control study," *Journal of the American Medical Association* 237:248–251 (1977).

Which Twin Has the High-C Vitamin?—paragraph 4:

18. S. Lewin, "Evaluation of potential effects of high intake of ascorbic acid," *Comprehensive Biochemistry and Physiology* 47: 681–695 (1973).

Hot Flashes, Impotence, and Libido in Men—paragraph 1:

19. J. M. Feldman, R. W. Postlewaite and J. F. Glenn, "Hot flashes and sweats in men with testicular insufficiency," *Archives of Internal Medicine* 136:606–608 (1976).

20. "Hot flash on male menopause," *Emergency Medicine*, Aug. 1976, pp. 66–67.

Hot Flashes, Impotence, and Libido in Men—paragraph 5:
21. "Male pill still elusive," *People magazine* 2(2), 1975.
Traditional Attitudes of Doctors—paragraph 1:
22. Letter from Dr. Michelle J. Harrison to Dr. J. Richard Crout, Jan. 13, 1977.

Index

Abortifacients, medical, 292–94
Abortion, 222, 248, 287–300
  complications of, 297–98
  definition of, 288
  by dilatation and curettage (D &
    C), 293–94, 298
  doctors' mismanagement of, 299–
    300
  emotional stress associated with,
    299
  incomplete, 289
  IUD insertion after, 205
  IUD pregnancies and, 193–95
  late (third trimester), 296–97
  laws against, 289
  maternal deaths due to, 287–88,
    296, 298
  medicinal or pharmacological
    methods of, 292–94
  by menstrual extraction, 295–96
  by menstrual regulation (mini-
    suction), 295
  physical methods of, 290–91
  psychogenic, 291–92
  by saline solution, 297–98
  septic, 194, 289–90
  spontaneous, see Miscarriages
  by suction (uterine aspiration),
    294–95
  surgical or mechanical methods
    of, 290
Aci-Jel, 34
Ackwell Industries, 309
Acne
  menstruation and, 177
  oral contraceptives and, 162–64
Acosta, Guadalupe, 281–84
Adams, P., 138
Adaptogen, ginseng as, 431–34
Adenocarcinoma in DES daughters,
  13–17, 28
  adenosis and, 31
  incidence of, 37
  treatment of, 38–39
Adenosis in DES daughters, 31–35
  treatment of, 33, 41, 45
Adolescents, see Teen-agers
Advertising
  for contraceptives, 243, 303–6
  for estrogen replacement therapy,
    341–42, 349, 353–54
Agency for International Develop-
    ment (AID), 89, 164,
    280–81, 307
Aging
  minerals and, 489–90
  See also Menopause

Agriculture, Department of: DES-
    fed animals and, 62, 65–71
Albright, Fuller, 386–87
Alcohol, ginseng and, 437–39
Aldosterone, 458
Allen, Willard, 49
Allen, William M., 10
Allergies to the pill, 127–28
Amatanango, 381
American Home Products Corp.,
    388–89
Amenorrhea after quitting the pill,
    168–72
American College of Obstetricians
    and Gynecologists (ACOG),
    22
  on IUDs, 194, 196
American Medical Association, 42,
    96, 103
Amino acids, vitamin B_6 and, 140
Ammonium chloride, 183
Anabolic steroids, 329, 503–4
Anderson, John, 502, 505
Anemia
  B_{12}-deficiency, 141–42, 156
  in IUD users, 188
Animal Health Institute, 62–63
Animals
  DES's effects on, 10, 12, 19,
    47–48
  estrogen products as carcino-
    genic in, 15, 116
  Flagyl's carcinogenicity in, 92
  ginseng research on, 430–31
  hormones fed to, 71–73
    See also Meat from DES-fed
      animals
  oral contraceptives' effects on
    sex drive of, 120–22
Anovulatory cycles, 263
Anticholinergic drugs, 181
Antidepressants, 343, 447, 449–50
Apgar, Virginia, 44
Arden, Elizabeth, 426
Aristotle, 239
Arthur, M., 403
Arthritis Foundation, 457
Arthritis-like symptoms, oral
    contraceptives and, 126
Ascorbic acid, see Vitamin C
Aspartame, 93–94
Aspirin, 141, 181
  See also Bufferin; Midol
Association for Voluntary
    Sterilization, 317
Asthma, the pill and, 127–28
Athletes, 502–5

ABOUT THE AUTHORS

In *Free and Female* (1972) BARBARA SEAMAN predicted that menopause estrogens were apt to cause cancer. In *The Doctors' Case Against the Pill* (1969) she identified many lethal side effects, including heart attacks and liver disease, that were not acknowledged until the mid-1970s. Formerly an Advanced Science Writing Fellow at Columbia University, Ms. Seaman was cited by the Department of Health, Education and Welfare as the author responsible for the first Patient Package Insert (on the pill), and by the Library of Congress as the author who raised sexism in health care as a worldwide issue.

GIDEON SEAMAN is Director of Graduate Medical Education and Director of Psychopharmacology at Creedmoor Psychiatric Center. He received his M.D. from the State University of New York, Downstate Medical Center, to which he returned after psychiatric residency, for two years additional training toward a Doctor of Medical Science degree in research. His scientific articles have been published in the *American Journal of Psychiatry* and the *Journal of Experimental Psychology*. He was one of the first psychiatrists to recognize that the pill causes widespread personality changes, including depression.

How's Your Health?

Bantam publishes a line of informative books, written by top experts to help you toward a healthier and happier life.

Bantam Book Catalog

Here's your up-to-the-minute listing of over 1,400 titles by your favorite authors.

This illustrated, large format catalog gives a description of each title. For your convenience, it is divided into categories in fiction and non-fiction—gothics, science fiction, westerns, mysteries, cookbooks, mysticism and occult, biographies, history, family living, health, psychology, art.

So don't delay—take advantage of this special opportunity to increase your reading pleasure.

Just send us your name and address and 50¢ (to help defray postage and handling costs).

BANTAM BOOKS, INC.
Dept. FC, 414 East Golf Road, Des Plaines, Ill. 60016

Mr./Mrs./Miss_____
(please print)

Address_____

City_____State_____Zip_____

Do you know someone who enjoys books? Just give us their names and addresses and we'll send them a catalog too!

_____

Mr./Mrs./Miss_____

Address_____

City_____State_____Zip_____

_____

Mr./Mrs./Miss_____

Address_____

City_____State_____Zip_____

FC—9/78